textbook of
OPHTHALMIC PLASTIC
and
RECONSTRUCTIVE
SURGERY

Lea & Febiger
Philadelphia 1988

ROGER KOHN, M.D.

Professor, Department of Ophthalmology
Division of Ophthalmic Plastic and Reconstructive Surgery
U.C.L.A. School of Medicine
Santa Barbara, CA

textbook of
OPHTHALMIC PLASTIC
and
RECONSTRUCTIVE
SURGERY

Lea & Febiger
600 South Washington Square
Philadelphia, PA   19106-4198
U.S.A.
(215) 922-1330

Library of Congress Cataloging-in-Publication Data

Kohn, Roger, 1946–
    Textbook of ophthalmic plastic and reconstructive
surgery.

    Includes bibliographies and index.
    1. Eye—Surgery.   2. Surgery, Plastic.   I. Title.
[DNLM: 1. Eye—surgery.   2. Surgery, Plastic.
WW 168 K79t]
RE87.K64   1988   617.7′1   87-26042
ISBN 0-8121-1112-5

PRINTED IN THE UNITED STATES OF AMERICA

Print number: 5   4   3   2   1

Dedicated to

BARBARA,
BRADLEY,
and ALLISON

FOREWORD

This book, *Textbook of Ophthalmic Plastic and Reconstructive Surgery*, is a sequel to the first edition of *Practical Ophthalmic Plastic and Reconstructive Surgery* by Reeh, Beyer, and Shannon. Begun by us in 1974 for publication in 1976, this project was dedicated to a bright star in this surgical field, Margaret F. Obear, M.D., whose career was cruelly interrupted by a disabling illness. We had hoped, in a limited way, to carry on her ideals.

Dr. Shannon later suffered a fatal heart attack. Were he present, I am sure that he would join Dr. Beyer and me in wishing this book a bright future in its mission of helping patients in need of ophthalmic plastic surgical care.

Work in this field in the 1930s and 1940s was, with some exceptions, poor and chaotic. I came to the spe-

cialty first as a general surgeon, but had the good fortune to be taken in hand by Colonel Walcott Denison when I was a First Lieutenant in the Army Medical Corps, assigned to the eye, ear, nose, and throat. Through his mentorship, and later that of Dr. Brittain F. Payne of New York, I was able to combine my knowledge of surgery with ocular anatomy and physiology for the correction of eyelid anomalies.

From a beginning of 16 members of the American Academy of Ophthalmology, who were responsible for teaching ophthalmic plastic surgery, we now have the American Society of Ophthalmic Plastic and Reconstructive Surgery. The members of this society have been most helpful to us in the past, and I am certain that they will support this beautiful volume equally well in the future.

Merrill J. Reeh, M.D., F.A.C.S.
Clinical Professor of Ophthalmology and Pathology,
University of Washington
Seattle, Washington

A textbook is meaningful if it is concise and complete in its context, is well organized, and has clear illustrations. It should reflect the author's experience in his field. Most of all, it should be practical and within a suitable price range.

These were our objectives when we wrote our text under a similar heading about 10 years ago. Dr. Kohn has applied these principles in this publication. His *Textbook of Ophthalmic Plastic and Reconstructive Surgery* incorporates all these objectives in admirable form. Anatomy and physiology are effectively combined to provide the average ophthalmologist, as well as the experienced oculoplastic surgeon, with a fine dissertation on all per-

tinent subjects in ophthalmic plastic surgery. Dr. Kohn has expanded on the previous text by including clear chapters on craniofacial abnormalities by Andrew Choy, M.D., and orbital tumors by James Orcutt, M.D.

I am enamored of this book for its completeness and clarity of presentation, and I believe that it deserves a top position for its practicality and value in a highly competitive market.

With great pride I would like to add that, over a decade ago, Dr. Roger Kohn was my first postgraduate fellow in ophthalmic plastic and reconstructive surgery, and was thus also the first fellow in the named specialty at the Massachusetts Eye and Ear Infirmary. He was and is a winner and so is his book.

Charles K. Beyer-Machule, M.D., F.A.C.S.
Clinical Associate Professor of Ophthalmology
Harvard Medical School;
Surgeon, Massachusetts Eye and Ear Infirmary
Boston, Massachusetts

PREFACE

Textbook of Ophthalmic Plastic and Reconstructive Surgery is the sequel to *Practical Ophthalmic Plastic and Reconstructive Surgery*, written by Merrill J. Reeh, M.D., Charles K. Beyer, M.D., and the late Gerard M. Shannon, M.D. in 1976. As such, it has a tradition of excellence to uphold. For 10 years the Reeh, Beyer, and Shannon text stood at the forefront of books in the field of ophthalmic plastic and reconstructive surgery. Its practical descriptions of relevant anatomy and operative procedures gave clear guidance to surgeons working in this area. All three authors are respected for their many contributions and innovations within this surgical field. Scores of residents and fellows have been professionally and personally enriched by the authors' scientific curiosity and insightful teaching. The untimely death of Dr. Shannon was a loss to us all. I sincerely appreciate the confidence that Doctors Reeh and Beyer have placed in me as the author of this sequel.

The intention of this textbook is to be comprehensive without being encyclopedic. The topics flow from an initial understanding of anatomy in the orbital and periorbital regions, along with basic principles of plastic and oculoplastic surgery. Congenital anomalies of the eyelid, socket, and craniofacial areas are then discussed. This is followed by specific chapters on various acquired abnormalities of the eyelids, socket, lacrimal system, and orbit.

Each subject is presented in terms of its clinical presentation, differential diagnosis, and surgical indications where relevant. The operative techniques depicted in this manuscript are those currently used in ophthalmic plastic and reconstructive surgery. Several additional procedures that I have published and used extensively are presented as author's technique. Emphasis is given to providing both functional and cosmetic improvement for the conditions discussed. Surgical complications are reviewed, along with measures available to avoid or manage such sequelae.

It is hoped that this volume will be a comprehensive guide for ophthalmologists and all other surgeons who work in this field. An extensive bibliography follows each chapter to provide references to the specific information that was the basis for this text.

Santa Barbara, CA   Roger Kohn, M.D.

ACKNOWLEDGEMENTS

I would like to express my sincere gratitude to James Orcutt, M.D. and Andrew Choy, M.D. for their significant contributions to this book. Dr. Orcutt's training in neuro-ophthalmology and orbital surgery are evident in the lucid and comprehensive approach he takes toward the complex subject of the orbit. Dr. Choy, as a member of craniofacial teams on both American coasts, has gained experience in surgical problems seen by few of us.

The superb medical illustrations for this textbook, all new, were created by David Hinkle, whose work has appeared in many publications of the Division of Ophthalmic Plastic and Reconstructive Surgery at U.C.L.A. His standard of excellence is evident here.

I am deeply indebted to my teachers in Ophthalmology and Ophthalmic Plastic and Reconstructive Surgery, David Shoch, M.D., Charles Beyer, M.D., and Alston Callahan, M.D., who provided me with a quality educational experience in an atmosphere of dignity and respect for the patient.

I wish to thank Bradley Straatsma, M.D. for his encouragement and support, which have been instrumental to the success of this project. The U.C.L.A. Department of Ophthalmology has been an extraordinary environment for development in this field.

Credit and thanks are also due to Mr. George H. Mundorff, Executive Editor for Lea & Febiger, for the effective manner in which he brought this sequel together. The secretarial assistance of G. Joanne Whelden and photographic contributions of James Hawe are also sincerely appreciated.

Most of all, I would like to thank my wife, Barbara, and children, Bradley and Allison, for their understanding through the long hours required for this project.

CONTRIBUTORS

ANDREW CHOY, M.D.
Clinical Associate Professor
Member, Craniofacial Surgical Unit
U.C.L.A. School of Medicine
Los Angeles, California

JAMES ORCUTT, M.D., PH.D.
Assistant Professor of Ophthalmology
Director, Neuro-Ophthalmology/Orbit and
  Ocular Plastic Service
University of Washington School of Medicine
Adjunct Assistant Professor of Otolaryngology
Chief, Opthalmology Section,
Seattle Veterans Administration Medical Center
Seattle, Washington

Illustrations by David Hinkle

CONTENTS

1

ANATOMY AND PHYSIOLOGY

To apply diagnostic and therapeutic skills successfully within the scope of ophthalmic plastic and reconstructive surgery, one must have a thorough knowledge of relevant anatomy and physiology. Surgical correction of oculo-plastic disorders strives to maintain or re-establish normal anatomy and physiology within the orbital and periorbital regions whenever possible.

As subspecialists, we are indebted to the pioneering work of Lester Jones, M.D. in this area. We are also grateful for the excellent collation of information by Marcos Doxanas, M.D. and Richard Anderson, M.D. in their textbook, *Clinical Orbital Anatomy.*

BONY ORBIT

The paired orbits are located in comparable positions on either side of the sagittal plane of the skull (Fig. 1–1). Each orbit is a deep, bony cavity lined with periorbita,

constructed to protect the globe and facilitate its function. Periorbita attaches to bony suture lines.

The orbit is comprised of seven bones (frontal, sphenoid, zygomatic, maxillary, ethmoid, lacrimal, and palatine), which compose the four orbital walls (superior, lateral, inferior, and medial). Structures contiguous with the orbit include the frontal sinus and anterior cranial fossa (superiorly), the temporal fossa and middle cranial fossa (laterally), the maxillary antrum and sinus (inferiorly), and the ethmoid sinus (medially).

The orbital margins assume a relatively rectangular configuration, curved somewhat at each of the four corners. Orbital rims afford firm, anterior support for the thinner bones of the four orbital walls located posteriorly. The superior, inferior, and lateral orbital walls are triangular, while the medial wall is rectangular. All orbital walls extend to the orbital apex except the inferior wall (orbital floor), which extends two-thirds of the orbital depth.

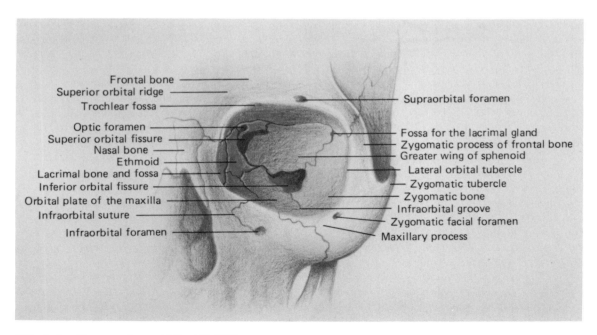

FIG. 1–1. Bony anatomy of the left orbit.

SUPERIOR ORBITAL MARGIN AND WALL

The superior orbital margin (Fig. 1–2) is comprised of the inferior portion of the frontal bone. Its contour is rounded medially and sharply angulated laterally; the junction of the medial and lateral sections delineates the supraorbital notch. The supraorbital vessels and nerve traverse this point. A smaller notch medial to this is formed by the supratrochlear vessels and nerve.

The superior orbital wall (orbital roof) (Fig. 1–2) is formed principally by the orbital plate of the frontal bone, which comprises the larger anterior component. A smaller posterior component is derived from the lesser wing of the sphenoid bone. The anterior portion of this wall is thick and forms the floor of the frontal sinus. Posteriorly, the wall thins somewhat, serving to separate the orbit from the anterior cranial fossa.

The orbital roof joins the lateral wall at the zygomaticofrontal suture anteriorly and at the superior orbital fissure posteriorly. At the posterior aspect of the superior orbital wall is the obliquely oriented frontosphenoid suture.

The orbital roof joins the medial wall at its junction with the lacrimal and ethmoid bones and the orbital plate of the sphenoid bone. The optic foramen is positioned at the apex of the orbital roof.

A concavity in the anterior portion of the superior orbital wall is the fossa for the lacrimal gland. The trochlea attaches medial to the supraorbital notch and 4 mm posterior to the supraorbital rim.

LATERAL ORBITAL MARGIN AND WALL

The lateral orbital rim (Fig. 1–3) is the strongest orbital margin and is formed by a fusion of the frontal process of the zygoma with the zygomatic process of the frontal bone. Their interface is near the superior portion of this rim at the zygomaticofrontal suture. Approximately 10 mm below this suture is the lateral orbital tubercle, which serves as the insertion of the lateral ocular retinaculum. The latter is comprised of the lateral canthal tendon, Lockwood's suspensory ligament, the lateral horn of the levator aponeurosis, and the check ligament of the lateral rectus muscle.

The zygomatic bone and the greater wing of the sphenoid comprise the lateral orbital wall (Fig. 1–3). Its posterior extent is demarcated by the superior and inferior orbital fissures. The anterior portion of the lateral orbital wall owes its strength to the zygomatic bone. This gradually weakens as it extends posteriorly to articulate with the greater wing of the sphenoid. Likewise, the sphenoid wing thins posteriorly, affording a small bony separation between the orbit and the middle cranial fossa.

Within the lateral wall is the zygomatico-orbital foramen, which extends into the zygomaticofacial and zygomaticotemporal canals. These transmit nerves and vessels of the same names (Fig. 1–4). The lacrimal branch of the zygomaticotemporal nerve also exits through the lateral wall before uniting with the lacrimal nerve.

INFERIOR ORBITAL MARGIN AND WALL

The infraorbital rim (Fig. 1–5) is formed by fusion of the maxilla medially with the zygoma laterally. Their interface at the zygomaticomaxillary suture is in the central aspect of the orbital margin. Approximately 10 mm below and somewhat medial to this suture is the infraorbital foramen, through which pass the infraorbital nerve (the main branch of the maxillary division of the trigem-

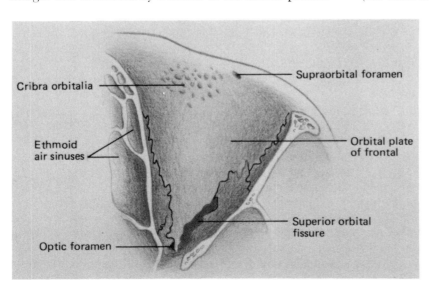

FIG. 1–2. Left superior orbital margin and wall.

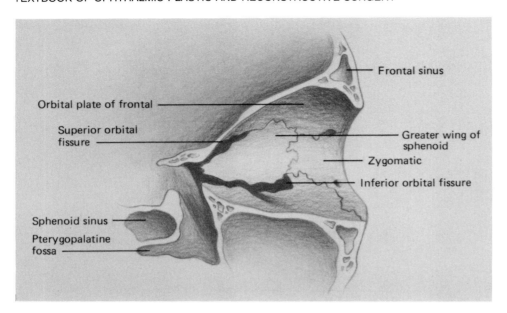

FIG. 1–3. Left lateral orbital margin and wall.

inal nerve) and the infraorbital artery (a branch of the internal maxillary artery).

Three bones comprise the inferior orbital wall (orbital floor): maxillary, zygomatic, and palatine bones (Fig. 1–5). The palatine makes a minor contribution, while the largest segment of the floor is composed of the orbital plate of the maxilla. The orbital floor serves as the roof of the maxillary sinus. The floor is thin, particularly medial to the infraorbital sulcus. It is thinnest at its posterior extent.

The infraorbital sulcus extends from the lateral aspect of the orbital apex toward the central aspect of the in-

fraorbital rim, becoming a canal in the process. This canal emerges on the maxilla anteriorly as the infraorbital foramen. Through this canal pass the infraorbital artery and nerve.

MEDIAL ORBITAL MARGIN AND WALL

The medial orbital margin (Fig. 1–6) is comprised of the maxillary process of the frontal bone, the lacrimal bone, and the frontal process of the maxilla. This rim is

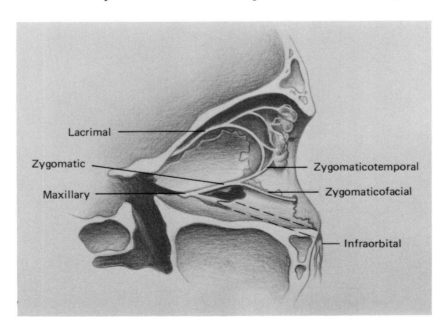

FIG. 1–4. Zygomatico-orbital foramina of the left lateral orbital wall with zygomaticofacial and zygomaticotemporal nerves emerging.

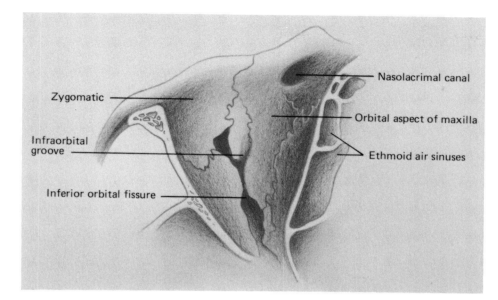

Zygomatic

Infraorbital groove

Inferior orbital fissure

Nasolacrimal canal

Orbital aspect of maxilla

Ethmoid air sinuses

FIG. 1–5. Left inferior orbital margin and wall.

discontinuous inferiorly, forming the lacrimal fossa. The superior portion of the medial orbital margin extends inferiorly to form the posterior lacrimal crest. The inferior portion of the medial orbital margin (frontal process of the maxilla) extends superiorly to form the anterior lacrimal crest. The concavity between the crests defines the lacrimal fossa. An opening at the inferior portion of the lacrimal fossa denotes the beginning of the nasolacrimal canal.

The medial wall (Fig. 1–6) is the thinnest wall of the orbit. Four bones comprise the medial orbital wall: the frontal process of the maxilla, the lacrimal bone, the lamina papyracea of the ethmoid, and the sphenoid bone. The lacrimal fossa is formed by the frontal process of the maxilla and the lacrimal bone. The latter is thin anterior to the posterior lacrimal crest, subjacent to the lacrimal sac. This bone is somewhat thicker posterior to the posterior lacrimal crest, where it interfaces with the lamina papyracea and the ethmoid air cells.

The ethmoid bone contains the anterior and posterior ethmoidal foramina. Through these small foramina emerge the respective anterior and posterior ethmoidal vessels. The ethmoid bone affords an extremely thin barrier separating the medial orbit from the ethmoid sinus,

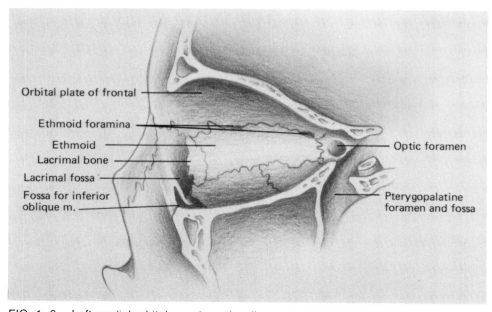

Orbital plate of frontal

Ethmoid foramina

Ethmoid

Lacrimal bone

Lacrimal fossa

Fossa for inferior oblique m.

Optic foramen

Pterygopalatine foramen and fossa

FIG. 1–6. Left medial orbital margin and wall.

predisposing this area to invasion from various organisms or tumors.

ORBITAL APEX

The superior orbital fissure (Fig. 1–2) comprises the gap between the greater and lesser wings of the sphenoid (between the orbital roof and the lateral orbital wall). Through this fissure emerge the superior and inferior divisions of the oculomotor nerve, trochlear nerve, abducens nerve, and nerve branches arising from the ophthalmic division (CN V_1) of the trigeminal nerve (lacrimal, frontal, and nasociliary). Also traversing the superior orbital fissure are the ophthalmic vein (formed by the fusion of the superior and inferior ophthalmic veins), the orbital artery (orbital branch of the middle meningeal artery), and a branch of the ophthalmic artery.

Likewise, the inferior orbital fissure (Fig. 1–5) comprises the gap between the greater wing of the sphenoid and the maxillary and palatine bones. This fissure is long, extending from the orbital apex to within 15 to 20 mm of the inferior orbital rim. The inferior orbital fissure transmits a portion of the maxillary division (CN V_2) of the trigeminal nerve and its zygomatic and alveolar branches. Other structures included are the infraorbital nerve and artery, and the inferior ophthalmic vein.

The optic foramen and canal (Fig. 1–1) are formed inferolaterally by the attachment of the lesser wing of the sphenoid to the body of the sphenoid bone (optic strut). Its medial extent is defined by the sphenoid sinus and ethmoid air cells. This foramen connects the middle cranial fossa to the orbital apex. Transmitted through the optic foramen are the optic nerve, ophthalmic artery, and ocular sympathetic nerves. The length of the canal varies and the structures contained therein are firmly confined.

ORBITAL CONNECTIVE TISSUE

A complex and diffuse connective tissue matrix supports the globe and the other orbital structures to maximize functional integrity (Figs. 1–7 through 1–9). This connective tissue framework is composed of three components: Tenon's capsule, fibrous tissue septae, and fascial sheaths of the extraocular muscles.

Tenon's capsule is located in the anterior orbit, surrounding the globe and extraocular muscles (Figs. 1–7 and 1–8). This extends from the limbus to the optic nerve, penetrated anteriorly by the oblique muscles and posteriorly by the rectus muscles. The latter penetration divides Tenon's capsule into its anterior and posterior portions. Tenon's capsule separates the globe from both intraconal and extraconal retrobulbar fat.

Fibrous tissue septae connect Tenon's capsule to the anterior periorbita (Fig. 1–9). This surrounds and stabilizes the globe within the central orbit.

Extraocular muscle fascial sheaths produce a connective tissue framework in the posterior orbit. This network connects the respective extraocular muscle (including the levator palpebrae superiorus) to its adjacent orbital wall (Fig. 1–9). The fascial sheaths coalesce anteriorly to form the intermuscular fibrous septae and the medial and lateral check ligaments. Thus, these sheaths support both the independence and interdependence of the extraocular muscles.

EXTRAOCULAR MUSCLES

The four rectus muscles originate from the region of the annulus of Zinn (Fig. 1–10). The annulus is a fibrous ring that surrounds the optic foramen and medial portion of the superior orbital fissure. At its base the annulus of Zinn is continuous with the dura mater of the middle cranial fossa.

The portion of the orbital apex encompassed by the annulus is designated the oculomotor foramen. All nerves and vessels entering the orbit through the optic foramen and the medial portion of the superior orbital fissure enter the oculomotor foramen on their course to the muscle cone (Fig. 1–10). Transmitted through the optic foramen are the optic nerve, the ophthalmic artery, and the ocular sympathetic nerves. Transmitted through the medial aspect of the superior orbital fissure are the superior and inferior divisions of the oculomotor nerve, the abducens nerve, the nasociliary branch of the ophthalmic division of the trigeminal nerve, the sensory root of the ciliary ganglion, and the superior ophthalmic vein.

The levator palpebrae superiorus muscle originates at the orbital apex above the superior rectus muscle, extrinsic to the annulus of Zinn (Fig. 1–11). The superior oblique muscle originates from a short tendon superomedial to the annulus, close to the frontoethmoidal suture. Approximately 10 to 15 mm posterior to the orbital margin the superior oblique changes from a muscle to a tendon, before passing through the trochlea. The inferior oblique muscle originates in the anterior nasal portion of the orbital floor.

The lateral rectus muscle is supplied by the abducens nerve (CN VI) (Fig. 1–10). The inferior rectus is supplied by the inferior division of the oculomotor nerve (CN III), while the medial and superior rectus muscles are sup-

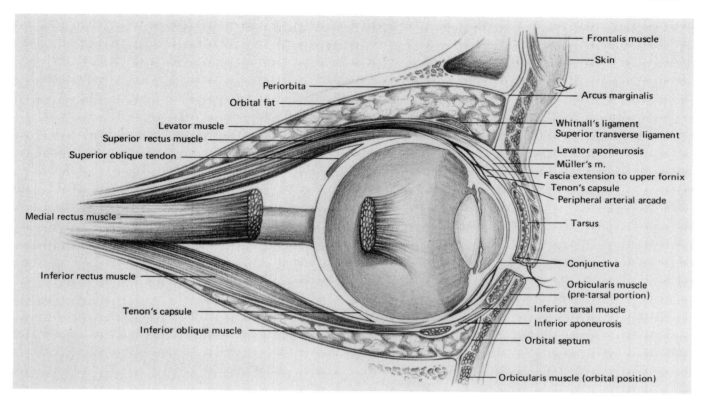

FIG. 1–7. Sagittal view of the anatomy of the left orbit, demonstrating the supportive connective tissue matrix.

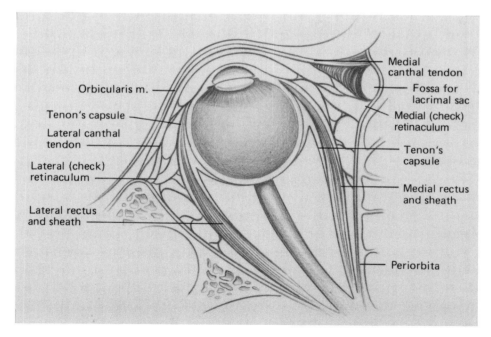

FIG. 1–8. A-P view of the left orbit depicting the interrelationship between extraocular muscle fascial sheaths and Tenon's capsule.

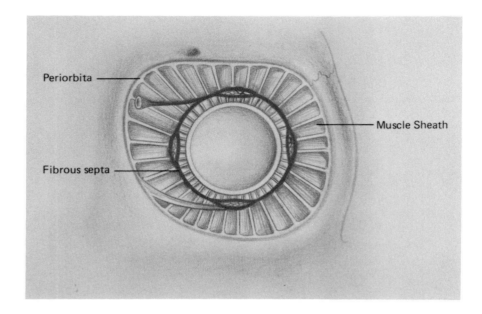

FIG. 1–9. Coronal view of the left orbit depicting the interrelationship between extraocular muscle fascial sheaths and fibrous tissue septae.

plied by the superior division of the oculomotor nerve (CN III).

The superior oblique muscle is supplied by the trochlear nerve (CN IV). The inferior oblique muscle is supplied by the inferior division of the oculomotor nerve (CN III).

Principal arterial supply to the extraocular muscles is derived from the muscular branches of the ophthalmic artery (Fig. 1–12). The superior muscular branch perfuses the lateral rectus, superior rectus, superior oblique, and levator palpebrae superiorus muscles. The inferior muscular branch supplies the medial rectus, inferior rectus, and inferior oblique muscles. In each rectus muscle, the muscular branches become the anterior ciliary arteries. Two anterior ciliary arteries are present in each, except for the lateral rectus muscle, which contains one.

Minor arterial contributions to the extraocular muscles are also derived from the lacrimal and infraorbital arteries. The lacrimal artery sends branches to both the superior and lateral rectus muscles, while the infraorbital artery sends a branch to the inferior oblique muscle.

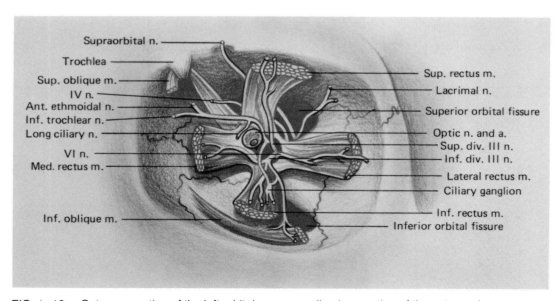

FIG. 1–10. Cutaway section of the left orbital apex revealing innervation of the extraocular muscles.

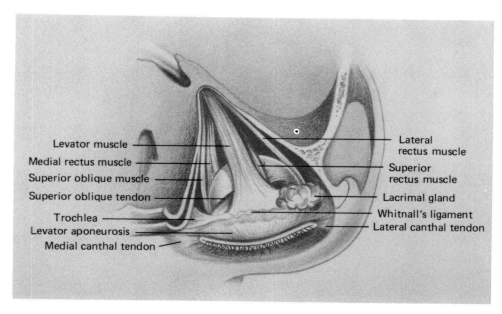

FIG. 1–11. A-P view of the left superior orbit.

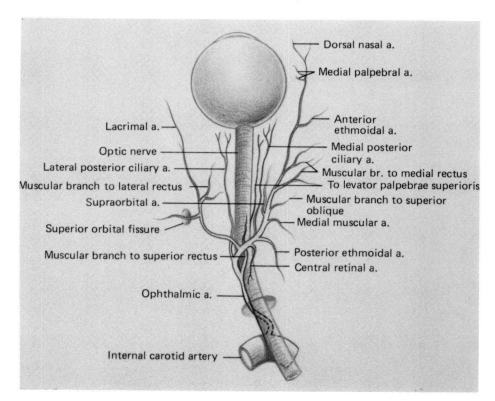

FIG. 1–12. Anatomy of the ophthalmic artery and its tributaries.

ORBITAL NERVE SUPPLY

Oculomotor Nerve. The oculomotor nerve (CN III) innervates the levator palpebrae superiorus, superior rectus, inferior rectus, medial rectus, and inferior oblique muscles. It also transmits parasympathetic fibers to the globe.

After exiting the intracranial space, the oculomotor nerve enters the superolateral portion of the cavernous sinus. As it courses forward it shifts to an inferior position, entering the superior orbital fissure. Within the fissure, the nerve divides into superior and inferior branches (Fig. 1–10).

The superior division enters the orbit through the annulus of Zinn, passing medial to the optic nerve. It sequentially supplies the superior rectus and levator palpebrae superiorus muscles. The inferior division also enters the orbit through the annulus, passing medial and inferior to the optic nerve. It further subdivides into three additional branches, supplying the medial rectus, inferior rectus, and inferior oblique respectively. This latter branch contains the orbital parasympathetic fibers at the orbital apex.

Trochlear Nerve. The trochlear nerve (CN IV) enters the cavernous sinus inferolateral to the oculomotor nerve (CN III). It then passes superiorly over the oculomotor nerve, entering the orbit through the superior orbital fissure external to the annulus of Zinn. The nerve passes along the orbital roof diagonally across the origins of the levator muscle and the superior rectus muscle, entering the posterior superior portion of the superior oblique muscle (Fig. 1–10).

Abducens Nerve. The abducens nerve (CN VI) is located near the lateral wall of the cavernous sinus. It enters the superior orbital fissure within the annulus of Zinn. Within the orbit, the abducens nerve enters the lateral rectus muscle along its inner surface (Fig. 1–10).

Trigeminal Nerve. The trigeminal nerve (CN V) is primarily a sensory nerve, although it does have a minor motor component. Within the cavernous sinus, the trigeminal ganglion sends off its three divisions: ophthalmic (V_1), maxillary (V_2), and mandibular (V_3).

The ophthalmic nerve (V_1) is situated at the lateral wall of the cavernous sinus. Posterior to the supraorbital fissure, it divides into three branches: lacrimal, frontal, and nasociliary (Fig. 1–13).

The lacrimal nerve enters the orbit through the lateral portion of the superior orbital fissure (Fig. 1–10). It is joined by a branch of the zygomaticotemporal nerve to provide parasympathetic secretomotor fibers to the lacrimal gland (Fig. 1–13). The lacrimal nerve also extends forward through the orbital septum as the lateral palpebral nerve to provide sensory fibers to the superior lateral portion of the upper eyelid (Figs. 1–10, 1–13, 1–14, and 1–15).

The frontal nerve enters the orbit through the superior orbital fissure as well. It courses near the periosteum and above the levator muscle to divide into a large supraorbital nerve and a small supratrochlear nerve (Fig. 1–13). Along with the supraorbital vessels, the supraorbital nerve exits the orbit through the supraorbital foramen to provide sensory innervation to the forehead (Fig. 1–15). Along with the supratrochlear vessels, the supratrochlear nerve exits medially in the region of the trochlea to innervate the medial portion of the upper eyelid and the lower portion of the forehead.

The nasociliary nerve enters the orbit through the annulus of Zinn within the oculomotor foramen. It crosses the optic nerve with the ophthalmic artery, sending branches to the medial orbital wall (Fig. 1–13). These branches form the posterior ethmoidal, anterior ethmoidal, and infratrochlear nerves (Fig. 1–15). The latter innervates the medial portion of the upper eyelid, inner canthus, medial conjunctiva, and lateral aspect of the nose.

A small sensory branch of the nasociliary nerve remains lateral to the optic nerve, passing through the ciliary ganglion. This continues forward to the globe as the short ciliary nerves (Fig. 1–14).

Two or three long ciliary nerves extend from the nasociliary nerve, bypass the ciliary ganglion, and proceed forward to the globe (Fig. 1–13) in consort with the short posterior ciliary nerves. The long ciliary nerves carry sensory information from the iris, ciliary muscle, and cornea, and also provide sympathetic input from the superior cervical ganglion to the iris dilator muscle.

Branches of the maxillary division (V_2) that traverse the orbit (Figs. 1–13 and 1–14) are the zygomatic nerve and the branches of the alveolar nerve.

The zygomatic nerve enters the orbit through the inferior orbital fissure, dividing into zygomaticotemporal and zygomaticofacial branches. The former carries secretomotor fibers from the trigeminal ganglion to the lacrimal gland. The latter extends along the inferolateral aspect of the orbit to innervate the cheek.

The posterior superior alveolar nerve (Fig. 1–14) enters the infraorbital groove, while the middle and anterior superior alveolar nerves reside within the infraorbital canal before extending inferiorly to innervate the teeth.

The maxillary nerve enters the infraorbital canal as the infraorbital nerve. Its terminal extensions are the inferior

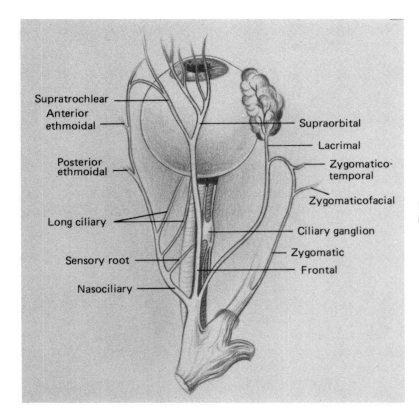

FIG. 1–13. A-P view of the trigeminal nerve and its branches.

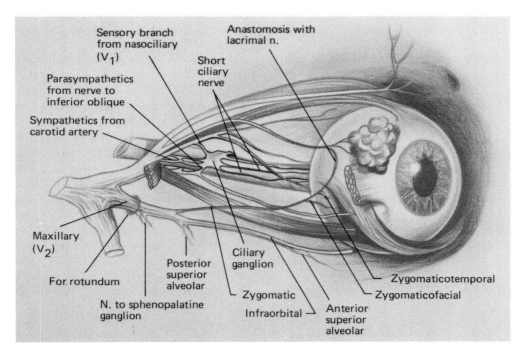

FIG. 1–14. Sagittal view of the trigeminal nerve and its branches.

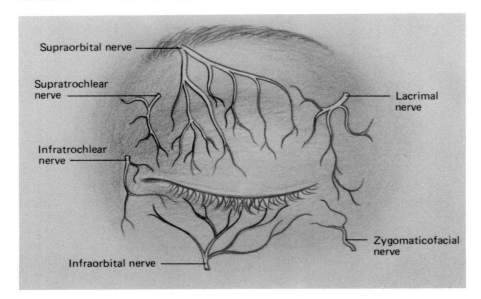

FIG. 1–15. Sensory innervation of the eyelid and periorbital area.

palpebral, external nasal, and superior labial nerves. These branches supply the lower eyelid (Figs. 1–15 and 1–16), nasal septum, and upper lip respectively.

Facial Nerve. The facial nerve (CN VII) exits from the styloid canal in the mastoid process of the temporal bone, emerging behind the sternocleidomastoid muscle. It passes below the external auditory canal, entering the posterior portion of the parotid gland. Within the gland, it divides into an upper (temporofacial) branch and a lower (cervicofacial) branch. The upper branch subdivides into temporal and zygomatic branches. The lower branch subdivides into buccal, mandibular, and cervical branches. These branches all course toward their respective facial muscles of innervation. This innervation varies somewhat among patients and between both sides of the face in the same patient.

Autonomic Nerves. Parasympathetic innervation to the orbit synapses at the ciliary ganglion. The ganglion is situated approximately 1 cm anterior to the orbital apex, temporal to the optic nerve (Figs. 1–10, 1–13, and 1–14). This provides fibers to the iris sphincter muscle, ciliary body, as well as secretomotor fibers to the lacrimal, submandibular, and sublingual glands. A sympathetic root passes from the sympathetic plexus within the cavernous sinus through the ciliary ganglion. The sympathetic system supplies fibers to the iris dilator muscle and sympathetic muscles of the upper and lower eyelids and lacrimal glands.

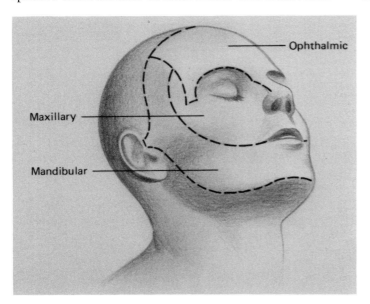

FIG. 1–16. Topographical distribution of sensory innervation from the trigeminal nerve.

Optic Nerve. The intracanalicular portion of the optic nerve is 5 mm long. It emerges through the optic foramen within the annulus of Zinn at the orbital apex (Fig. 1–10). Its intraorbital course is somewhat S-shaped. This accommodates the 30 mm long optic nerve within the 20 mm posterior orbit. Within the orbit, the nerve is surrounded by dura, arachnoid, and pia mater. The dura becomes continuous with sclera anteriorly and periosteum at the orbital apex. The central retinal artery enters the optic nerve 10 mm posterior to the globe on the inferomedial surface of the nerve (Fig. 1–12).

ORBITAL VASCULAR SUPPLY

Within the orbit, the major arteries and veins are incorporated into the walls of the connective tissue matrix.

Arterial System. The principal arterial supply to the orbit is derived from the ophthalmic artery (Fig. 1–12). This is a branch of the internal carotid artery with some minor contributions from the external carotid artery.

The internal carotid artery enters the cavernous sinus just medial to the abducens nerve. The artery assumes an S-shaped configuration within the sinus, designated the carotid siphon. Upon exiting the cavernous sinus, the internal carotid artery gives off its first major branch; the ophthalmic artery. The opthalmic artery remains below the optic nerve throughout its intracranial and intracanalicular course. It enters the orbit through the optic foramen, inferolateral to the optic nerve.

The ophthalmic artery divides, forming the central retinal artery, posterior ciliary arteries, anterior ciliary arteries, and optic nerve collateral arteries.

The central retinal artery is the first branch of the ophthalmic artery. It is located below the optic nerve, penetrating the dura of the nerve on its inferomedial surface 10 mm posterior to the globe (this distance varies from 5 to 15 mm). The central retinal artery continues forward within the substance of the nerve.

The two posterior ciliary arteries subdivide to form approximately 15 to 20 short posterior ciliary arteries. These penetrate the sclera near the optic nerve, perfusing the choroid and optic nerve head. Two of these vessels proceed anteriorly as the long posterior ciliary arteries, perfusing the ciliary muscle, iris, and anterior choroid.

The anterior ciliary arteries are derived from the muscular branches of the ophthalmic artery. They extend through the rectus muscles and penetrate the limbal sclera to supply the anterior uveal tract.

The small collateral branches to the optic nerve further

support the vascular supply throughout the course of the nerve.

The lacrimal artery (Figs. 1–12 and 1–17) is also derived from the ophthalmic artery and, in conjunction with the lacrimal nerve, courses along the lateral orbital wall to supply the lacrimal gland through its glandular branch. After supplying the gland, the lacrimal artery gives off the two lateral palpebral arteries. These go on to unite with the corresponding medial palpebral arteries to become the arterial (marginal) arcades of the eyelids.

The supraorbital artery is derived from the ophthalmic artery and passes with the supraorbital nerve to the supraorbital foramen. This artery perfuses the eyebrows and forehead.

Extraorbital branches of the ophthalmic artery include the posterior ethmoidal, anterior ethmoidal, medial palpebral, supratrochlear, and dorsal nasal arteries.

The posterior ethmoidal artery penetrates the posterior ethmoidal foramen to supply the posterior ethmoidal air cells. The anterior ethmoidal artery courses with its corresponding nerve through the anterior ethmoidal foramen. This supplies the remainder of the ethmoidal air cells, frontal sinus, lateral wall of the nose, and a portion of the dura of the anterior cranial fossa.

The two medial palpebral arteries arise from the ophthalmic artery below the trochlea. They course around the medial canthal tendon to enter the medial aspect of the upper and lower eyelids. Here they merge with the corresponding lateral palpebral arteries to form the marginal arcades. These arcades are located either within or just anterior to the tarsal plates. In the upper eyelid they are located approximately 4 mm from the eyelid margin; while in the lower eyelid they are located approximately 2 mm from the eyelid margin.

The supratrochlear artery pierces the orbital septum, extending superiorly with the supratrochlear nerve to supply the scalp. The dorsal nasal artery extends above the medial canthal tendon to fuse with the angular artery. This establishes a communication between the internal and external carotid artery networks. The dorsal nasal artery supplies the forehead and scalp near the midline.

Only a few branches of the external carotid artery perfuse the orbit (Fig. 1–17). One such branch is the superficial temporal artery, which gives off the zygomatic artery. This vessel extends over the zygomatic arch to supply the orbicularis oculi muscle, and then joins the lacrimal and palpebral branches of the ophthalmic artery. This establishes an additional communication between the two carotid systems. A frontal branch of the superficial temporal artery supplies the eyebrows and forehead. Biopsy of this vessel is often used to support the diagnosis of giant cell arteritis.

The other external carotid branch that supplies the

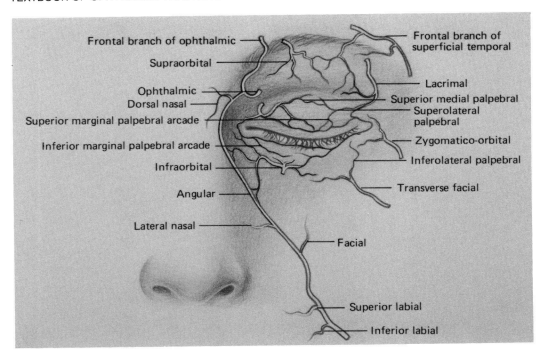

FIG. 1–17. Arterial system of the eyelid and periorbital area.

orbit is the internal maxillary artery (Fig. 1–17). This becomes the infraorbital artery. The infraorbital and orbital arteries are derived from the middle meningeal branch of the internal maxillary artery. As the terminal branch of the internal maxillary artery, the infraorbital artery enters the orbit through the infraorbital fissure. It passes through the infraorbital groove and canal, emerging through the infraorbital foramen. It contributes to the perfusion of the inferior rectus and inferior oblique muscles, as well as the lacrimal sac and the lower eyelid. The orbital artery enters the orbit through the supraorbital fissure, joining a recurrent branch of the lacrimal artery.

Venous System. The orbital venous system demonstrates limited correspondence with the arterial system. The most prominent vein within the orbit is the superior ophthalmic vein. Its superior root is an extension of the supraorbital vein. It extends from the superonasal portion of the orbital rim, along the orbital roof, to the medial portion of the levator palpebrae superiorus muscle. At this point the superior root joins the inferior root of this vein.

The inferior root is simply an extension of the angular vein. The superior ophthalmic vein courses along the superior rectus muscle to the superior orbital fissure. Before entering the fissure, it is joined by ciliary veins, superior vortex veins, lacrimal veins, and anterior and posterior ethmoidal veins. After entering the fissure in conjunction with the ophthalmic artery, the superior ophthalmic vein extends into the cavernous sinus.

The inferior ophthalmic vein originates along the orbital floor, supplied by venules from the lateral rectus, inferior rectus, and superior and inferior oblique muscles. Further contributions come from the inferior vortex veins, inferior conjunctiva, and lacrimal sac. The inferior ophthalmic vein joins the superior ophthalmic vein before entering into the cavernous sinus.

The central retinal vein courses in conjunction with the central retinal artery. It emerges from the optic nerve 10 mm (this varies from 5 to 15 mm) posterior to the globe, extending directly into the cavernous sinus.

Veins of the eyelids (Fig. 1–18) are subdivided into pretarsal and post-tarsal divisions. The pretarsal division joins the angular vein medially, the superficial vein temporally, and the lacrimal vein laterally. The post-tarsal division is deeper, joining various orbital veins, deep facial branches of the facial vein, and pterygoid plexus. The pre- and post-tarsal divisions also communicate with one another. The principal vein of the inner canthus is the angular vein, which is positioned just anterior to the medial canthal tendon.

Orbital Lymphatics. Orbital lymphatics comprise both a deep and a superficial system. Deep lymphatics form plexuses along the borders of the tarsal plates. These

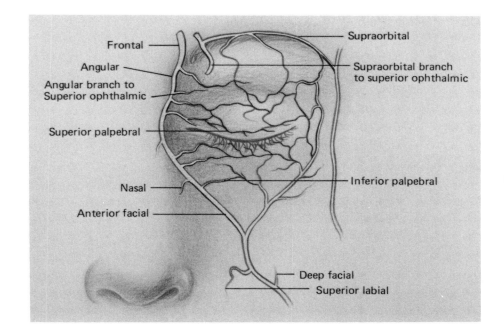

FIG. 1–18. Venous system of the eyelid and periorbital area.

drain the posterior lamella of the eyelid, principally the tarsoconjunctival region. Superficial lymphatics drain the anterior lamella of the eyelid, principally the skin and orbicularis oculi muscle. Lymphatic drainage from the medial portion of the eyelids and conjunctiva extends to the submaxillary nodes (Fig. 1–19). Lymphatic drainage from the lateral portion of the eyelids and conjunctiva extends to the preauricular and parotid nodes. The orbit itself contains no demonstrable lymph nodes or lymph vessels.

ANATOMY OF THE EYELIDS AND ADJACENT TISSUES

The eyelids and eyebrows are dynamic structures that provide for the functional integrity of the subjacent globe.

EYEBROW ANATOMY

The eyebrows are the lowest portion of scalp tissue, extending downward to the area of the supraorbital rim (Fig. 1–20). In males the brow usually overlies the rim, while in females it may be somewhat higher. The brow hairline is widest medially, tapering temporally with the follicles positioned obliquely in a lateral direction. The eyebrows are comprised of four layers: skin, muscle, fat, and aponeurosis. Eyebrow skin is thick, containing ir-

regularly spaced hair follicles surrounded by sebaceous and sweat glands. Four muscle groups (frontalis, procerus, corrugator superciliaris, and orbicularis oculi) comprise the muscular layer (Fig. 1–21).

The frontalis muscle is a downward extension of the anterior portion of the epicranius, inserting at the eyebrow without bony attachment. The frontalis elevates the brow, contributing significantly to facial expression.

The medial segment of the frontalis muscle attaches to the nasal bones as the procerus muscle. This structure pulls the medial portion of the brow inferiorly, resulting in a somewhat hostile facial expression.

The corrugator superciliaris muscle is positioned obliquely between the frontalis and orbicularis oculi muscles. It originates at the frontal bone near the superior orbital margin, extending laterally for 2 to 3 cm, where it merges with the orbicularis oculi and frontalis muscles. The corrugator pulls the brow in an inferomedial direction, resulting in vertical glabellar furrows. This muscle is innervated by upper branch fibers of the facial nerve (CN VII).

The superior portion of the orbicularis oculi muscle intermingles with the inferior portion of the frontalis muscle. The remainder of the orbicularis oculi muscle encircles the eyelid in its anterior lamellae.

The aponeurosis of the brow is an extension of the galea aponeurotica of the scalp. The galea splits to surround the frontalis muscle, inserting at the supraorbital margin, where it contributes to the arcus marginalis.

Fat within the brow is located between the muscular

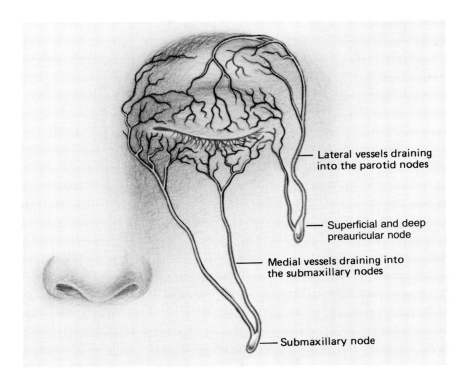

Lateral vessels draining
into the parotid nodes

Superficial and deep
preauricular node

Medial vessels draining into
the submaxillary nodes

Submaxillary node

FIG. 1–19. Lymphatic drainage from the eyelid and periorbital area.

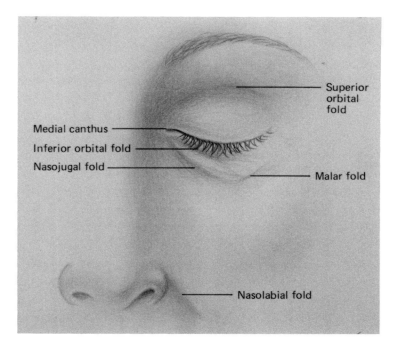

Superior
orbital
fold

Medial canthus

Inferior orbital fold

Nasojugal fold

Malar fold

Nasolabial fold

FIG. 1–20. Topographical anatomy of the eyelid and eyebrow demonstrating the natural folds contained therein.

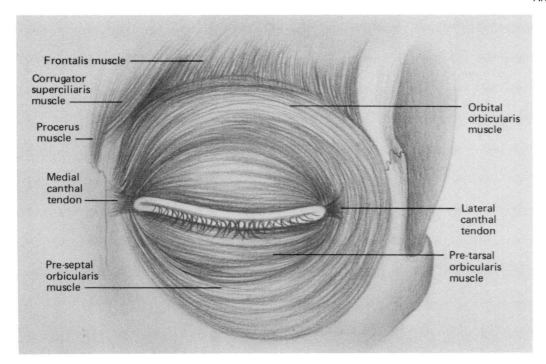

FIG. 1–21.   Musculature of the eyelid and eyebrow.

and aponeurotic layers; it augments brow mobility. A small portion of brow fat extends inferiorly into the eyelid, beneath the superior portion of the orbicularis oculi muscle.

EYELID ANATOMY

Anatomy Common to the Upper and Lower Eyelids. Eyelid skin is relatively thin and loose, in contrast to the surrounding brow, temple, and cheek skin. Eyelid skin is the thinnest in the entire body, having less developed sweat and sebaceous glands than elsewhere. The upper eyelid extends to the brow and lateral orbital rim, while the lower eyelid extends beyond the infraorbital rim to the nasojugal and malar skin folds (Fig. 1–20). In primary position (Fig. 1–22), the upper eyelid margin is positioned 1 to 2 mm below the superior limbus. In primary position, the lower eyelid margin is positioned at the inferior limbus.

The upper eyelid crease is formed by the attachment

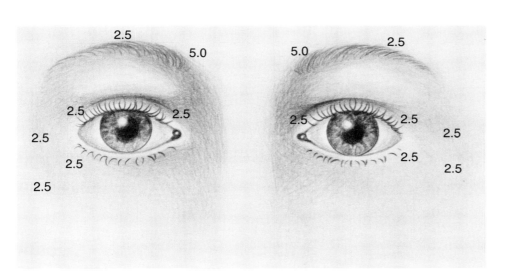

FIG. 1–22. Primary position—relationship between the eyelid margin and the limbus in a normal individual.

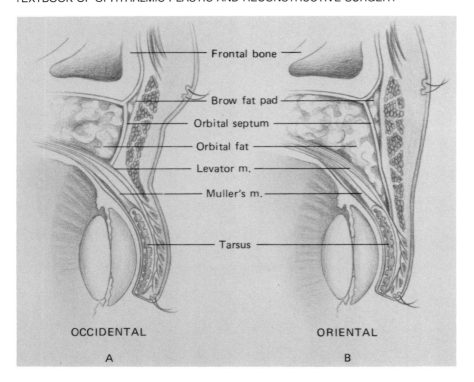

Frontal bone

Brow fat pad

Orbital septum

Orbital fat

Levator m.

Muller's m.

Tarsus

OCCIDENTAL

ORIENTAL

A

B

FIG. 1–23. A, Lateral view of an Occidental upper eyelid demonstrating the higher attachment between orbital septum and levator aponeurosis. This displaces the preaponeurotic fat to a higher position. B, Lateral view of an Oriental upper eyelid demonstrating the lower attachment between orbital septum and levator aponeurosis. This displaces the preaponeurotic fat to a lower position.

of levator aponeurosis fibers in the subcutaneous layer (Figs. 1–23A and 1–24). The crease is variably located from 7 to 11 mm above the eyelid margin. It denotes the division between loosely adherent preseptal skin and more adherent pretarsal skin.

In Oriental eyelids, the orbital septum fuses with the levator aponeurosis at a lower position than that found in Occidental eyelids (Fig. 1–23B). This displaces orbital fat to a lower level, impeding the subcutaneous attach-

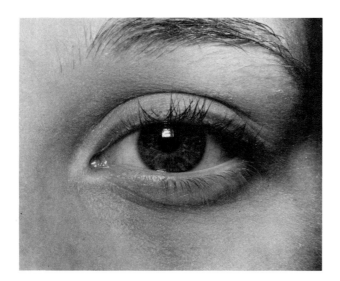

FIG. 1–24. Normal upper and lower eyelid crease.

ments of levator fibers. As a result, Oriental eyelids have a somewhat exaggerated upper eyelid skin fold that obliterates the eyelid crease and may obscure the upper eyelid margin.

The lower eyelid may demonstrate an eyelid crease (Fig. 1–24), particularly in children. This extends to within 3 mm of the eyelid margin medially, slanting downward to within 6 mm of the margin laterally.

The canthi represent the conjoined ends of the eyelids. The lateral (outer) canthus assumes a somewhat more acute angle than the medial (inner) canthus (Fig. 1–24). Subjacent to the medial canthus is the caruncle, which is composed of a blend of mucosal and cutaneous elements. The outer canthus is more mobile than the inner canthus.

Nasojugal and malar folds may be variably present (Fig. 1–20). The former appears between the lateral aspect of the nose and the inferomedial portion of the lower eyelid. The latter appears between the upper aspect of the cheek and the inferolateral portion of the lower eyelid. These folds result from the interface between thinner eyelid skin and coarser facial skin.

The eyelid margin affords the union of keratinized stratified squamous epithelium anteriorly with nonkeratinized stratified squamous and stratified columnar epithelium posteriorly (Fig. 1–25). This transition occurs at the gray line, which divides the eyelid margin into an anterior (ciliary) portion and a posterior (tarsal) portion. Within the ciliary portion reside the orbicularis oculi

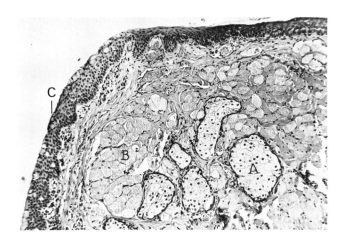

FIG. 1–25. Eyelid margin showing epithelial transition from squamous to stratified columnar type with goblet cells. A, Sections of a saccule of a meibomian gland; B, subtarsal part of muscle of Riolan; C, tarsal conjunctiva. (×150).

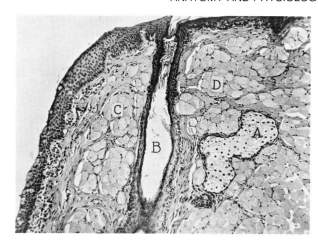

FIG. 1–27. Eyelid margin. A, Section of one lobule of meibomian glands; B, meibomian duct emptying at the muco-cutaneous junction; C, Subtarsal part of muscle of Riolan; D, ciliary part of the same muscle. (×150).

muscle and two or three somewhat irregular rows of cilia. The strip of orbicularis oculi muscle at the eyelid margin is designated the muscle of Riolan (Fig. 1–25). More cilia are found in the upper than in the lower eyelid.

Pilosebaceous glands supporting these cilia are located at the interface between the ciliary and tarsal segments of the eyelid margin. These are composed of the holocrine sebaceous glands of Zeis and the apocrine secretory glands of Moll (Fig. 1–26).

Within the tarsal portion reside the meibomian gland orifices (Fig. 1–27). Secretions from the meibomian glands, with minor contributions from the glands of Zeis and Moll, produce the outer (lipid) layer of the tear film.

Both the upper and lower eyelids are multilayered structures. The number of layers and specific composi-

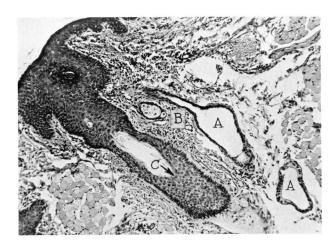

FIG. 1–26. Eyelid margin. A, Two portions of a gland of Moll and the first part of its duct; B, gland of Zeis; C, hair follicle. (×150).

tions vary with their respective positions from the eyelid margin. Near the margin the eyelid is composed of skin, orbicularis oculi muscle, tarsal plate, and conjunctiva.

In the upper eyelid, the levator aponeurosis forms a fifth layer at the junction of the lower and middle third of the tarsal plate (Fig. 1–7). Additionally, in the upper eyelid, the tarsal border serves as the site of attachment for both orbital septum and Müller's muscle. In the lower eyelid, the tarsal border serves as the point of attachment for both orbital septum and the inferior aponeurosis (capsulopalpebral head of the inferior rectus muscle). The latter is the lower eyelid retractor, analogous to the levator aponeurosis. Subjacent to the orbital septum are the orbital fat pads: two in the upper eyelid (medial and central) and three in the lower eyelid (medial, central, and lateral).

The orbicularis oculi muscle is concentrically positioned, surrounding the palpebral fissure, and is subdivided into orbital and palpebral segments. These muscle groups are continuous with one another and serve as the principal protractors of the eyelids.

The orbital portion of the orbicularis oculi muscle (Fig. 1–21) overlies the orbital rims, where it interfaces with the frontalis, procerus, and corrugator superciliaris muscles superiorly, and the temporalis muscle laterally.

The palpebral portion of the orbicularis oculi muscle is subdivided into preseptal and pretarsal segments, as defined by the subjacent structures (Fig. 1–28).

In each eyelid, the preseptal portion extends from the medial canthal tendon and anterior lacrimal crest to the lateral raphe overlying the lateral canthal tendon (Fig. 1–29). The deep heads of the preseptal muscle extend

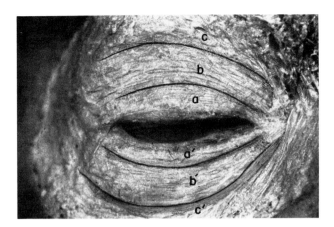

FIG. 1–28. Main subdivisions of the orbicularis oculi muscle. A and A′, Upper and lower pretarsal parts; B and B′, upper and lower preseptal parts; C and C′, orbital part.

over the lacrimal sac, contributing to the lacrimal pump mechanism (Fig. 1–30).

The pretarsal portion is composed of two heads, arising from the anterior and posterior limbs of the medial canthal tendon respectively (Fig. 1–21). In each eyelid, the pretarsal muscles fuse to form the lateral canthal tendon, which inserts into the lateral orbital tubercle.

The medial canthal tendon is composed of two heads. The more prominent superficial head attaches to the anterior lacrimal crest, while the smaller deep head (Horner's muscle) attaches to the posterior lacrimal crest. Within the lacrimal fossa, as defined by the lacrimal crests, is the lacrimal sac. The canaliculi are positioned just beneath the superficial head of the medial canthal tendon (Fig. 1–30).

The tarsal plates serve as the principal supportive structures of the eyelids. Composed of dense collagenous

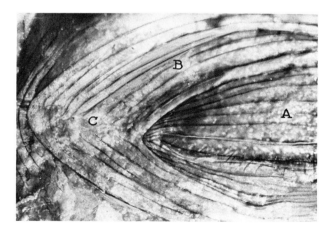

FIG. 1–29. Lateral part of palpebral muscle. A, Upper pretarsal part; B, upper preseptal part; C, lateral palpebral raphe. (Courtesy of Lester T. Jones, M.D.)

tissue, they extend from the punctum medially and to the outer canthus laterally. The tarsi end horizontally as tendinous expansions to the medial and lateral canthal tendons (Fig. 1–31). In the upper eyelid, the tarsus extends approximately 10 mm vertically, while in the lower eyelid, it extends 4 mm vertically. Conjunctiva firmly adheres to the posterior aspect of both tarsal plates as it lines the posterior lamella of each eyelid toward its respective fornix.

The orbital septum defines the anterior extent of the orbit (Fig. 1–7). The septum extends from the arcus marginalis (a thickening of periorbita) of the various orbital rims to the tarsal borders. At the medial orbital rim, the lacrimal crests afford the septum dual attachment to the arcus marginalis. This places the lacrimal sac outside the anatomic definition of the orbit. Laterally, the septum passes posterior to the lateral canthal tendon, fusing with the tendon and the lateral horn of the levator aponeurosis.

The orbital septum fuses with the levator aponeurosis in the upper eyelid and the inferior aponeurosis in the lower eyelid at a variable distance from the respective tarsal border (Fig. 1–7).

Preaponeurotic orbital fat is situated in the upper eyelid between the septum and levator aponeurosis. Similarly, in the lower eyelid it is situated between the septum and inferior aponeurosis.

The medial ocular retinaculum attaches to periosteum and bone posterior to the posterior lacrimal crest. Onto it attach the following structures: the medial end of the inferior transverse ligament, medial check ligament, deep head of the pretarsal muscle, medial horn of the levator aponeurosis, medial end of the superior transverse ligament, and the orbital septum.

The lateral ocular retinaculum attaches to the lateral orbital tubercle and zygomatic bone. Onto it attach the lateral end of the inferior transverse ligament, lateral check ligament, lateral canthal tendon, lateral horn of the levator aponeurosis fused with the lateral end of the superior transverse ligament, and the expansion of the superior rectus sheath designated the inferior ligament of Schwalbe.

Anatomy Unique to the Upper Eyelid. The levator palpebrae superiorus muscle and aponeurosis is the principal upper eyelid retractor. It originates above the annulus of Zinn at the orbital apex and extends horizontally along the superior portion of the orbit. Approximately 15 to 20 mm above the upper tarsal border, the levator muscle is redirected vertically by the superior transverse ligament (Whitnall's ligament) (Fig. 1–31). At this point, the levator gradually transforms into an aponeurosis as it extends forward.

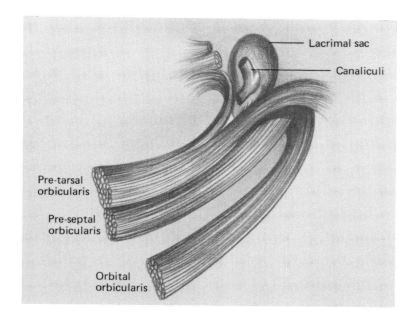

FIG. 1–30. Anatomic relationship between the orbicularis oculi muscle and the lacrimal sac and canaliculi.

Approximately 10 to 12 mm above the upper tarsal border, this eyelid retractor separates into two lamellae. The posterior lamella is composed of Müller's muscle (Fig. 1–7). This is designated as the superior tarsal muscle and ends in a somewhat tendinous insertion at the superior tarsal border. Müller's muscle functions by means of sympathetic innervation.

The anterior lamella is composed of levator aponeurosis (Figs. 1–7 and 1–31). This appears glistening and white beneath preaponeurotic fat during surgical dissection. The aponeurosis fuses with the orbital septum at a variable distance above the tarsal border.

The principal insertion of the levator aponeurosis is at the anterior surface of the tarsal plate, approximately 3 mm above the eyelid margin. Additional insertions go to pretarsal orbicularis oculi muscle and to subcutaneous tissue to form the eyelid crease. The levator muscle and aponeurosis function by means of innervation from the superior branch of the oculomotor nerve (CN III).

Medial and lateral extensions of the levator aponeurosis have been designated as its "horns" (Fig. 1–31). The prominent lateral horn extends through the lacrimal gland, separating the orbital and palpebral lobes. It attaches to the lateral orbital tubercle, contributing to the

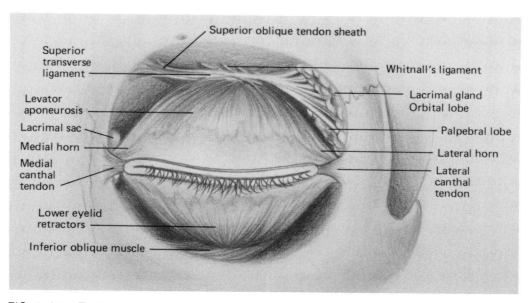

FIG. 1–31. Eyelid anatomy at the depth of the tarsal plates and eyelid retractors.

lateral canthal tendon and lateral retinaculum in the process. The medial horn is less developed as it passes in an inferomedial direction to contribute to the deep head of the medial canthal tendon.

The superior transverse ligament of Whitnall is a condensation of fascial sheaths. It extends from the trochlear region medially, through the lacrimal gland, to insert on the superior portion of the lateral orbital wall. Whitnall's ligament serves as a pulley, redirecting levator action from horizontal to vertical. It also supports the lacrimal gland within the orbit. As such, it is analogous to Lockwood's ligament in the lower eyelid. Both structures should be preserved during surgery.

Anatomy Unique to the Lower Eyelid. In the lower eyelid, the inferior aponeurosis (capsulopalpebral head of the inferior rectus) is the analog of the levator aponeurosis. This is a fibrous tissue extension of the inferior rectus sheath and muscle. As it travels forward toward the eyelid, it splits to surround the inferior oblique muscle (Figs. 1–7 and 1–31). Further anteriorly, it reunites, contributing to Lockwood's ligament. The inferior aponeurosis extends forward to fuse with the orbital septum and insert at or near the lower tarsal border. The somewhat rudimentary inferior tarsal muscle responds to sympathetic innervation and inserts at the lower tarsal border along with the inferior aponeurosis.

Lockwood's suspensory ligament is principally composed of fibers from the inferior aponeurosis and the inferior oblique fascia. Additional contributions are derived from Tenon's capsule, intermuscular fibrous septae, and the inferior rectus muscle fascia. Lockwood's ligament supports the orbital floor. This becomes particularly important after orbital floor ("blowout") fracture or Ogura orbital decompression.

LACRIMAL SYSTEM

The lacrimal system may be divided into three subsystems involving secretion, distribution, and drainage.

Lacrimal Secretory System. The lacrimal secretory system is composed of basic and reflex secretors.

Basic tear secretion provides mucin, lacrimal fluid, and lipid, composing the three layers of the tear film.

The innermost layer of the tear film is composed of mucin derived from conjunctival goblet cells. Additional contributions come from the crypts of Henle and the glands of Manz (Fig. 1–32). Henle's crypts are found along the entire length of the distal tarsal surface in each eyelid. The glands of Manz are circumferentially positioned within the perilimbal conjunctiva. This is the thinnest layer of the tear film and interfaces with corneal epithelium.

Lacrimal fluid provides the aqueous middle layer of the tear film. This is the thickest portion of the tear film. The principal basic lacrimal secretors are the glands of Krause and Wolfring, and the accessory lacrimal glands. They are exocrine glands, located subjacent to the conjunctiva near the fornix and tarsal border respectively. Approximately 20 to 40 glands of Krause occur in the upper fornix and 6 to 8 in the lower fornix. Approximately three glands of Wolfring occur at the superior tarsal border of the upper eyelid and one at the inferior tarsal border of the lower eyelid. All these accessory glands produce a serous fluid and drain directly onto the conjunctival surface.

Aqueous production is augmented by reflex tearing emanating from the main lacrimal gland.

The outermost layer of the tear film is composed of lipid derived principally from the meibomian glands. Approximately 25 such holocrine glands are present within the upper eyelid and 20 within the lower eyelid. The meibomian glands are positioned vertically within the tarsal plate. Their secretions emerge from orifices in the posterior lamella of the eyelid margins. Minor additional contributions to lipid production come from the holocrine glands of Zeis and the apocrine glands of Moll. These two glands are anatomically associated with the cilia. The resultant outer layer of the tear film serves to stabilize the inner layers and to minimize evaporation.

The main lacrimal gland comprises the reflex secretors. It is an exocrine gland with parasympathetic innervation.

The main lacrimal gland is located in the superolateral quadrant of the anterior orbit. It is situated in the lacrimal gland fossa, just posterior to the orbital rim and orbital septum. The lacrimal gland is pinkish-gray and glandular in appearance, distinguishing it from surrounding orbital fat. The lateral horn of the levator aponeurosis divides the gland into the larger, superiorly positioned orbital lobe and the smaller, inferiorly positioned palpebral lobe (Fig. 1–31).

The orbital lobe is approximately 20 mm long, 12 mm wide, and 5 mm deep, assuming a somewhat oval configuration. It extends inferiorly to the level of the zygomaticofrontal suture and its shape is, in part, molded by the subjacent globe. Two to six excretory ducts extend from the orbital portion of the lacrimal gland to the palpebral portion.

The palpebral lobe is situated between the lateral horn of the levator aponeurosis above and the palpebral conjunctiva below, to which it is firmly attached. It consists of 15 to 40 lobules, each with its own excretory duct.

The lacrimal gland receives its principal anatomic sup-

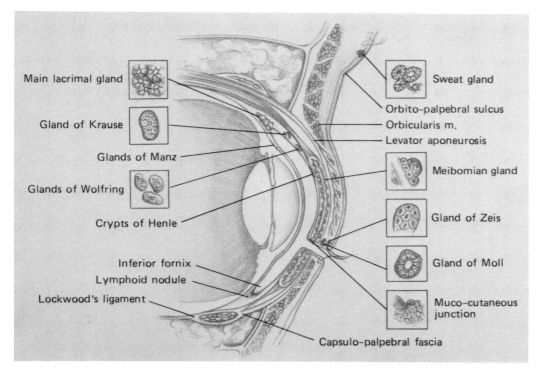

FIG. 1–32. Glandular structures of the eyelid.

port from Whitnall's ligament and the lateral horn of the levator aponeurosis. Minor additional support is provided by the suspensory ligament of Soemmering.

The lacrimal gland does not have a true capsule. It is surrounded by connective tissue that separates the various lobules of the gland. The gland is tubuloracemose, consisting of numerous lobules drained by tubules (Fig. 1–32). The secretory elements are the acini, which consist of cells surrounding a central lumen; these produce a serous fluid. The accumulated fluid then passes through a series of excretory ducts.

Lacrimal gland excretions flow sequentially into the intralobular ducts, interlobular ducts, and main excretory ducts. The lumen within this ductal system becomes progressively larger. Approximately 12 main excretory ducts carry secretions from both lobes of the lacrimal gland on the conjunctival surface. All ducts traverse the palpebral lobe before exiting approximately 5 mm above the superolateral tarsal border in the upper eyelid. Some duct orifices may also emerge at the outer canthus.

The main lacrimal gland provides reflex tearing through a reflex arc. It also responds to direct central nervous system stimulation. The afferent pathway of the reflex arc is by way of the trigeminal nerve (CN V) (Figs. 1–13 and 1–14), while the efferent pathway is by way of the facial nerve (CN VII). Afferent innervation is provided by the lacrimal nerve, a branch of the ophthalmic

division of the trigeminal nerve (V_1). The nerve contains a superior division that is sensory for the skin and conjunctiva of the lateral portion of the upper eyelid (Fig. 1–15). The inferior division joins the zygomaticotemporal branch of the zygomatic nerve to form a sensory nerve for the temple. Efferent innervation is mediated by parasympathetic fibers within the zygomaticotemporal branch of the maxillary nerve.

Stimulation of branches of the trigeminal nerve (to the cornea, uvea, conjunctiva, and nasal mucosa) results in reflex tearing. Interruption of the reflex arc causes loss of reflex tearing. Central stimuli from the retina, frontal cortex, basal ganglia, thalamus, hypothalamus, and cervical sympathetics may also trigger the main lacrimal gland.

Lacrimal Distribution System. Contraction of the orbicularis oculi muscle on blinking distributes the tear film vertically. This resurfaces the corneal epithelium, provides nutritional support for the anterior corneal layers, and removes debris and waste material from the eye.

A tear meniscus also forms at the lower eyelid margin. This moves horizontally and medially toward the lacrimal lacus and punctum through a lacrimal pump mechanism.

Lacrimal Drainage System. The lacrimal drainage sys-

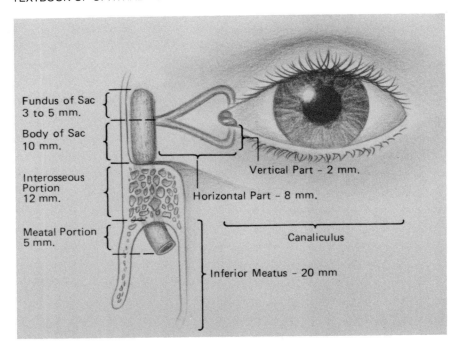

Fundus of Sac
3 to 5 mm.

Body of Sac
10 mm.

Interosseous
Portion
12 mm.

Meatal Portion
5 mm.

Vertical Part - 2 mm.

Horizontal Part - 8 mm.

Canaliculus

Inferior Meatus - 20 mm

FIG. 1–33. Schematic anatomy of the lacrimal drainage system.

tem (Fig. 1–33) is composed of the lower and upper puncta, lower and upper canaliculi, common canaliculus, lacrimal sac, and nasolacrimal duct. Tears pool at the lacrimal lacus, adjacent to the inner canthus. They enter the lacrimal drainage system at the punctum. The puncta are located at the mucocutaneous junction of the medial portion of each eyelid. Their location is defined by their position within a somewhat apical elevation of the eyelid margin, the lacrimal papilla. Each punctum is approximately 0.3 mm in diameter, surrounded by a ring of fibroelastic tissue.

Gravitational factors result in greater quantities of fluid passing through the lower punctum than the upper one. Efficiency of the lower punctum is further augmented by its somewhat posterior orientation. Tears then flow through their respective canaliculi, joining at the common canaliculus before entering the lacrimal sac. Each canaliculus extends vertically for approximately 2 mm to the ampullae, then medially for approximately 8 mm. The canalicular lumen is 1 to 2 mm in diameter.

The canaliculi unite either just above the lateral wall of the lacrimal sac as the common canaliculus (90%), or at the lacrimal sac wall as the internal common punctum (10%). The internal common punctum is subjacent to the medial canthal tendon. The entrance into the lacrimal sac is angulated, producing the valve of Rosenmüller. This minimizes reflux from the lacrimal sac into the canalicular system.

Histologically, the puncta and canaliculi are lined with nonkeratinizing, stratified squamous epithelium.

The lacrimal sac and nasolacrimal duct are a continuous

membranous tube lined with modified, nonciliated, respiratory epithelium. The lacrimal sac resides within the lacrimal sac fossa between the superficial and deep heads of the medial canthal tendon. Its dome (fundus) extends 4 mm above the superior aspect of the superficial head of the medial canthal tendon. The body of the lacrimal sac extends from the fundus to its junction with the nasolacrimal duct at the bony nasolacrimal canal. The nasolacrimal duct is approximately 12 mm long and extends vertically and somewhat laterally, entering the nose at the inferior meatus beneath the inferior turbinate. Within the meatal opening is a fold of nasal mucosa, the valve of Hasner. This valve is inferolateral to the inferior turbinate.

Jones and Wobig have described a lacrimal pump mechanism that actively moves tears into the nose through the nasolacrimal system. In this process, contraction of the pretarsal orbicularis oculi muscle with blinking compresses the canaliculus, closing its vertical portion (ampulla). The puncta move medially in the process. Contraction of the preseptal orbicularis oculi muscle expands the lacrimal sac to which it is attached. This creates negative pressure (suction) within the sac. The periorbita at the lateral wall of the sac functions as a lacrimal diaphragm. Its lateral pull creates additional negative pressure within the sac. This draws tears from the ampulla and canaliculus into the lacrimal sac. Therefore, closing the eyelids will siphon tears into the lacrimal sac.

Opening the eyelids expands the canaliculus and ampulla, siphoning tears into the canaliculus in preparation for the next blink. Further passage of tears through the nasolacrimal duct results from gravity. Reflux of tears is impeded by the valve of Rosenmüller.

A modification of this lacrimal pump theory has been recently postulated by Doane (1981).

BIBLIOGRAPHY

Anderson, R.: Medial canthal tendon branches out. Arch. Ophthalmol. 95:2051, 1977.

Anderson, R. and Beard, C.: The levator aponeurosis. Attachments and their clinical significance. Arch. Ophthalmol. 95:1437, 1977.

Anderson, R. and Dixon, R.: The role of Whitnall's ligament in ptosis surgery. Arch. Ophthalmol. 97:705, 1979.

Beard, C. and Quickert, M.: Anatomy of the Orbit. Birmingham, Aesculapius, 1977.

Bergen, M.: Spatial aspects of the orbital vascular system. In Duane, T. and Jaeger, E. (eds.): Biomedical Foundations of Ophthalmology. Philadelphia, Harper and Row, 1982.

Doane, M.: Interactions of eyelids and tears in corneal wetting and the dynamics of the normal human eyeblink. Am. J. Ophthalmol. 89:507, 1980.

Doane, M.: Blinking and the mechanics of the lacrimal drainage system. Ophthalmology. 88:844, 1981.

Doxanas, M. and Anderson, R.: Clinical Orbital Anatomy. Baltimore, Williams and Wilkins, 1984.

Harris, F. and Rhoton, A.: Anatomy of the cavernous sinus. A microsurgical study. J. Neurosurg. 45:169, 1976.

Hawes, M. and Dortzbach, R.: The microscopic anatomy of the lower eyelid retractors. Arch. Ophthalmol. 100:1313, 1982.

Hayreh, S.: The ophthalmic artery. III. Branches. Br. J. Ophthalmol. 46:212, 1962.

Hayreh, S.: Arteries of the orbit in the human being. Br. J. Surg. 50:938, 1963.

Hayreh, S. and Dass, R.: The ophthalmic artery. I. Origin and intra-cranial and intra-canalicular course. Br. J. Ophthalmol. 46:65, 1962.

Hayreh, S. and Dass, R.: The ophthalmic artery. III intra-orbital course. Br. J. Ophthalmol. 46:165, 1962.

Holly, F. and Lemp, M.: Tear physiology and dry eyes. Surv. Ophthalmol. 22:69, 1977.

Hugo, N. and Stone, E.: Anatomy for a blepharoplasty. Plast. Reconstr. Surg. 53:381, 1974.

Jones, L.: The anatomy of the lower eyelid and its relation to the cause and cure of entropion. Am. J. Ophthalmol. 49:29, 1960.

Jones, L.: The lacrimal secretory system and its treatment. Am. J. Ophthalmol. 62:47, 1966.

Jones, L.: A new concept of the orbital fascia and rectus muscle sheaths and its surgical implications. Trans. Am. Acad. Ophthalmol. 72:755, 1968.

Jones, L. and Wobig, J.: Surgery of the Eyelids and Lacrimal System. Birmingham, Aesculapius, 1976.

Koornneef, L.: New insights in the human orbital connective tissue: Results of a new anatomic approach. Arch. Ophthalmol. 95:1269, 1977.

Koornneef, L.: Orbital septa: Anatomy and function. Ophthalmology. 86:876, 1979.

Koornneef, L.: Orbital connective tissue. In Duane, T. and Jaeger, E. (eds.): Biomedical Foundations of Ophthalmology. Philadelphia, Harper and Row, 1982.

Lempke, B. and Stasior, O.: The anatomy of eyebrow ptosis. Arch. Ophthalmol. 100:981, 1982.

Miller, N.: Walsh and Hoyt's Clinical Neuro-Ophthalmology, 4th Ed. Baltimore, Williams and Wilkins, 1983.

Reeh, M., Beyer, C., and Shannon, G.: Practical Ophthalmic Plastic and Reconstructive Surgery. Philadelphia, Lea & Febiger, 1976.

Umansky, F. and Nathan, H.: The lateral wall of the cavernous sinus: With special reference to the nerves related to it. J. Neurosurg. 56:228, 1982.

Walsh, F. and Hoyt, W.: Clinical Neuro-Ophthalmology, 3rd Ed. Baltimore, Williams and Wilkins, 1969.

Warwick, R.: Eugene Wolff's Anatomy of the Eye and Orbit. 7th Ed. Philadelphia, W.B. Saunders, 1976.

Wolff, E.: The Anatomy of the Eye and Orbit. 6th Ed. London, Lewis, 1968.

2

BASIC
PRINCIPLES

The primary goal in ophthalmic plastic and reconstructive surgery is the maintenance of vision by protecting the globe and establishing proper function of the orbital adnexa. Cosmesis, although important, is secondary to a functioning eye and orbit.

Optimal oculoplastic surgical care requires the integration of adequate preoperative evaluation, proper patient selection, and correct choice of treatment with effective execution. A basic understanding of wound healing is integral to this process.

WOUND HEALING

Vasoconstriction and blood coagulation from transected capillaries trigger the healing process following surgery or trauma. Wound healing may be subdivided into a continuum of four overlapping stages: inflammation (latent), fibroblast proliferation, scar contraction, and scar maturation.

Inflammation follows tissue insult in which vasodilatation facilitates accumulation of leukocytes, macrophages, and other cellular elements within the wound. Chemotactic substances further attract these cellular elements. This cleanses the area of debris, necrotic tissue, and bacteria while preparing the wound for the later fibroblastic and scar maturation stages. Interstitial serum and fluid accumulate within the wound. Capillary buds appear between the fourth and fifth days, providing additional strength and nutritional support. Inflammation wanes after 4 to 6 days.

Fibroblasts appear at approximately the seventh day. This leads to collagen deposition, which begins on the ninth day and persists from 2 to 4 weeks. At this point, wound strength rapidly increases as the scar becomes relatively hypertrophic. This process generates a framework for tissue reconstruction. Toward the end of the fibroblastic stage, collagenase is produced, balancing collagen production with degradation.

The period of scar contraction follows. Although contraction occurs in all directions, it is most manifest vertically. It is, therefore, important to initially produce a slightly everted skin closure, which will yield a level scar over time. The greatest degree of contraction occurs in the areas of loosest tissue support (i.e., in free skin grafts, untreated trauma).

After approximately 1 month, the fibroblasts leave the wound and the maturation stage begins. The collagen becomes less hydrated and more organized, resulting in a stronger, less prominent scar.

Adjacent tissue further contributes toward closing a defect. Within several hours of tissue injury, cutaneous epithelium begins to migrate from the wound margins to fill the defect and form a barrier to infection. The epidermis expands by mitotic growth, while the subjacent dermis stretches, rendering dermal elements (glands, follicles) more widely spaced.

Foreign material that cannot be absorbed or removed during the acute inflammatory phase stimulates chronic inflammation. This is manifested by deposition of collagen, epithelioid cells, and foreign body giant cells to form a granuloma. This same process may occur around absorbable sutures (Fig. 2–1). Fibrous capsules surrounding nonabsorbable sutures and alloplastic materials are an additional source of chronic inflammation (Fig. 2–2).

The entire process of wound healing lasts approximately 2 months, although the scar continuously matures for several years.

Chemical mediators are involved in initiating and end-

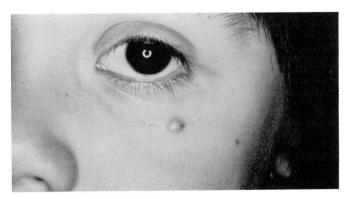

FIG. 2–1.   Foreign body giant cell granulomatous response to a chromic catgut suture.

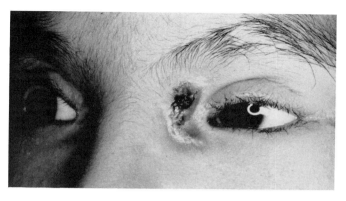

FIG. 2–2. Chronic inflammatory reaction stimulated by a Supramid suture.

ing the wound healing process. They serve to attract cells into the wound and cleanse the site of debris, necrotic tissue, and bacteria. The mediators may be inhibited by steroid use, immunosuppression, and intercurrent infection. The abundant vascularity of the periorbital area makes infection relatively uncommon. A large inoculum of bacteria, the presence of foreign material, an excessively large wound dead space, steroid treatment, or immunosuppression, however, may retard wound healing and predispose to infection.

SURGICAL PRINCIPLES

Informed Consent. All potential surgical candidates should be clearly informed about their disorder and the benefits and risks of the various medical and surgical treatment modalities available, including anesthetic risk. They must be apprised of all available alternatives (including non-treatment). The contents of this discussion should be documented in the patient's office record. From this information, patients will be in an optimal position to choose the approach with which they are psychologically comfortable and that they feel will be in their best interest. Before surgery, the various discussions between surgeon and patient should engender confidence and realistic expectations.

Photography. Photographs are essential in ophthalmic plastic and reconstructive surgery. They form an accurate record of the patient's condition, providing a chronicle of evolving changes and a reminder of the preoperative condition for surgeon and patient alike. Insurance companies now frequently request evidence of the patient's preoperative status, which can best be presented through photography.

A 35 mm camera with macro lens and forward-mounted flash is optimal. When the flash unit is not placed forward, the lens may cast a shadow over the field. Smaller camera systems have been effectively adapted for this purpose. Exposure settings are based on experience, or may be preset as in some commercially available units (e.g., those of Lester Dine, Inc.). Preoperative and postoperative photographs should be taken with the same settings and focal distances to maximize comparability. Videotaping certain conditions (blepharospasm, anomalous third nerve reinervation, Marcus Gunn jaw-winking) may also be beneficial in capturing dynamic dysfunction.

Tissue Preparation for Surgery. The most effective surgical preparatory solution is povidone-iodine (Betadine). It has a germicidal effect against gram-positive and gram-negative bacteria, as well as fungi, yeast, viruses, and protozoa. It may be used on both the skin and conjunctival cul-de-sac, and may also be used on open wounds if subsequently irrigated out. It is relatively nonirritating, but can cause severe allergic reactions in patients with iodine sensitivity. Hexachlorophene (pHisohex) and chlorhexidine gluconate (Hibiclens) are reasonable alternative solutions, particularly in patients with iodine sensitivity.

Anesthesia. Preparation of the patient for the anesthetic should be done with close coordination between the operating surgeon, surgical assistant, anesthesiologist or anesthetist, and members of the nursing staff.

General anesthesia is necessary in all oculoplastic procedures performed on children. In adults, general anesthesia is required in orbital surgery, correction of craniofacial anomalies, major socket surgery, open reduction and internal fixation of periorbital fractures, most lacrimal procedures, major eyelid reconstruction, and facial nerve avulsion for blepharospasm. Most other cases within the scope of this subspecialty lend themselves to local anesthesia. This can be enhanced by monitored local anesthesia arrangement for patients requiring additional medical monitoring or additional medications to relax the patient. Local anesthesia without anesthesia monitoring may proceed effectively in young, healthy patients, supplemented if necessary by selected sedatives.

In all cases, an intravenous line should be established to afford rapid and painless administration of supplementary medication. Patients under either local or monitored local anesthetic conditions may require either oxygen delivery (through nasal prongs), or carbon dioxide suction, or open-face draping to minimize claustrophobia. If oxygen is used, caution must be exercised to avoid combustion from cautery. Continuous monitoring of vital signs is essential to ensure patient safety.

Local anesthesia is usually in the form of direct infiltration subjacent to the surgical site. In some cases, this may be supplemented by regional nerve blocks. This combination results in analgesia, while not distorting tissue within the surgical field. Such blocks should not be used when dynamic eyelid movement is necessary to achieve optimal results. Thus, the supraorbital, supratrochlear, or infratrochlear nerves should not be blocked in blepharoptosis surgery because the anesthetic agent will partially penetrate into the orbit, resulting in a partial retrobulbar nerve block. This temporarily diminishes levator action and impedes surgical quantification.

The local anesthetic mechanism of action is through stabilization of the nerve membrane, preventing depolarization by inhibiting sodium ion entrance. Nerve conduction is thereby temporarily impaired. Lidocaine hydrochloride 2% (Xylocaine) is an ideal agent for local anesthesia. Lidocaine with epinephrine enhances hemostasis and the duration of anesthetic action. The use of epinephrine, however, should be judicious (or perhaps avoided) in patients with hypertension or organic heart disease. Combined use of halothane (Fluothane) with either epinephrine or cocaine may predispose to significant cardiac arrhythmias. Likewise, the combined use of epinephrine and cocaine should be judicious because resultant high catecholamine levels may exacerbate hypertension or induce cardiac arrhythmias. Epinephrine is not recommended in blepharoptosis surgery or in cases requiring free skin grafts. In the former situation, the effect of epinephrine on Müller's muscle artifactually raises the eyelid and may influence the surgeon toward a more limited correction. In the latter situation, epinephrine may transiently diminish the vascular support subjacent to a free skin graft. Although bupivacaine hydrochloride (Marcaine) has been used for its longer duration of action, cases of respiratory depression (and arrest) have occurred following its retrobulbar infiltration.

Allergy to local anesthetics is uncommon. Should a patient's history clearly document sensitivity, a shift from the amide to the ester group of anesthetics, or vice versa, is mandated. Cross-sensitivity between these two groups has not been reported.

Periorbital Nerve Blocks. The supratrochlear and infratrochlear nerves are located through their juxtaposition to the trochlea (Fig. 2–3). The trochlea is palpable beneath the medial portion of the supraorbital rim, medial to the supraorbital notch. These nerves can be reached by placing a long 25-gauge needle 2 cm deep along the orbital roof in the region of the trochlea. The supratrochlear nerve is blocked by injecting an anesthetic just temporal to the trochlea; the infratrochlear

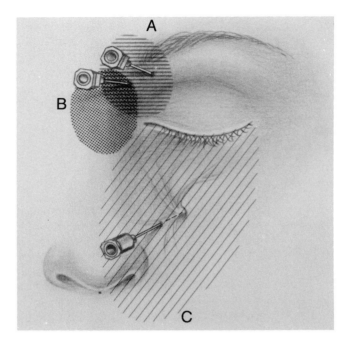

FIG. 2–3. Anatomic areas of sensory block from the A, supratrochlear nerve, B, infratrochlear nerve, and C, infraorbital nerve.

nerve is blocked by injecting the anesthetic just nasal to the trochlea. Blocking these nerves anesthetizes the inner canthus and the medial one-fourth of the upper eyelid and brow.

The infraorbital nerve exits the maxilla through the infraorbital foramen in conjunction with the infraorbital artery and vein (Fig. 2–3). This point is usually found midway along the vertical line between the angle of the mouth and the lower eyelid margin, just lateral to the nasal ala. The infraorbital nerve may be blocked by anesthetic infiltration into the foramen or around its point of emergence. The canal may be entered by following its contour and by directing a 25-gauge needle 20 degrees in a superolateral direction. In locating the foramen, care must be taken to ensure that the needle does not extend to or beyond the infraorbital rim toward the globe. Blocking this nerve will anesthetize the entire lower eyelid, cheek, and lateral aspect of the nose. Sensation to the upper teeth and gums may, on occasion, be transiently affected.

The supraorbital nerve is located by means of its relationship to the supraorbital notch (Fig. 2–4). The notch is located where the sharply angled lateral portion of the supraorbital rim joins the bluntly angled medial portion of the rim. This occurs at the junction of the medial third and the lateral two-thirds of the rim. A short 25-gauge needle is all that is needed to infiltrate the supraorbital

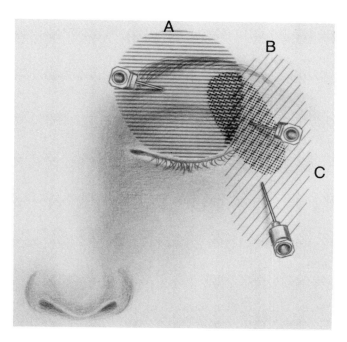

FIG. 2–4. Anatomic areas of sensory block from the A, supraorbital nerve, B, lacrimal nerve, and C, zygomaticofacial nerve.

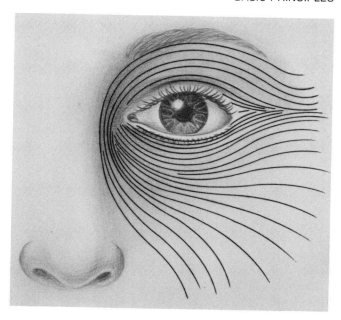

FIG. 2–5. Langer's lines in the periorbital area, representing the direction of normal skin tension (wrinkle lines).

nerve at the notch. Blocking this nerve anesthetizes the medial three-fourths of the upper eyelid and brow.

The lacrimal nerve emerges directly above the lateral canthal tendon at the lateral orbital rim (Fig. 2–4). Its infiltration with anesthetic will block sensation at the lateral aspect of the upper eyelid and the upper portion of the outer canthus.

The zygomaticofacial nerve emerges through the zygomaticofacial foramen (Fig. 2–4). This nerve is located along the zygoma, 1 cm inferior to the inferotemporal angle of the bony orbit. Its infiltration blocks the remainder of the outer canthus, lateral orbital floor, and adjacent temple.

Surgical Incision and Dissection. When the surgeon has a choice, the incisions (and hence the suture lines at closure) should be camouflaged. This can be achieved by placing the incision in conformity with Langer's lines (the lines of normal skin tension) (Fig. 2–5), in existing folds (such as the upper eyelid crease), or at the junction of facial landmarks (such as the upper border of the brow). Following these guidelines limits both the extent and perception of scarring. The attainment of symmetry should be a coexistent surgical goal. What might appear as a satisfactory unilateral result might represent a deformity when compared with the contralateral side.

All intended surgical sites should be delineated with either a fine methylene blue line or a marking pen. Mark-

ing the incision before local anesthetic infiltration is generally preferable, because this ensures accuracy and avoids tissue distortion. Incisions are carried out with a sharp scalpel (#64 Beaver blade or #15 Bard Parker blade) or scissors (sharp Stevens) and, with the exception of the eyebrow, should not be beveled. This diminishes resultant scarring. The incision is extended from the lowest segment to the highest segment, permitting gravity to keep any accrued blood away from the advancing blade. Traction on the tissue facilitates motion of the scalpel. The incision is extended through the dermis and should remain continuous to avoid skin irregularities.

Deeper dissections are achieved with scissors (sharp or blunt Stevens for periorbital tissue, small Metzenbaum for facial tissue). Using the scissors for spreading, rather than cutting, minimizes bleeding and helps to safeguard vital structures during careful dissections. Applicator sticks can also be used for meticulous dissection during some procedures.

Careful and gentle handling of tissue is important, as well as evaluation of the elasticity of the tissues to be used in surgical reconstruction. Fine-toothed Castroviejo forceps (0.5 mm, 0.3 mm, 0.12 mm) are effective and gentle for use in the periorbital area, while Adson forceps may be required for use in thicker adjacent facial tissue. Wound exposure can be augmented by placing fine bipronged skin hooks or by placing specialized retractors (self-retaining lacrimal retractor in lacrimal surgery, orbital or malleable retractor in orbitotomy, Desmarres retractor in posterior approach blepharoptosis surgery).

The surgical dissection in complex procedures should be carefully approached. To maintain proper tissue identification when surgical planes become obscure, it may be helpful to label structures with temporary sutures. This facilitates later wound closure.

In operating on the eyelids or orbit, protection of all underlying tissues must be sustained. A protective type of contact lens (protective shell) or lid plate is always used. Care in protecting the globe is essential. This may entail protecting the subjacent globe from cautery used on the overlying eyelid, or protecting the adjacent globe from the Stryker saw used in lateral orbitotomy procedures, the Hall drill used in lacrimal procedures, or the Wright needle used in frontalis suspension and transnasal wiring procedures. Intermittent irrigation of the cornea with a balanced salt solution prevents its desiccation and epithelial disruption.

Consideration must be given to protecting structures adjacent to the orbit. Be aware, in lacrimal procedures, of the close anatomic relationship to the maxillary antrum, the ethmoid sinus, and the cribriform plate. Orbital roof surgery should be evaluated in view of this structure's relationship to the frontal lobe of the brain. Function of the optic nerve and various extraocular muscles must be preserved in orbital surgery for tumor removal, fracture repair, or decompression.

Hemostasis. Maintaining adequate hemostasis is essential in ophthalmic plastic surgery. Intraoperative bleeding appreciably diminishes surgical visualization. Any blood retained postoperatively may retard wound healing, increase scarring, and predispose to infection.

The use of epinephrine in the local anesthetic mixture significantly augments hemostasis. As noted in the section on anesthesia, its use must be selective and may be limited by underlying medical conditions or particular surgical goals. To be effective, lidocaine (Xylocaine) with epinephrine should be infiltrated 10 to 15 minutes before the first incision to optimize vasoconstriction. The anesthesiologist should be apprised when epinephrine is used so that he can monitor its potential cardiac and hypertensive effects and avoid using any agents with which it might adversely interact.

In surgical procedures extending into the nose, cocaine nasal packing may further assist hemostasis. This should be used judiciously because significant cardiac effects may result, particularly when such packing is used in conjunction with epinephrine.

Pressure may effectively eliminate minor bleeding sites. More extensive bleeding requires electrocautery. Both the unipolar Bovie cautery with microtip and the bipolar Wetfield cautery with fine forceps work exceedingly well. The Bovie cautery has the advantage of al-lowing direct application of cautery tip to the bleeding site. The Wetfield cautery has the advantage of being effective under water or blood, and having limited systemic effect because it does not require grounding. The choice of modalities rests with the surgeon's preference. In patients who bleed profusely, placing of hemostats may also be necessary. Cauterization of the clamped tissue is established by touching the cautery to the hemostat. Skin should always be protected from cautery. Additionally, cautery may penetrate more deeply than expected. When the globe is subjacent, it should be protected by a surgical conformer (shell) or lid plate.

Suture ligatures are rarely required in ophthalmic plastic surgery. In certain circumstances, epinephrine-laden cotton pledgets, thrombin, a gelatin sponge (Gelfoam), microfibrillar collagen hemostat, or MCH (Avitene), and bone wax (for persistent bony bleeding) may prove helpful. Epinephrine causes effective vasoconstriction, but may be contraindicated in patients with hypertension or organic heart disease. Thrombin augments clotting by converting soluble fibrinogen into the insoluble fibrin form. The gelatin sponge (Gelfoam) stimulates thromboplastin release, augmenting this precursor of coagulation. MCH (Avitene) creates a mechanical matrix supporting clot formation. Care must be exercised in the use of MCH. After hemostasis is established, all of the MCH should be removed from the surgical site. Several cases have been reported whereby appreciable residual MCH has caused wound necrosis. Bone wax establishes a mechanical tamponade for minor cancellous bone bleeding.

Suture Materials. Suture material available for ophthalmic plastic surgical application encompasses a wide, diverse group of materials of various sizes. All have been modified for various surgical applications.

In general, the suture material should be fine, have good tensile strength, and form a flat knot when tied. Attention should be paid to the absorbability of the sutures and their specific absorption times.

The suture material should effect a wound closure that eliminates all dead space and wound irregularities. Sutures must not interfere with the circulation of the wound.

Sutures are categorized as absorbable and nonabsorbable. Absorbable sutures may be synthetic (Vicryl and Dexon) or nonsynthetic (catgut or chromic catgut). Catgut sutures are derived from sheep intestinal submucosa. When they are processed by soaking in a chromic salt solution, the protein coagulates, resulting in a firmer, less reactive material (chromic catgut).

Absorbable sutures are used for wound closures below skin level. Synthetic absorbable sutures (Vicryl or

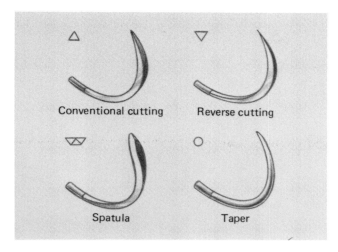

FIG. 2–6. Needles most applicable in ophthalmic plastic surgery.

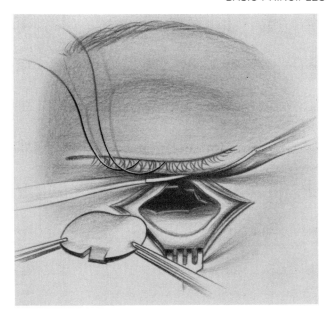

FIG. 2–7. Supramid sheeting fashioned for reconstruction of an orbital floor defect.

Dexon) are stronger than catgut or chromic catgut and last longer than nonsynthetic absorbable sutures (6 weeks for Vicryl and Dexon versus 3 weeks for catgut and chromic catgut). They also produce less inflammation. As a result of these properties, Vicryl and Dexon are excellent for wound closure below the skin surface. Catgut and chromic catgut are appropriate for closure of mucosal surfaces and for skin closure in young children when suture removal may be precluded.

Silk is an ideal skin suture because it is soft, pliable, and ties easily as well as being minimally reactive with the surrounding tissue. Prolene is effective as a subcuticular "pull-out" suture because it slides easily, which enhances its removal. Steri-strips secured with tincture of benzoin are useful in supporting traction sutures in the early postoperative period and also in approximating small and superficial wounds in young children. They are relatively ineffective for other purposes.

Supramid and Mersilene are useful when strong sutures are needed, particularly in reconstructing or repositioning a canthal tendon. Larger Supramid sutures and wire are effective in supporting the closure of bony defects. Supramid is a cable polyfilament suture that is nonbiodegradable and will retain its tensile strength.

Needles and Needle Holders. Four types of needles are used in ophthalmic plastic surgery: conventional cutting, reverse cutting, spatula, and taper (Fig. 2–6). Spatula needles have a flat bottom and sharp tip, which allow them to penetrate tissue with ease. They are useful in engaging skin, tarsal plate, or sclera. Cutting needles have a triangular tip and a sharp cutting edge facing their concave surface. They are effective for both skin and deep suturing. Reverse cutting needles have a triangular tip and a sharp cutting edge facing their convex surface. They are effective for penetration of firmer tissue. Taper needles have a round, tapered body, led by a cutting tip. They are somewhat less effective for cutaneous closure. The most commonly used configuration is three-eighths circle, while small half-circle needles facilitate closure of anastomotic flaps in dacryocystorhinostomy.

The Castroviejo needle holder is excellent for needles ranging from 4-0 to 10-0 size. Larger needles require a standard plastic surgery needle holder such as the Webster.

Alloplastic Materials. Nonporous implants are impervious to host tissue invasion. A fibrous membrane develops around such implants, permitting partial isolation. Porous implants accommodate tissue invasion, resulting in connective tissue attachment between implant and host tissue.

Orbital floor implants in blowout fracture repair may be made of Teflon, Silastic, or Supramid (Fig. 2–7). The last is preferable because it comes in sheets of variable thickness; it is easy to work with because it is more pliable than the other materials.

Orbital contouring for longstanding depressed fractures can be performed with proplast, precast silicone, or RTV silicone (Room Temperature Vulcanizing). Proplast is a relatively porous Teflon/carbon material that allows fibrous tissue to enter its substance, thereby enhancing tissue binding (Fig. 2–8). It may be prefabri-

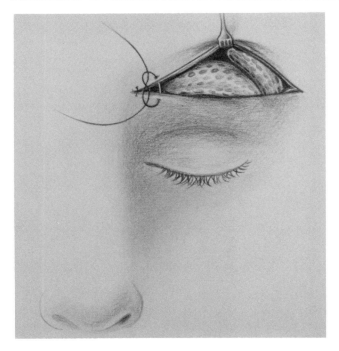

FIG. 2–8. Proplast fashioned to fill bony defect at the supraorbital rim.

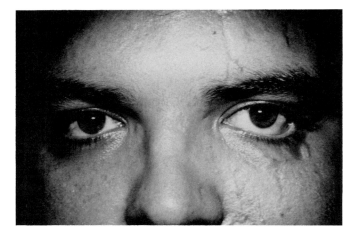

FIG. 2–9. Traumatic "tatooing" from incomplete removal of dirt and other foreign material during prior laceration repair.

cated and further fashioned and shaped intraoperatively with a scalpel blade and/or burr.

Cranioplast is a polymer that can be used to correct periorbital deformities. Care must be taken in the mixing process because it generates a highly exothermic reaction that may injure soft tissue. It solidifies to extreme hardness and may be fixated between periosteum and bone.

Before implantation, these materials should be soaked in an antibiotic solution and irrigated to remove nonadherent particles. They are placed in a snug pocket between periosteum and bone. The softer materials may also be directly sutured. Postoperative use of oral antibiotics for the first week may help avoid infection.

Primary enucleation or evisceration spheres may be composed of Teflon, Silastic, methylmethacrylate, titanium, or glass. Of these, Teflon and Silastic are preferable because they are softer and less apt to predispose tissue to pressure necrosis.

WOUND APPROXIMATION

The choice of surgical approach and instrumentation should always be based upon the most effective and least invasive method possible.

In traumatic cases, all necrotic, devitalized, or infected tissue should be excised. Purulent material may be sent for culture and antibiotic sensitivity studies. This may

provide valuable information if an infection later becomes manifest. Contaminated wounds should also be irrigated with an antibiotic solution, such as gentamicin (Garamycin). Foreign material, including dirt, is meticulously removed from the wound to maximize cosmesis and minimize infection and possible resultant "tatooing" (Fig. 2–9). Skin tags and irregular wound borders may be conservatively trimmed to convert the defect to a more regular configuration. This should always be carried out with a goal of maximum tissue conservation to minimize later tissue insufficiency.

In wound closure, particularly after trauma, it is essential to first re-establish bony landmarks. This is comparable to an architect structuring a building around the foundation and frame. Bone approximation, if necessary, should be carefully performed with properly sized wire or Supramid suture. If the chosen materials are inadequate, the closure is inadequate. For most purposes, 27-gauge wire or 2-0 Supramid satisfy the bony reconstruction needs in the periorbital area.

In complex soft tissue and cutaneous closure after trauma, it is also helpful to re-establish major anatomic landmarks (e.g., canthi, eyelid margin, canaliculi, levator aponeurosis, tarsus) and wound angles first (Figs. 2–10 to 2–12). The intervening tissue may then be more easily and accurately reconstructed.

In wound approximation, a primary consideration is proper tissue layer approximation. Poor cutaneous or subcutaneous apposition often leads to disfiguring scars and deformity (Figs. 2–13 and 2–14). In a shallow wound, this may cause an elevated scar, while in a deep wound it may result in a depressed scar.

It is important that tissue layers be closed separately (i.e., the tarsoconjunctival layer, the muscular or subcutaneous layer, and the skin layer) (Fig. 2–15). If the

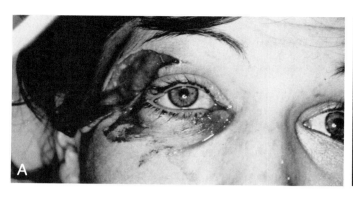 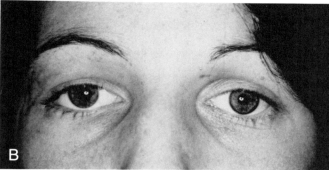

FIG. 2–10. A, Shelved laceration involving the outer canthus and upper eyelid. B, Appearance of patient 6 weeks postoperatively.

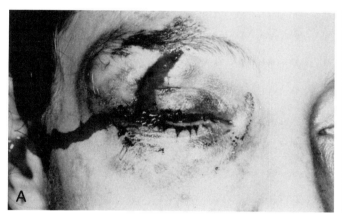 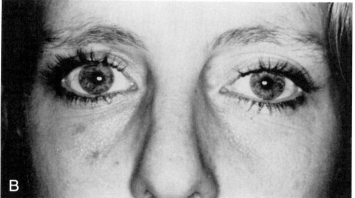

FIG. 2–11. A, Full-thickness laceration of the upper eyelid, including the margin. The eyelid margin was re-established first. B, Appearance of patient 6 weeks postoperatively.

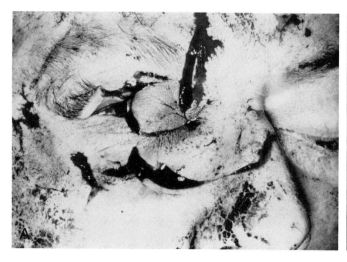 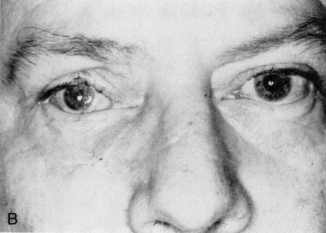

FIG. 2–12. A, Complex laceration of the right eye, right upper and lower eyelids, and right canthi. After repair of the globe, the canthi and eyelid margins were re-established. B, Appearance of patient 8 weeks postoperatively.

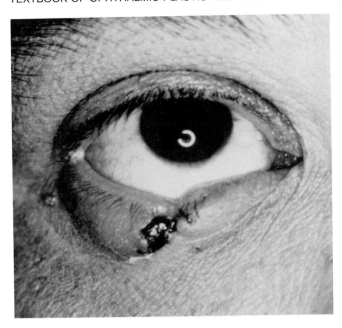

FIG. 2–13. Eyelid margin notch deformity resulting from unrepaired dog bite.

incision is perpendicular to the direction of orbicularis oculi muscle pull, a traction suture may be placed to counterbalance vectors of cicatrization that might otherwise result in notching.

Deep wounds may require closure in two or three layers (Fig. 2–16). In a three-layer closure, the deepest tissues should be approximated with vertical mattress sutures of an absorbable material (Fig. 2–17). Vicryl is an excellent choice because of its tensile strength and retention time of approximately 6 weeks. These sutures are placed so that the knot is buried, tying it at the suture's lowest point to minimize any elevation of overlying skin. Vertical mattress sutures eliminate dead space in the wound and provide strength to the closure,

thereby maximizing apposition of the more superficial layers. The subcutaneous tissues can be closed with interrupted horizontal mattress sutures (Fig. 2–17). Although this imparts some strength to the closure, it serves principally to optimize skin apposition and reduce tension on the overlying cutaneous suture line. Residual tension widens the scar and may predispose toward breakdown of the cutaneous suture line. Vicryl is again an excellent choice for the subcutaneous layer.

As a general rule, the smallest possible suture material that will adequately support the wound closure should be used to minimize the resultant scar.

The skin may be closed with either silk or Prolene. Silk appears to yield the best results in situations calling

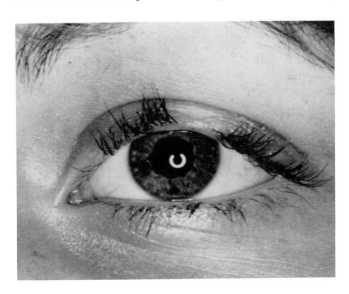

FIG. 2–14. Eyelid margin notch and area of permanent lash loss from poorly repaired upper eyelid margin.

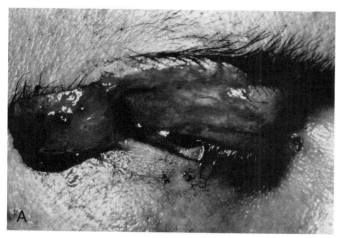 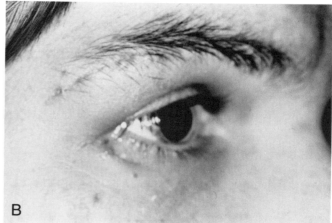

FIG. 2–15. A, Shelved laceration of the upper eyelid. B, Appearance 10 days after layer-by-layer wound closure.

for running sutures (with or without lock), while Prolene is most effective as a subcuticular "pull-out" suture (Fig. 2–18). In the eyelids, most skin sutures are ideally placed 1 mm from the skin edge and 2 mm apart. At closure, the skin margin should be slightly everted to compensate for vertical postoperative contraction. The depth and quantity of tissue incorporated within each bite should generally remain uniform.

Exceptions to these principles include cicatricial entropion repair by means of the Wies procedure, in which differing eyelid layers are intentionally united to achieve a rotation effect. Another exception is closure of a cutaneous "dog ear," in which the suture bites must be wider on the side of the wound with the most skin (Fig.

2–19). Other methods of eliminating a dog ear include elliptical excision of the dog ear or oblique extension of the skin incision followed by excision of a triangular skin segment.

Skin sutures should be tied with secure apposition. If sutures are tied too tightly, wound necrosis may occur. If they are tied too loosely, an excessively wide scar may result.

In general, silk and Prolene sutures should be removed on the fourth to sixth postoperative day. Any resultant wound gaping may be closed by placing Steri-strips, supported by tincture of benzoin.

In situations calling for a two-layer closure, the wound may be reunited as noted above, deleting the deeper vertical mattress sutures (Fig. 2–20).

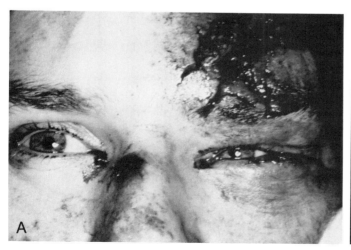 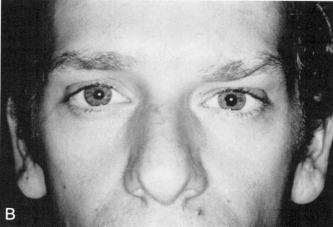

FIG. 2–16. A, Deep laceration of the brow and forehead. B, Appearance 6 weeks after three-layer wound closure.

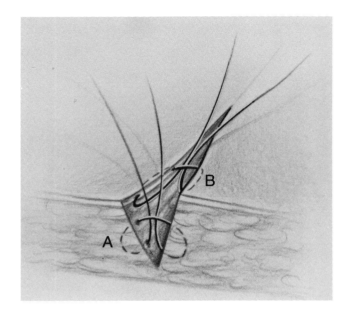

FIG. 2–17. Illustration of proper placement of A, vertical mattress suture and B, horizontal mattress suture.

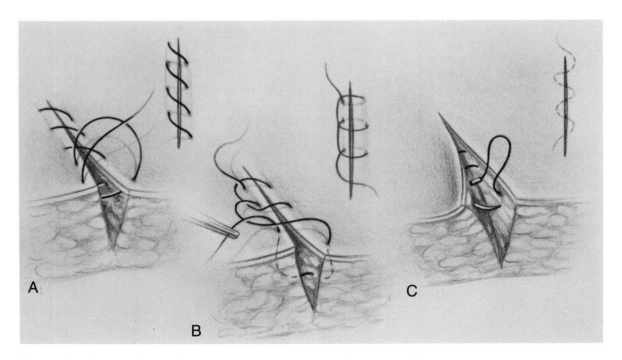

FIG. 2–18. Views of three skin closure techniques portrayed from two different perspectives: A, running suture, B, running locking suture, C, subcuticular "pull-out" suture.

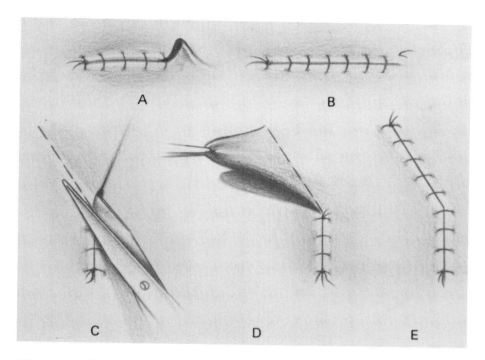

FIG. 2–19. Cutaneous "dog ear" (A) and the various techniques available to avoid or eliminate this redundant tissue, (B) wider suture bites on one side of the wound, (C, D, E) oblique extension of the skin incision followed by excision of a triangular segment of skin. Direct elliptical excision of the "dog ear" may also be used.

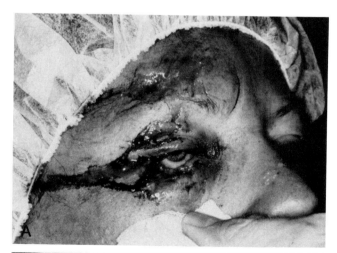

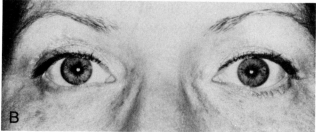

FIG. 2–20. A, Laceration of the right upper and lower eyelid and outer canthus. B, Appearance 6 weeks after two-layer wound closure.

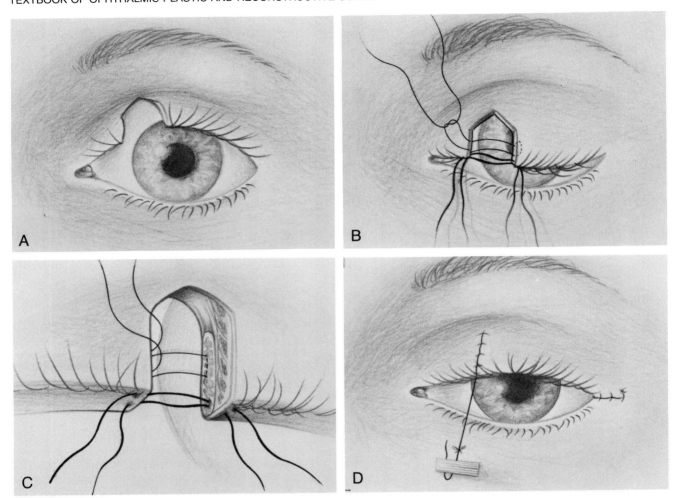

FIG. 2–21. A, Upper eyelid margin defect. B, 4-0 silk sutures positioned within tarsus to re-establish the eyelid margin and gray line; 5-0 suture placed posterior to gray line. C, Enlargement of B demonstrating suture location within tarsus. A third eyelid margin suture may be added if tissue size and integrity permit. D, Following closure of the eyelid margin and tarsal plate, the skin is approximated with running 7-0 silk. If a cantholysis is required, a simple canthoplasty reapproximates the outer canthus.

SPECIAL WOUND CLOSURE TECHNIQUES

EYELID MARGIN DEFECTS

Small defects involving the eyelid margin require careful reformation to avoid later marginal notching (Fig. 2–21A). The central eyelid margin suture of 4-0 silk is inserted in the center of the gray line, engaging each side of the defect (Fig. 2–21B). Immediately posterior to the gray line a 5-0 silk suture is placed, engaging both sides of the defect. If sufficient tissue is available immediately anterior to the gray line, a similar 5-0 silk

suture is placed. Each suture should penetrate 2 mm deep into the tarsus and emerge 2 mm from each cut edge of the eyelid margin (Fig. 2–21C). Placement of the anterior suture should carefully avoid damage to the nearby eyelash follicles. As each suture is placed, it should be tied temporarily with a slip knot to assess the accuracy of apposition. Any suture that does not achieve optimal approximation should be replaced. The two posterior-most sutures should be tied first and then tunnelled anteriorly underneath the anterior suture, which is tied last. This minimizes corneal epithelial disruption by the eyelid margin suture line. These sutures should be left long and secured to the opposing cheek or brow to minimize any postoperative notching tendency (Fig. 2–21D). The tarsus is approximated with 6-0 Vicryl mattress sutures followed by skin closure with running 7-0 silk. The skin sutures may be removed 6 days postoperatively, while the eyelid margin sutures should remain under mild traction for 10 days.

Defects involving loss of 30 to 50% of the eyelid margin may additionally require a lateral canthotomy with lysis of the appropriate crus of the lateral canthal tendon (Fig. 2–22). Defects greater than 50% may be reconstructed with Mustarde or Tenzel rotation flaps, or Hughes or Cutler-Beard eyelid sharing flaps, as described in Chapter 10.

DEFECTS NOT INVOLVING THE EYELID MARGIN

Small defects not involving the eyelid margin are often amenable to primary reapproximation. An elliptical defect is effectively approximated. This may sometimes require undermining to enhance mobilization. If possible,

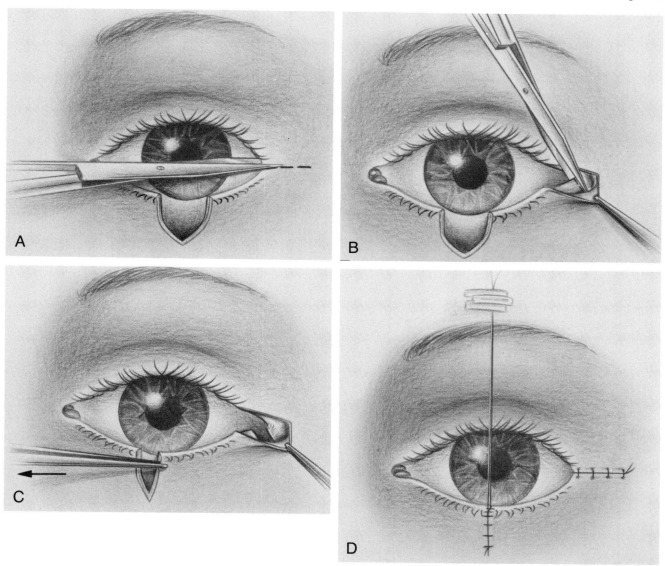

FIG. 2–22.   Lower eyelid margin defect of left eye requiring canthotomy with lysis of the inferior crus of the lateral canthal tendon. A, Canthotomy site designated by either marking pen or crush from a straight hemostat. B, Inferior crus of the lateral canthal tendon is isolated and severed. C, Increased medial mobility of the lateral portion of the eyelid afforded by canthotomy and cantholysis. D, Closure of the eyelid margin defect and canthotomy site.

these closures should be oriented to conform to Langer's lines. Such horizontal suture lines, however, should not be allowed to create vertical tissue insufficiency and ectropion.

Larger defects such as those resulting from trauma, burns, tumor removal, severe dermatitis (ichthyosis), or overzealous cosmetic surgery away from the eyelid margin may result in relative or absolute tissue insufficiency. These situations may require sliding, advancement, rotation or transposition flaps (Fig. 2–23), or free skin grafts to cover the defect and relieve tissue tension. Flaps are segments of skin and subcutaneous tissue transposed from one site to another while retaining their original blood supply through an unaltered base. The transposed tissue does not depend entirely on the recipient bed for its nutritional support. This makes it ideal for reconstruction in areas of compromised soft tissue or vascularity. Flaps have other advantages over free skin grafts. Because flaps generally have more substantial vascular support, they are less prone to infection. Flaps also tend to contract less, both circumferentially and vertically. A flap with a muscular component is designated a myocutaneous flap (Fig. 2–24).

As a general rule, flap length should be no longer than three times the size of its base. This ratio can be extended somewhat (up to five to one) for flaps with demonstrable and significant arterial support. Flaps are mobilized by undermining in the subcutaneous layer.

Sliding flaps consist of tissue that has been undermined and pulled forward to close a subjacent defect (such as an elliptical closure) (Fig. 2–23). Advancement flaps are three-sided sliding flaps, undermined and advanced usually in a rectangular shape to close an adjacent defect (such as the Cutler-Beard flap). Rotation flaps consist of undermined tissue rotated to close an adjacent defect (such as the Mustarde and Tenzel flaps). Transposition flaps are rotation flaps, undermined and moved to cover a nonadjacent defect (such as the midline forehead flap).

These various flaps are able to survive in the periorbital area due to their substantial vascular support. In these techniques, however, cautery should be judicious to avoid further vascular compromise. The surgeon should handle flaps carefully, particularly avoiding traumatizing the tips that have the least perfusion. These tissues should be sutured smoothly to avoid kinking at the vascular base.

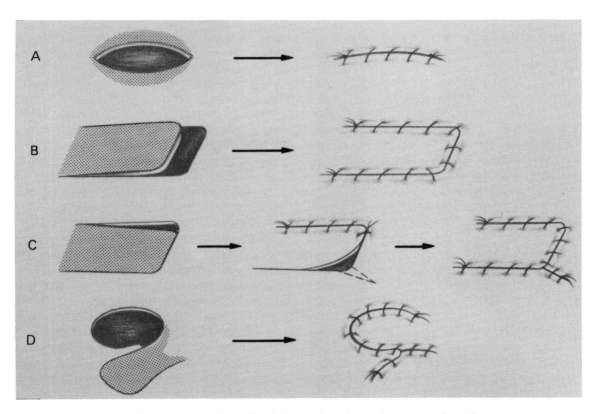

FIG. 2–23.   Flap techniques commonly applicable to ophthalmic plastic surgery: A, sliding, B, advancement, C, rotation, D, transposition.

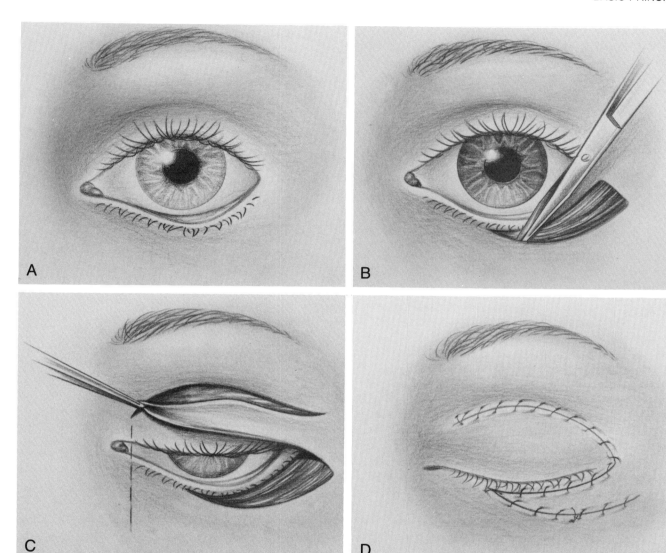

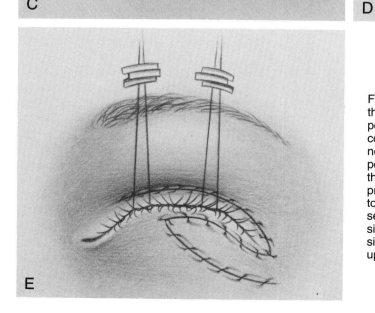

FIG. 2–24. A, Cicatricial ectropion of the lateral portion of the lower eyelid before repair using myocutaneous transposition flap. B, Lower eyelid incision is extended through the contracture to the level of the orbital septum. C, Myocutaneous pedicle is fashioned from the upper eyelid. This is positioned at the upper eyelid fold and is long enough to fill the lower eyelid defect. The base of the pedicle must be properly oriented to facilitate transposition and wide enough to support the entire pedicle. D, Pedicle sutured in place with several buried 6-0 Vicryl mattress sutures and running 7-0 silk. Donor site also closed with running 7-0 silk. E, Two 4-0 silk-modified Frost sutures are placed for 10 days under mild upward tension to minimize postoperative contracture.

Flap Techniques

Z-plasty. The Z-plasty is a classic transposition flap used to relieve lines of tension (Fig. 2–25). Additional applications include lengthening tissue in a desired direction (Figs. 2–26 and 2–27), interrupting the continuity of a long scar (Fig. 2–28), and transposing tissue to its proper position (i.e., canthal Z-plasty in vertical canthal malposition or ectopic brow hairline [Figs. 2–29 and 2–30]).

The crossbar of the Z (the central line) is at the position of the line of greatest tension. The two side arms are offset at 60-degree angles, allowing rotation of the flaps (Fig. 2–25). Although larger angles further lengthen the line at the crossbar, this is technically difficult to accomplish. The crossbar and two arms should all be the same length.

After the central incision line has been made across the scar tissue, this tissue is removed (if necessary) and the flaps to be transposed are effectively fashioned and undermined. The two resultant triangular flaps are then rotated and sutured into position with minimal tension. This transposition rotates the crossbar 90 degrees and affords a 30% increase in length along the central line of tension.

In Z-plasty, the larger flap angle, the greater the tissue lengthening. It should also be recognized that the longer the crossbar, the more prominent the resultant scar. This may be obviated somewhat by performing multiple, adjacent, small Z-plasties in reconstruction. A modification of the Z-plasty, when combined with canthal tendon repositioning, is an effective means of treating vertical displacement of the canthi.

Bilobed Flap. The bilobed flap closes the primary defect with a "lobe" of tissue directly transposed from an adjacent perpendicular area composed of more lax tissue (Fig. 2–31). The first lobe fills the primary defect, while the secondary defect (the donor site for the first lobe) is closed by a second, smaller lobe. The donor site for the second lobe is closed directly. This technique involves marking the flaps, incising and undermining tissue, and mobilizing the resultant flaps. After all flaps are properly positioned, they may be secured with either 6-0 or 7-0 silk sutures in a running fashion.

Rhomboid Flap. Rhomboid defects may be closed by inwardly rotating a triangular flap. The base of this rotation flap should be positioned to afford maximum skin extensibility. In marking this flap, a short diagonal is placed with its length corresponding to the length of the shortest axis of the defect. From this diagonal, a second incision is marked, extending backward at a 60-degree angle (Fig. 2–32A). The tissues are incised and effectively undermined, thereby converting the triangle into a rhomboidal configuration to fill the defect (Fig. 2–32B). If significant wound tension is manifest, several Vicryl (5-0 or 6-0) horizontal mattress sutures may be required. The corners of the cutaneous defect should be secured with interrupted silk sutures (5-0 or 6-0) and the wound may be further closed with running silk sutures (6-0 or 7-0).

O- to Z-Plasty. This flap uses lax skin surrounding a round defect to achieve closure in a Z-like configuration. Two curvilinear lines are marked extending from opposite poles of the defect. Corresponding incisions are made and the flaps are undermined (Fig. 2–33A). The flaps are slid into position and closed with Vicryl and silk sutures as noted above (Fig. 2–33B).

Y- to V-Plasty. These flaps are effective in mobilizing tissue or closing defects as an advancement flap (Y- to V-plasty) (Fig. 2–34) or in releasing a tight scar (V- to Y-

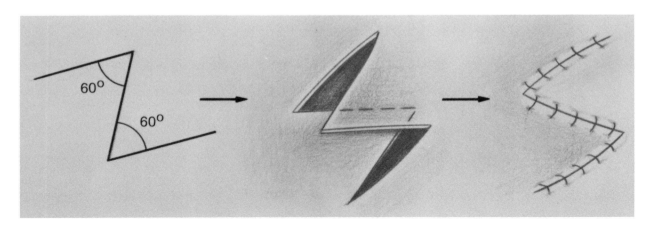

FIG. 2–25. Classic Z-plasty configuration.

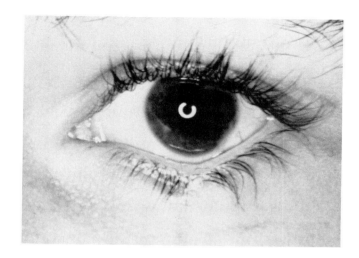

FIG. 2–26. Cicatricial ectropion resulting from a vertical scar in the lower eyelid, including the margin. Such cases lend themselves well to Z-plasty, which changes the orientation of the scar.

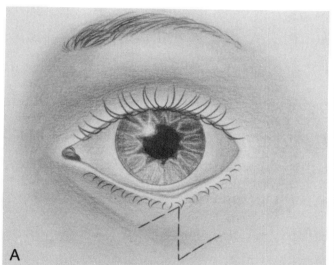

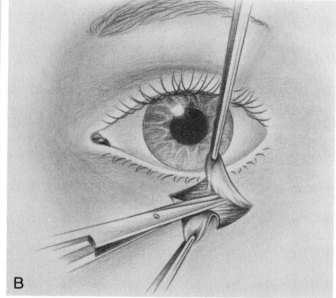

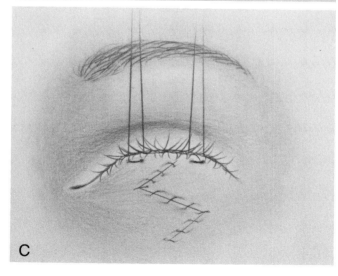

FIG. 2–27. Repair of segmental cicatricial ectropion with Z-plasty. A, Placement of the Z-configuration with the central line (crossbar of the Z) along the meridian of greatest tension. B, Resultant triangular flaps are undermined and rotated into position. C, Appearance at wound closure with transposition completed. Modified Frost traction sutures minimize later contracture.

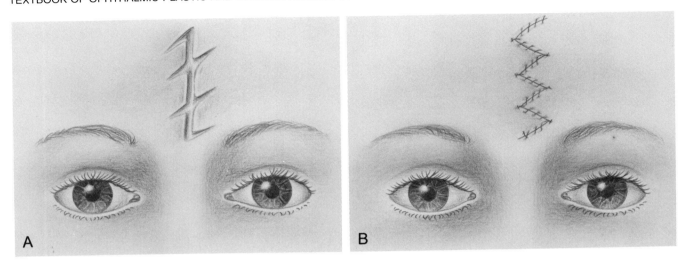

FIG. 2–28. Series of Z-plasties used to interrupt the continuity of a long scar. A, Appearance before transposition of flaps. B, Appearance following transposition of flaps.

plasty) (Fig. 2–35A). The latter technique contributes tissue to the long axis of the Y, while diminishing tissue perpendicular to this axis. In either version, the surgeon marks the configuration (Fig. 2–35B), makes a corresponding incision, and undermines and mobilizes the flap (Fig. 2–35C). The edges may be trimmed somewhat to fit the new configuration. Vicryl horizontal mattress sutures are helpful in supporting these flaps. Skin closure is usually amenable to interrupted 6-0 silk sutures combined with running 7-0 silk (Fig. 2–35D).

W-Plasty. The W-plasty technique is used to change the direction of a linear scar. Its principal applications are in brow, forehead, temple, and cheek closures. After scar excision, multiple contiguous small triangles are marked on both sides of the defect. They are positioned to interdigitate in a saw-toothed manner (Fig. 2–36A). Corresponding incisions are made and the small flaps are mobilized. The wound is then closed with 6-0 or 7-0 silk sutures (Fig. 2–36B). This technique does not lengthen a contracted scar, but rather breaks up a long scar and may be used to position the small scars more in conformity with Langer's lines.

Grafting Procedures

Autogenous Grafts. For all grafts, the recipient bed must have sufficient vascular support. The highly vascular eyelid and periocular tissue suitably fit this prerequisite. Previous irradiation will diminish this nutritive support. Autogenous donor material may include full-thickness or split-thickness skin, fascia lata, postauricular cartilage, mucous membrane, and dermis fat.

Full-Thickness Skin Grafts. Full-thickness skin grafts contain both epidermal and dermal elements. These grafts may variably include sweat glands, sebaceous glands, and hair follicles, depending upon the donor site. They may be taken from the upper eyelid (only when tissue is abundant and symmetry is maintained), the retroauricular area, the supraclavicular area, and the upper inner arm (Fig. 2–37). This order of preference should be maintained to ensure optimal color and texture conformity of the donor graft to the recipient bed.

Although the upper eyelid provides the best tissue match, it is not uniformly useful because it is often coexistently foreshortened, and if used additionally requires a contralateral upper blepharoplasty to achieve postoperative upper eyelid symmetry. As a result, retroauricular full-thickness skin grafts are used more commonly. In most situations these grafts should be 25% larger than their recipient bed to allow expected postoperative shrinkage. The effect of the elastic fibers contained in the graft causes graft shrinkage during the second postoperative week. In circumstances in which excessive shrinkage is expected (ichthyosis, burns, recurrent cicatricial ectropion), the graft should be 50% larger than its bed. Additionally, intermarginal adhesions can be placed for 2 months or longer to minimize postoperative shrinkage. Technical details on full-thickness graft harvesting and placement are contained in Chapter 7.

Split-Thickness Skin Grafts. Split-thickness grafts are thinner and tolerate poor circulation and infection better than full-thickness grafts. A split-thickness graft consists of epidermis and a portion of dermis. Abundant donor sites include the arm, leg, and abdomen. The thickness of the graft and choice of donor site determine the quan-

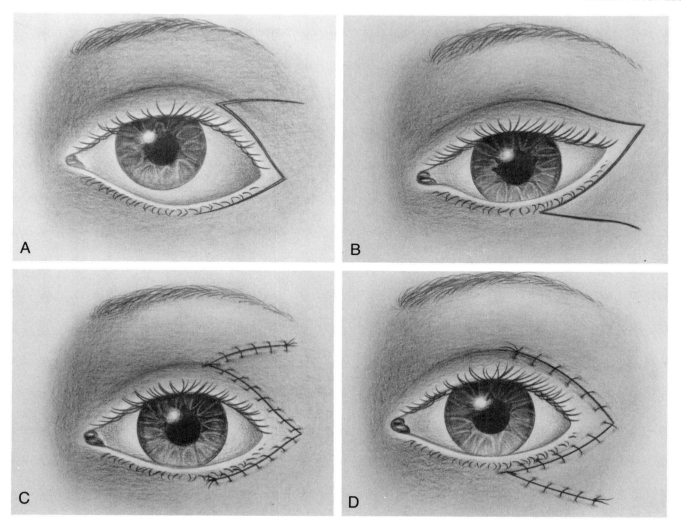

FIG. 2–29. Z-plasty used to treat A, inferior or B, superior displacement of the outer canthus. When combined with canthal tendon repositioning, this effectively restores normal canthal placement (C and D).

tity of sweat glands, sebaceous glands, and hair follicles. Despite this, split-thickness grafts are rarely used in ophthalmic plastic surgery because they contract excessively in comparison to full-thickness grafts. Split-thickness grafts also produce an insufficient color match to donor tissue and further darken over time. They are abundantly available, however, require less vascular support than do full-thickness grafts, and are therefore useful in lining orbital bone following exenteration. Split-thickness grafts are sutured in the same manner as full-thickness grafts.

For split-thickness grafts, the donor site is prepared with povidone iodine (Betadine) and the graft configu-ration is marked. A dermatome is used to obtain grafts of varying thickness. Dermatome settings between .01 and .015 inches usually result in split-thickness grafts of adequate thickness. This may be facilitated by spreading a thin layer of mineral oil over the skin. Even pressure should be maintained to afford graft uniformity. As the graft emerges from the dermatome, it should be grasped with forceps to prevent re-engagement by the cutting blades. After an adequate graft has been fashioned, the dermatome is stopped and separated from the graft. The graft is then detached from the donor site, placed on a flat surface, irrigated with an antibiotic solution, and kept moist with the epithelial surface facing upward. Either

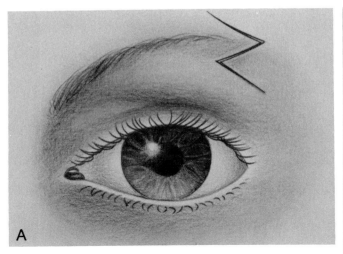 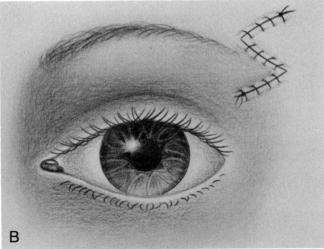

FIG. 2–30. A, Z-plasty used to infraplace an ectopic brow hairline. B, Appearance following transposition of flaps.

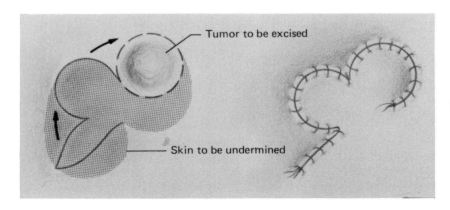

FIG. 2–31. Configuration of the bilobed flap.

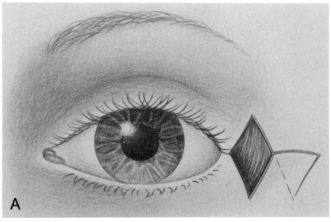 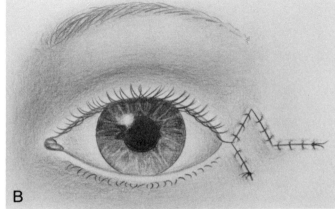

FIG. 2–32. Rhomboid flap, A, before rotation and, B, after rotation.

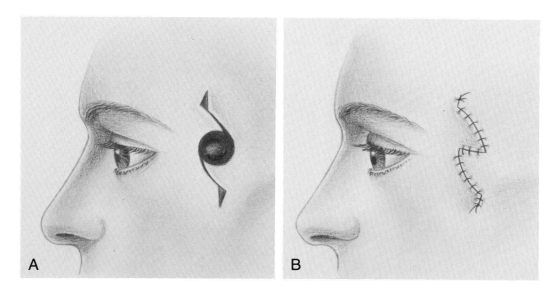

FIG. 2–33. O- to Z-plasty, A, before advancement and, B, after advancement.

a Teflon dressing or nitrofurazone (Furacin) gauze patch effectively covers the donor site and promotes epithelialization.

In any grafted eyelid, placing several modified Frost traction sutures in the eyelid margin, secured under mild tension, helps to stretch the graft and maximize apposition to the underlying nutritive recipient bed. Meticulous hemostasis is essential to prevent graft separation.

Plasma and red blood cells absorbed through the undersurface provide initial nourishment to these grafts. Vascular channels subsequently enter this surface through a fibrinous network that binds the graft to its recipient bed. Larger vascular channels later develop.

Composite Grafts. Composite grafts may occasionally be used to reconstruct a limited portion of the eyelid margin (Fig. 2–38). They should be approached with great care because of their fragile initial blood supply. This is reviewed in more detail in Chapter 10.

Conjunctival Defects

Conjunctiva may be reconstructed with transposition conjunctival flaps, free conjunctival grafts, buccal mucous membrane grafts, or composite nasal septal cartilage and mucous membrane grafts. The composite grafts are thick and thereby applicable principally when upper eyelid tarsus and conjunctiva require replacement. The details of mucous membrane graft placement are in Chapter 8.

Harvesting Grafts of Buccal Mucosa. Buccal mucous membrane is the principal conjunctival replacement material used in socket, fornix, and posterior lamellar eyelid reconstruction.

Under general anesthesia, the area surrounding the mouth is effectively prepped and draped. Two large towel clamps are placed at the ends of the lower lip and the lip is everted (Fig. 2–39). The vermilion border is clearly marked with methylene blue or a marking pen

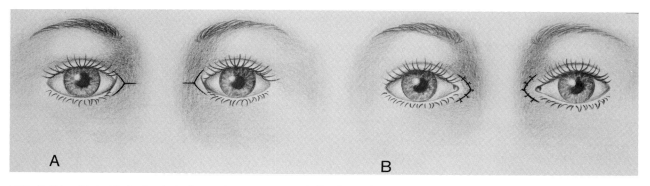

FIG. 2–34. Y- to V-plasty, A, before advancement and, B, after advancement.

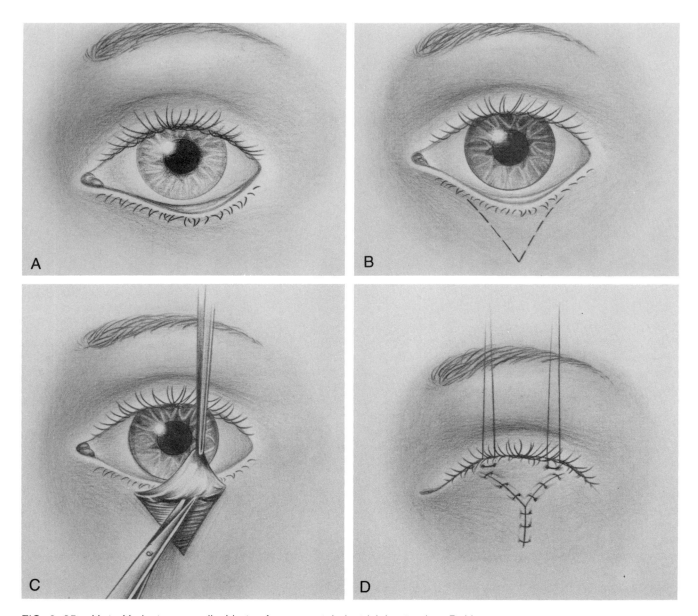

FIG. 2–35.   V- to Y-plasty as applicable to, A, segmental cicatricial ectropion. B, V-configuration is marked along the same axis as the contracture. C, The incision is made and the flap is undermined and mobilized. D, The flap is recessed into a Y-configuration, releasing the contracture. Temporary placement of modified Frost sutures may lessen the chance of recurrence.

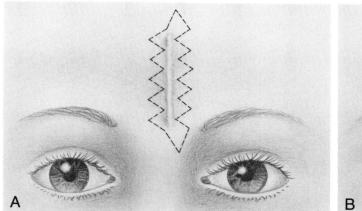 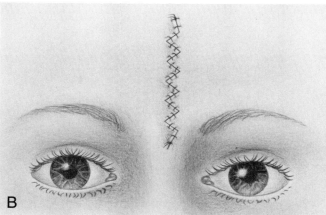

FIG. 2–36. A, W-plasty marked around a hypertrophic forehead scar. B, The multiple triangles are brought together to interdigitate in a saw-toothed manner.

to delineate the junction between mucous membrane and stratified squamous epithelium. The mucosal surface is infiltrated with normal saline through a 25-gauge short needle. Enough saline must be injected to swell the lower lip sufficiently so that the mucosal surface is tense, broad, and relatively flat.

A Castroviejo mucotome set at 0.3 mm thickness is used to harvest the graft. A thinner setting causes the graft to partially shred, while a thicker setting causes dissection into the fat layer of the lip and scar. Obtaining a mucous membrane graft of 0.3 mm thickness affords

ideal thickness and graft integrity, while allowing the lip to heal without scarring. The same site can therefore be used again if additional grafting is later required.

The head of the mucotome must remain in firm contact with the lip mucosa at all times to ensure graft uniformity. As the graft emerges from the mucotome, it should be grasped with forceps to prevent reengagement by the cutting blades. After an adequate graft has been fashioned, the mucotome is stopped and separated from the graft. The graft is then detached from the donor site, placed on a flat surface, irrigated with an antibiotic so-

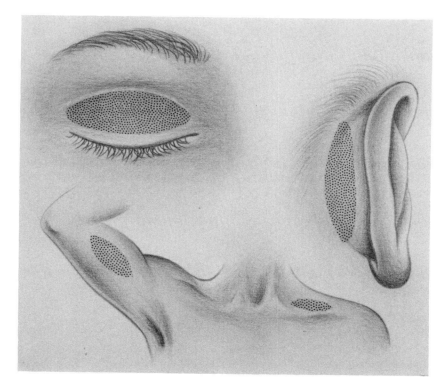

FIG. 2–37. Sources of autogenous full-thickness skin grafts: A, upper eyelid, B, retroauricular area, C, supraclavicular area, and D, upper-inner arm.

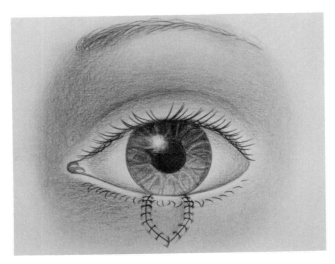

FIG. 2–38. Composite grafts may be used to reconstruct a limited full-thickness eyelid defect that is too large for primary closure and cantholysis.

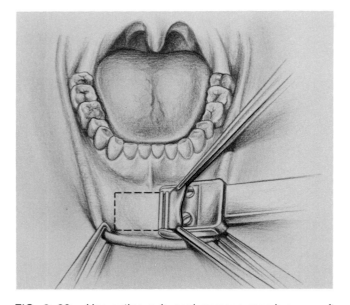

FIG. 2–39. Harvesting a buccal mucous membrane graft with a Castroviejo mucotome (0.3 mm setting). Under general anesthesia, the lip is secured with two towel clips. The vermilion border is designated with a marking pen. The mucosal surface is infiltrated with normal saline to create a firm flat surface for the mucotome to traverse. As the graft emerges from the mucotome, it is grasped with forceps.

lution, and kept moist with the epithelial surface facing upward. Petroleum gauze effectively covers the donor site and promotes epithelialization.

The upper lip and inner aspect of the cheek may also be used for donor buccal mucosa. These grafts are less optimal and technically more difficult. Grafts taken from the cheek undersurface must be removed in a free-hand manner and tend to be more irregular (Fig. 2–40). The parotid duct should be left undisturbed.

Harvesting Composite Grafts of Nasal Septal Cartilage and Mucosa. A composite graft of nasal septal cartilage and mucosa may sometimes be useful in reconstructing the posterior lamella of the upper eyelid. It is too thick as a substitute for the more rudimentary tarsus of the lower eyelid.

Under general anesthesia, the side of the nasal septum serving as the donor site is packed with cocaine. Infiltration of lidocaine with epinephrine on this side adds vasoconstriction and expands the mucosa, facilitating surgical dissection. A properly oriented nasal speculum and fiberoptic headlight provide optimal exposure. An alar flap may, at times, enhance visualization.

The mucous membrane should be incised 1 cm behind the anterior edge of the cartilaginous septum (Fig. 2–41) to preserve support for the anterior strut and bridgeline of the nose. For larger grafts, the incision may extend from the top of the cartilaginous septum down to the maxillary bone. The goal should be to cleave the cartilage in a lamellar fashion, preserving some cartilage and the contralateral mucosa. Dissection is facilitated by using a periosteal elevator. Final detachment of the graft requires a scalpel blade. Grafts up to 30 mm × 15 mm may be obtained in this manner. The graft is soaked in an antibiotic solution and any attached bone should be removed from the graft before its implantation. If the cartilage is too thick, it may be trimmed before positioning in the recipient bed. In the entire process, it is imperative that mucosa remain in complete union with the underlying cartilage.

Bleeding is usually moderate, despite vasoconstriction, and is effectively controlled by using a combined suction-cautery unit. Effective hemostasis should be achieved by this means, and at the completion of graft harvesting the nose should be firmly packed with petroleum gauze imbricated with an antibiotic ointment. The pack may be removed on the first or second postoperative day.

Once harvested and trimmed to fit the recipient bed, the conjunctiva or mucous membrane graft should be secured with 7-0 chromic catgut sutures, interrupted at the corners and running throughout the remainder of the suture line. It is helpful to bury the knots to minimize

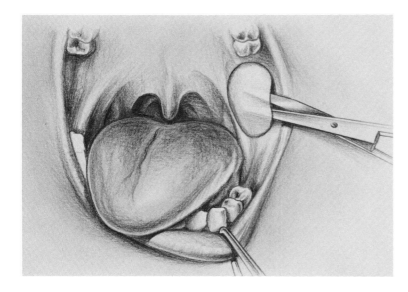

FIG. 2–40. Harvesting a free-hand buccal mucous membrane graft removed from the cheek undersurface. The parotid duct must be left undisturbed.

corneal erosion. In many instances, a stent, either in the form of a conformer, symblepharon ring, or rubber bolster, should be placed over the graft to help maintain pressure and tissue apposition during the early healing phase. Unlined mucous membrane grafts (i.e., without cartilage) undergo slight shrinkage (25%) and must be made slightly larger than their recipient beds.

Bone Grafts. Bone grafts for ophthalmic plastic surgery are obtained from the anterior iliac crest. Antibiotic coverage is important to safeguard against infection in such grafts.

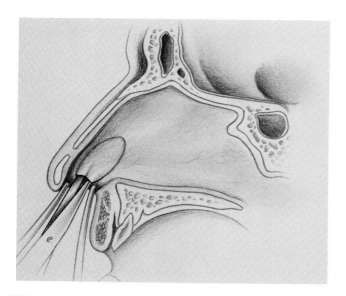

FIG. 2–41. Harvesting a composite graft of nasal septal cartilage and mucosa. This should be incised 1 cm behind the anterior edge of the cartilaginous septum to preserve proper structural support for the nose.

Homografts. Homografts used in oculoplastic surgery are sclera and fascia lata. Sclera originates from enucleated donor eyes, processed and stored to ensure sterility and minimal tissue reactivity. It is available through larger eye banks. Homogenous fascia lata is available through the Hospital for Sick Children in Toronto (J.S. Crawford, M.D.) and is an alternative to autogenous fascia lata, particularly in children. Heterogenous fascia lata (bovine) is processed by Ethicon. This material is somewhat less efficacious because of its tendency to enhance tissue inflammation.

POSTOPERATIVE CARE

ANTIBIOTICS AND DRESSINGS

At surgical closure, an antibiotic ointment should be applied to all suture lines, and to the globe if indicated. The ointment should be applied daily for several days beyond the time of suture removal. Unless previous culture and sensitivity findings dictate otherwise, the surgeon should choose an agent that has broad spectrum coverage and is compatible with the patient's allergic history. Prophylactic systemic antibiotics are useful in larger procedures, contaminated wounds, operations in which the nose or adjacent sinuses are entered, or situations in which autogenous or foreign substances are placed. Systemic antibiotics should be continued through the time of suture removal.

Many oculoplastic surgical procedures require no postoperative dressing. This affords maximum wound observation. In larger operations in which a dressing is required, it should remain for only 1 day (36 hours in cases involving placement of a free skin graft).

Pressure dressings are not particularly effective in inhibiting hemorrhage. Instead, they may delay observation of ongoing bleeding and may predispose to infection by loculating bacteria within a warm and moist environment.

Pressure dressings are effective in two situations: placement of a free skin graft and enucleation/evisceration surgery. The pressure is achieved by covering the surgical site with an eye pad covered with a fluff dressing, secured with a 2-inch elastic bandage (Elastoplast) and tincture of benzoin.

SUTURE REMOVAL

Removal of skin sutures should be carried out as early as possible to minimize fibrosis and cutaneous scarring. In the eyelids, the skin is thin and heals rapidly; therefore, the skin sutures in the periorbital area can be removed in approximately 4 to 6 days. Sutures extending into the thicker skin of the face should remain for 5 to 7 days, and in some situations even longer. Sutures used to effect tissue rotation or to establish an eyelid fold should remain for 10 days.

All traction sutures that have been placed in either the tarsal plate or the periosteum should remain for 10 to 14 days.

MANAGEMENT OF COMPLICATIONS

The three most generally encountered complications in ophthalmic plastic and reconstructive surgery are hemorrhage, infection, and excessive scarring.

Hemorrhage. A postoperative hematoma increases the tension on the skin edges and may predispose to excessive scarring. It may also provide an excellent culture medium, leading to postoperative infection. Subjacent to a free skin graft, a hemorrhage may appreciably separate the graft from its potential blood supply. Any significant blood accumulation in the first 24 to 48 hours postoperatively should therefore be managed by opening up the wound, evacuating the clot, and cauterizing the bleeding source. Drains will rarely be required (except in the orbit) and skin grafts should have fenestrations to provide drainage. Persistent bleeding requires evaluation to rule out a pre-existing bleeding diathesis (Fig. 2–42). Tests should include a study of platelet quantity and quality, along with evaluation of prothrombin time (pro-time) and partial thromboplastin time (PTT).

Keloids and Hypertrophic Scars. Following surgery,

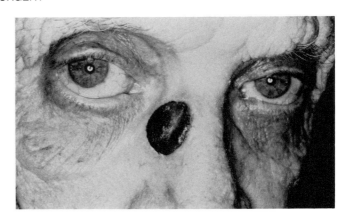

FIG. 2–42. Persistent hemorrhage beneath a properly fenestrated full-thickness skin graft. Despite two attempts to expose and cauterize the graft bed, the bleeding persisted. A work-up was initiated and the patient was found to have a bleeding diathesis from a myeloproliferative disorder. His platelet count was 3,000,000, with significant cellular atypia.

melanogenesis may induce hyperpigmentation in the surgical site. This process is facilitated by ultraviolet radiation. Patients should be advised to avoid direct sunlight and to use effective sunscreens for the first 6 months after surgery.

Hypertrophic scars and keloids can compromise even the most meticulously closed wounds. They represent different degrees of exaggeration of the wound-healing process. Hypertrophic scars often become less prominent over time. Keloids, on the other hand, are ropy overgrowths that may expand into surrounding tissues and evolve over months to years. Although keloids are most common in blacks, they may occur in any racial or ethnic group. In suspected keloid formers, it may be helpful preoperatively to inspect other scars.

Patients predisposed to hypertrophic scarring should have a triamcinolone acetonide (Kenalog) injection (10 mg/ml) placed along the suture line at surgical closure. This can be accomplished by using a 27-gauge needle and a small syringe. Several additional injections may be required within the first 2 months following surgery. Tissue atrophy and/or depigmentation may follow higher steroid concentrations (40 mg/ml) or intradermal injection.

Older keloids may become dense collagenous scars that hinder extravasation of the steroid, even through the finest needles. This may require injection of triamcinolone acetonide (Kenalog) through an "air-gun" mechanism (Panjet or Medajet). The tissue being injected should always be retracted over a bony prominence to protect the globe from the force of injection. Unintentional steroid penetration into the globe is otherwise possible.

It may be necessary to excise larger, older keloids and provide meticulous wound closure and steroids as outlined above. Although hypertrophic scarring will probably occur again, this approach might produce a less aggressive (and less unsightly) tissue response.

BIBLIOGRAPHY

Borges, A.: Elective Incisions and Scar Revision. Boston, Little, Brown and Company, 1973.

Bullock, J., Koss, N., and Flagg, S.: Rhomboid flap in ophthalmic plastic surgery. Arch. Ophthalmol. 90:203, 1973.

Callahan, M. and Callahan, A.: Ophthalmic Plastic and Orbital Surgery. Birmingham, Aesculapius, 1979.

Freeman, B.: Synthetic materials in orbital and surrounding tissue. In Soll, D. (ed.): Management of Complications in Ophthalmic Plastic Surgery. Birmingham, Aesculapius, 1976.

Grabb, W. and Myers, M.: Skin Flaps. Boston, Little, Brown and Company, 1975.

Iliff, C., Iliff, W., and Iliff, N.: Oculoplastic Surgery. Philadelphia, W.B. Saunders, 1979.

Ketchum, L., Robinson, D., and Masters, F.: Follow-up on treatment of hypertrophic scars and keloids with triamcinolone. Plast. Reconstr. Surg. 3:256, 1971.

Reeh, M., Beyer, C., and Shannon, G.: Practical Ophthalmic Plastic and Reconstructive Surgery. Philadelphia, Lea & Febiger, 1976.

Shannon, G. and Connelly, J.: Oculoplastic Surgery and Prosthetics. Boston, Little, Brown and Company, 1970.

Silver, B.: Local Anesthesia. In Soll, D. (ed.): Management of Complications in Ophthalmic Plastic Surgery. Birmingham, Aesculapius, 1976.

Stewart, W.: Ophthalmic plastic and reconstructive surgery. San Francisco, American Academy of Ophthalmology, 1984.

Wilkins, R. and Kulwin, D.: Wound healing. Ophthalmology 86:507, 1979.

Wilkins, R. and Kulwin, D.: Skin and tissue techniques. In McCord, C. (ed.): Oculoplastic Surgery. New York, Raven Press, 1981.

3

CONGENITAL ANOMALIES OF THE EYELIDS AND SOCKET

This chapter chronicles the principal congenital and developmental anomalies of the eyelids and socket. These varied disorders represent tissue deficiencies, structural abnormalities, and tumors. Uncomplicated congenital blepharoptosis and congenital nasolacrimal dysfunction are discussed in Chapters 5 and 13.

CONGENITAL EYELID COLOBOMAS

Congenital eyelid colobomas typically manifest as full-thickness deletion defects in a triangular configuration (Fig. 3–1). They may occasionally assume a quadrilateral, W, or irregular shape, while partial-thickness colobomas may occur in the lower eyelid. These partial-thickness defects may retain orbicularis oculi muscle, tarsal elements, cilia, or glandular structures. Such retained tissues are usually malformed and malpositioned. The coloboma edge is rounded and covered with conjunctiva. Defect size may range from a small indentation at the eyelid margin to absence of almost the entire eyelid, suggesting ablepharon.

Colobomas are most frequently encountered at the medial aspect of the upper eyelid or the lateral aspect of the lower eyelid. Typically unilateral, colobomas may also be bilateral, with occasional involvement of all four eyelids. Symmetrical defects are not uncommon, and multiple colobomas may occur on one eyelid.

Since their initial description by Jacques Guillemeau in 1585, eyelid colobomas have been associated with a myriad of ocular, periorbital, and facial defects. Associations have included microphthalmos, corneal opacification (from exposure), corectopia, coloboma of the iris or choroid, anterior polar cataract, lens subluxation, epibulbar dermoid, caruncle malformation, symblepharon, nasolacrimal obstruction, eyebrow malformation, orbital dermoids, Treacher Collins syndrome, (Fig. 3–2), Goldenhar's syndrome, and cleft lip and palate.

The pathogenesis of congenital eyelid coloboma results from delayed or incomplete union of mesodermal sheets of the frontonasal and maxillary processes. Although colobomas are rarely hereditary, a dominant pedigree is occasionally observed.

Timing of surgery should be determined by the degree to which the cornea is threatened by desiccation. Upper eyelid colobomas are more prone to cause corneal exposure, while lower eyelid colobomas frequently cause trichiasis. Exposure becomes a significant factor when more than one-third of either eyelid is missing. The clinically apparent size of a coloboma may be misleading. The disrupted orbicularis oculi muscle causes the surrounding normal eyelid elements to retract horizontally away from the defect, much like the effect of cutting a stretched rubber band. This artifactually expands the

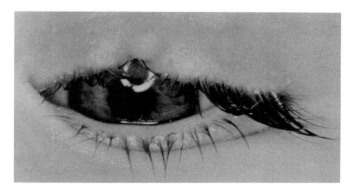

FIG. 3–1. Typical coloboma, full thickness, having triangular configuration.

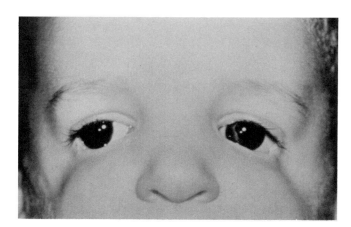

FIG. 3–2. Coloboma of the lateral aspect of the lower eyelid in Treacher Collins syndrome.

coloboma. The true extent of the defect may be determined simply by approximating the defect's edges.

Most colobomas are small, allowing surgery to proceed electively during the first 4 years of life if Bell's phenomenon is intact. During this interval, medical management is essential to avoid exposure. In mild cases, frequent application of lubricating ointment and drops such as Lacri-Lube and polyvinyl alcohol (Liquifilm Forte) may prove sufficient. In more severe cases, a moisture chamber or bandage soft contact lens may also be required. Surgery becomes urgent if significant corneal exposure ensues despite these measures.

Most colobomas involve less than 30% of the eyelid, allowing reconstruction by simply freshening the margin of the defect, converting it to a pentagonal configuration (Fig. 3–3A), and closing it by direct approximation. All normal eyelid tissue should be preserved to minimize the scope of reconstruction.

Eyelid reformation is structured around reformation of the eyelid margin. Although three margin sutures would be ideal for this purpose, the small anatomy of young children often allows placement of only two such sutures (Fig. 3–3B). The anterior eyelid margin suture of 7-0 silk (or chromic catgut) is inserted just anterior to the gray line, engaging each side of the defect. Immediately posterior to the gray line, a similar 7-0 silk (or chromic catgut) suture is placed, engaging both sides of the defect. Each suture should penetrate 2 mm deep into the tarsus and emerge 2 mm from each cut edge of the eyelid margin (Fig. 3–3C). Placement of the anterior suture should carefully avoid damage to the nearby eyelash follicles. As each of these sutures is placed, it should be temporarily tied with a slip knot to determine the accuracy of apposition. Any suture that does not achieve optimal approximation should be replaced. The posterior suture should be tied first and then tunneled anteriorly underneath the anterior suture, which is tied last. This minimizes corneal epithelial disruption by the eyelid margin suture line. These sutures should be left long and secured to the opposing cheek or brow, respectively, to minimize any postoperative notching tendency (Fig. 3–3E). The tarsus is then approximated with 7-0 Vicryl mattress suture followed by skin closure with 7-0 silk (or chromic catgut). The skin sutures may be removed 6 days postoperatively, while the eyelid margin sutures should remain under mild traction for 10 days.

Colobomas involving 30 to 50% of the eyelid additionally require a lateral canthotomy with lysis of the appropriate crus of the lateral canthal tendon (Fig. 3–3D). Defects greater than 50% are rare, but can be preferentially reconstructed with Mustarde or Tenzel rotational flaps described elsewhere in the text. Hughes or Cutler-Beard eyelid sharing flaps are not recom-

mended because they cover the globe for 3 months and may predispose to deprivation amblyopia in young children.

MICROBLEPHARON AND ABLEPHARON

Microblepharon is a rare vertical foreshortening of full-thickness eyelid tissue. Either eyelid can be affected, although the upper eyelid is more commonly involved. Lagophthalmos and corneal desiccation are often mild when Bell's phenomenon is intact. Marked degrees of microblepharon may approach ablepharon, with rudimentary cutaneous nodules in place of the eyelid. The globe may vary from normal to vestigial. Microblepharon has been additionally associated with absent eyelashes and eyebrows and with auricular, oral, and genital abnormalities.

Speculation on the pathogenesis of microblepharon suggests four possible causes: (1) primary growth failure of eyelid tissue, (2) normal initial formation with subsequent destruction and absorption of eyelid tissue, (3) temporary fusion of the eyelids during fetal development, or (4) a widespread coloboma.

Management should be based on the specific tissue deficiencies of each patient and the functional integrity of the globe. Cheek rotation flaps, eyelid sharing advancement flaps, pedicle rotation flaps, and full-thickness retroauricular skin grafts, applied alone or in partial combination, may prove useful.

EURYBLEPHARON

Euryblepharon is an anomalous bilateral, symmetrical enlargement of the palpebral aperture associated with enlarged eyelids. Horizontal palpebral fissure length may be 35 mm in this condition, compared with 25 to 30 mm in normal individuals. Although euryblepharon is stable, the extreme flaccidity of the eyelids may, in time, cause lateral ectropion of the lower eyelids, decreased blink response, and lagophthalmos.

The etiology is unknown, although speculation has centered around hypoplasia of the orbicularis oculi muscle. Hereditary associations documented in euryblepharon have not fallen into clear autosomal or sex-linked categories. It may occasionally present as a manifestation of Down's syndrome.

Patients with euryblepharon may benefit surgically from horizontal shortening of the lateral aspect of the upper and lower eyelids. The wound closure should in-

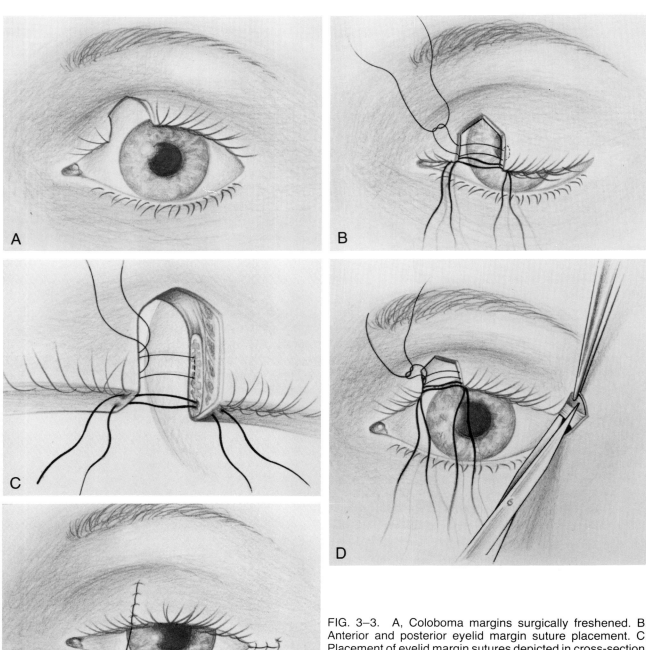

FIG. 3–3. A, Coloboma margins surgically freshened. B, Anterior and posterior eyelid margin suture placement. C, Placement of eyelid margin sutures depicted in cross-section. D, Lateral cantholysis to enhance coloboma closure. E, Eyelid margin sutures secured to cheek to minimize postoperative notching.

corporate a lateral canthoplasty to further shorten the palpebral fissure.

CRYPTOPHTHALMOS

Cryptophthalmos is a rare failure of eyelid fold formation (from mesodermal and ectodermal nondifferentiation). This disorder is subdivided into three groups. In typical (complete) cryptophthalmos, the most common form, skin replaces the eyelids, passing smoothly from the forehead to the cheek, completely covering and attaching to the subjacent globe. Eyebrow hair and lashes are absent. Partial (incomplete) cryptophthalmos occurs when facial skin fuses with the medial aspect of the globe, replacing the eyelid in that region. The lateral eyelid is normal in this form. In congenital (abortive) symblepharon, the upper eyelid is fused to the upper aspect of the globe while the cornea is covered by keratinized stratified squamous epithelium. The superior punctum is absent and xerosis of the globe may occur.

This disorder is typically bilateral and symmetrical, although unilateral and asymmetrical cases have been reported. Its occurrence is sporadic, with occasional autosomal recessive or dominant pedigrees elicited.

Associated ophthalmic features may include microphthalmos, small or absent anterior chamber, absent trabecular meshwork and Schlemm's canal, subluxated lens, iris and lens either absent or adherent to corneal endothelium, atrophic ciliary body, variable choroidal colobomatous cysts, dermoids, supernumerary brow, absent hair follicles, and absent lacrimal and accessory lacrimal glands. These associated findings often render the visual prognosis poor.

Associated nonophthalmic features may include dyscephaly (including meningomyelocele), mental retardation, otolaryngologic malformations (inner, middle, and outer ear anomalies, deafness, preauricular tags, nasal clefts, abnormal nares, cleft lip and palate, and laryngeal atresia), genitourinary malformations (hypospadias, undescended testes, clitoral hypertrophy, renal agenesis), cardiac malformations, syndactyly, umbilical hernia, and anal atresia, frontal and temporal bone flattening, and abnormal hair distribution.

Histopathologic examinations in cryptophthalmos have demonstrated metaplastic changes from the corneal epithelium to the skin. The orbicularis oculi and levator palpebrae superiorus muscles are well represented, while the tarsal plate and conjunctiva are rudimentary or absent.

Treatment is directed toward functional and cosmetic eyelid reconstruction. The palpebral aperture must be promptly parted in the neonate to allow any potential

for formed vision. In parting the eyelids, the subjacent globe must be carefully protected and preserved. The opening should be made at the point of eyelid fusion. If this landmark is indistinct, the incision should run along the horizontal axis as defined by the angles of the medial and lateral orbital rims.

SYNDROME OF BLEPHAROPTOSIS, BLEPHAROPHIMOSIS, EPICANTHUS INVERSUS, AND TELECANTHUS (KOHN-ROMANO SYNDROME)

Four varieties of epicanthal fold may be present in the inner canthus: epicanthus supraciliaris, epicanthus palpebralis, epicanthus tarsalis, and epicanthus inversus. Epicanthus supraciliaris is a fold arising from the region of the brow, terminating over the lacrimal sac. Epicanthus palpebralis is a fold arising in the upper eyelid, terminating in the lower eyelid. Epicanthus tarsalis arises from the tarsal eyelid fold and terminates in the inner canthus.

Epicanthus inversus arises in the lower eyelid, extending upward to partially obscure the inner canthus. It is seen almost exclusively as part of a congenital syndrome in conjunction with blepharoptosis, blepharophimosis, and telecanthus (Kohn-Romano syndrome).

In this condition, blepharoptosis is usually severe, demonstrating a levator palpebrae superiorus that is hypoactive and fibrotic (Fig. 3–4). One case with dehiscence of the levator aponeurosis has also been noted (Fig. 3–5). These patients have hypoplasia of the tarsal plate with absence of the eyelid fold and smooth overlying skin, which correlates with the very poor levator function commonly found. Vertical brow width is increased from constant use of the frontalis muscle for eyelid lifting. To compensate for the severe blepharoptosis, the head may assume a backward tilt while the chin arches upward (Fig. 3–4).

Blepharophimosis is a diminution of horizontal palpebral fissure length from a normal 25 to 30 mm to 18 to 22 mm (Fig. 3–4).

Epicanthus inversus folds originate in the lower eyelid and sweep superiorly and medially over the inner canthus (Fig. 3–4). This may diminish the normal canthal depression. The caruncle and plica semilunaris are hypoplastic and secluded beneath the epicanthus inversus fold.

Telecanthus, as defined by Mustarde, denotes increased distance between the inner canthi (Fig. 3–4). This is subdivided into primary and secondary forms based upon radiologic evidence of hypertelorism. In this

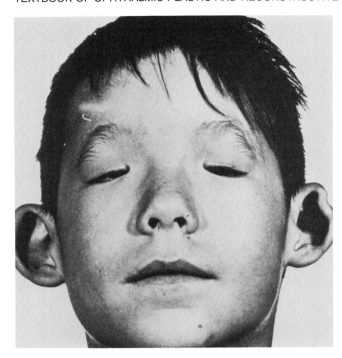

FIG. 3–4. Characteristic features of the syndrome of blepharoptosis, blepharophimosis, epicanthus inversus, and telecanthus (Kohn-Romano syndrome). (From Kohn, R. and Romano, P.: Blepharoptosis, blepharophimosis, epicanthus inversus, and telecanthus—a syndrome with no name. Published with permission from Am. J. Ophthalmol., 72:625–632, 1971. Copyright by the Ophthalmic Publishing Company.)

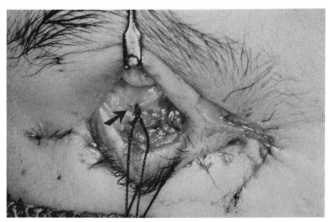

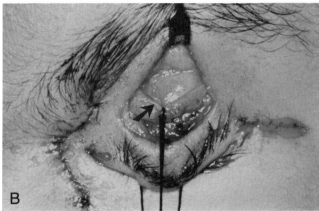

FIG. 3–5. Dehiscence of the levator aponeurosis in the Kohn-Romano syndrome (arrow). A, Right upper eyelid. B, Left upper eyelid.

syndrome, the length of the medial canthal tendon is increased from a normal 8 to 9 mm to 13 mm.

Additional eyelid features include the upper eyelid margin with a characteristically S-shape and the lower eyelid margin with a downward concavity, particularly laterally, which may result in ectropion. Trichiasis was additionally present in several reports. The lacrimal system is often affected. The lower punctum is uniformly laterally displaced, while the upper punctum is medially displaced. Posterior ectopia of the lower punctum (Fig. 3–6) and aplasia of the upper punctum have also been described. Other variations may include stenosis of all canaliculi, elongation of the horizontal canaliculi, and punctal reduplication.

Additional ophthalmic features include microphthalmos, exotropia, esotropia, underaction of the superior rectus muscle with limitation of upgaze, underaction of the inferior rectus muscle with limitation of downgaze, nystagmus, and optic disc colobomas.

Additional facial features include a broad and flat nasal bridge with a bony deficiency at the supraorbital rim and brow. The palate may be high-arched (Fig. 3–7) and the ears low-set and cupped with an overhanging helix (Fig. 3–4). Despite appearance, mental status is normal, although some patients have developed secondary psychological problems from their cosmetic handicap. This condition is quite stable over time (Fig. 3–8).

The syndrome is associated with an increased incidence of amenorrhea in women. This correlates with the autosomal dominant hereditary pattern with essentially 100% penetrance, occurrence more commonly in men, and expression more commonly through male lineage (Fig. 3–9). Sporadic cases are occasionally found. All chromosomal studies have proven normal.

Management is often deferred until the preschool years when the patient's anatomy becomes larger and easier to work with. The surgery is based on a medial canthoplasty that eliminates the epicanthus inversus while reducing the blepharophimosis.

Traditional approaches to the inner canthoplasty have included Y- to V-plasty and Mustarde's quadrilateral flaps. In Y- to V-plasty, a Y-shaped configuration is marked just medial to each inner canthus, avoiding the canaliculi in the process (Fig. 3–10A). A skin-muscle incision mobilizes the flaps medially into a V-shaped configuration (Fig. 3–10B). The Y- to V-plasty has several notable disadvantages. In this technique, the leading edge of the V is maximally advanced, while the remain-

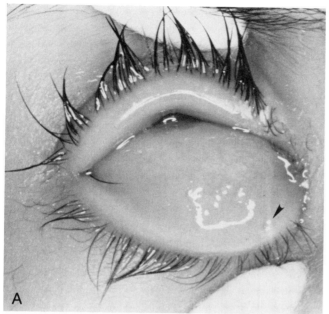

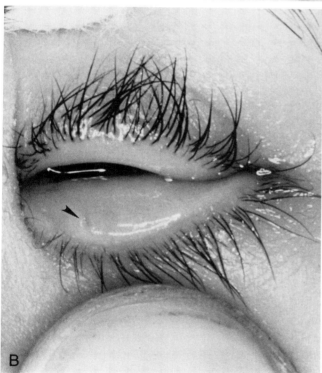

FIG. 3–6. Posterior and lateral ectopia of the lower punctae (arrow). A, Right lower punctum, B, Left lower punctum.

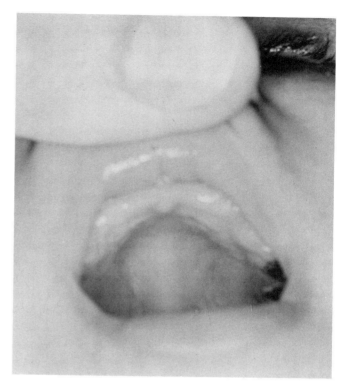

FIG. 3–7. High-arched palate is variably present in this syndrome.

der of this flap is advanced progressively less. A second disadvantage results from the prominent V-shaped scar, which does not conform well to Langer's lines (Fig. 3–11).

In Mustarde's flaps, a double Z-plasty is superimposed upon the Y- to V-configuration (Fig. 3–10C). This produces two pairs of flaps that are positionally transposed (Fig. 3–10D). The double Z-component does not contribute further to reduction of the epicanthus inversus fold, but does accentuate the resultant scar because considerable suture material is placed in a small region (Fig. 3–12). For this reason, quadrilateral flaps have proven less efficacious than Y- to V-plasty.

In either technique, the superficial head of the medial canthal tendon is shortened. Most cases require transnasal wiring, although occasional mild cases may benefit from simply resecting the medial canthal tendon and securing it to periosteum or bone at the anterior lacrimal crest.

I have recently made two modifications in the surgical technique for this disorder. A C- to U-plasty is used rather than Y- to V-plasty. This provides appreciable advancement of the entire flap, not just at the apex, and conforms to Langer's lines. Additionally, severing the insertion of the antagonist lateral canthal tendon results

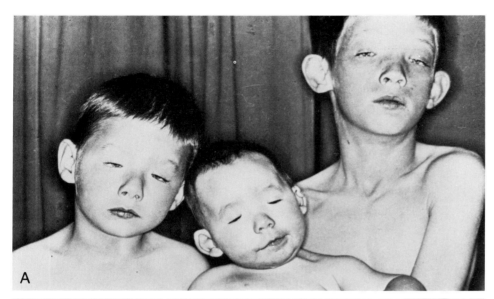

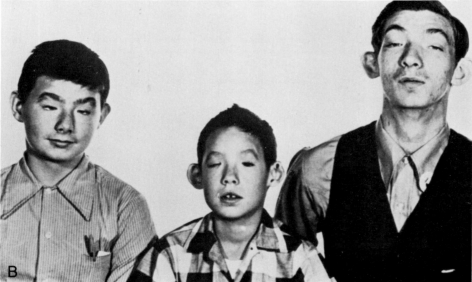

FIG. 3–8.   A, B, The stability of this condition is demonstrated by the 7-year interval between photographs of these siblings. (From Kohn, R. and Romano, P.: Blepharoptosis, blepharophimosis, epicanthus inversus, and telecanthus—a syndrome with no name. Published with permission from Am. J. Ophthalmol., 72:625–632, 1971. Copyright by the Ophthalmic Publishing Company.)

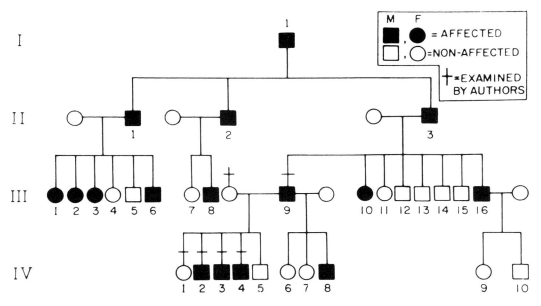

FIG. 3–9. Pedigree demonstrating autosomal dominance, strong penetrance, and dispro-portionate expression through male lineage. (From Kohn, R. and Romano, P.: Blephar-optosis, blepharophimosis, epicanthus inversus, and telecanthus—a syndrome with no name. Published with permission from Am. J. Ophthalmol., 72:625–632, 1971. Copyright by the Ophthalmic Publishing Company.)

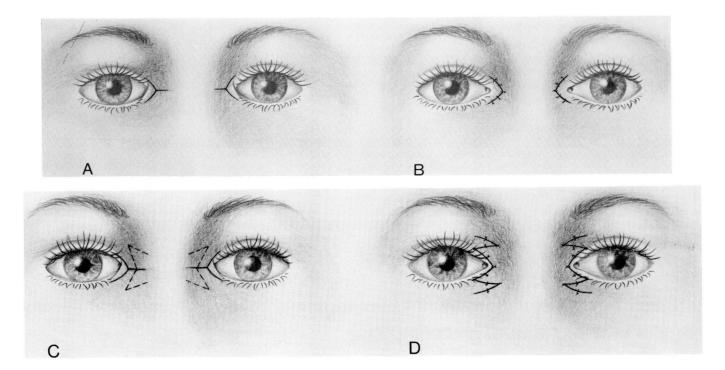

FIG. 3–10. Y- to V-plasty. A, Incision site marked in Y-shaped configuration. B, Flaps mobilized into V-configuration. Mustarde's quadrilateral flaps. C, Incision site marked. Note that this is a Y- to V-plasty with a superimposed double Z-plasty. D, Flaps mobilized.

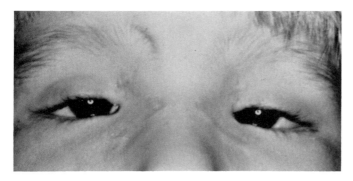

FIG. 3–11. Y- to V-plasty 1 year postoperatively, demonstrating prominent scar and limited medial mobilization.

in more effective advancement of the medial canthal tendon in transnasal wiring. This is comparable to the augmentative effect of recession and resection in strabismus surgery. The medial advancement of the medial canthus and eyelids appears to prevent rounding of the lateral canthus from lysis of its tendon.

Author's Surgical Technique. The inner canthal incision site should be marked bilaterally with methylene blue. This mark should assume a C-shaped configuration with approximately 7 mm of tissue incorporated within the defined skin-muscle excision site (Fig. 3–13A, B). The size can be modified somewhat to accentuate or lessen the excision from one case to another. The C should be placed approximately 5 mm medial to the inner canthus and should not approach the nearby canalicular system. Skin and muscle should be excised according to these lines (Fig. 3–13C, D). The incision is carried to the anterior lacrimal crest, where the superficial head of the medial canthal tendon is isolated and resected with one side secured with either a 27-gauge wire or a 2-0 Supramid suture.

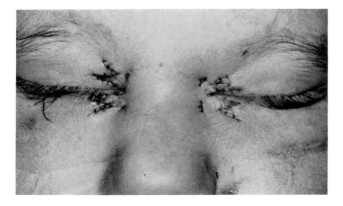

FIG. 3–12. Quadrilateral flaps demonstrating considerable amount of suture material placed within a small anatomic region.

A 3 mm horizontal incision is made just lateral to the outer canthus, overlying the lateral orbital rim. Through this incision, the lateral canthal tendon is isolated at the lateral orbital tubercle and is completely disinserted. Skin at the outer canthus is closed with running 7-0 silk (or chromic catgut). The medial mobility of the medial canthal tendon will now be appreciably enhanced.

In mild cases, the resected superficial head of the medial canthal tendon may be secured to periosteum or bone at the anterior lacrimal crest. Most cases, however, require transnasal wiring.

In wiring, a bony window is fashioned in the posterior lacrimal and anterior ethmoidal areas. The lacrimal sac should be displaced somewhat laterally to avoid damage. Sufficient bone should be removed to accommodate a Wright needle for wire or suture passage. The Wright needle enters the bony window on the side without suture or wire. It is then passed through the orbital septum, emerging through the opposite bony window (Fig. 3–13E). Some pressure is required to penetrate the septum. Careful attention must be focused to prevent momentum from carrying the needle immediately through the second window because the medial globe is in close proximity. The Supramid suture or wire should be placed through the eyelet opening of the Wright needle. This material becomes properly positioned as the Wright needle is withdrawn. The Supramid or wire is then secured to the second medial canthal tendon to provide maximal advancement of the medial canthal structures (Fig. 3–13F, G). Tightening should be snug and secure, but not so tight that tendon necrosis and suture disengagement ensue. The suture material gains some stability from its passage through the orbital septum. Medial advancement is enhanced by the previous lysis of the lateral canthal tendons.

The C-shaped skin-muscle flap is mobilized medially and may be further tailored to reduce the epicanthal fold and telecanthus. This is secured with three interrupted 5-0 Vicryl horizontal mattress sutures to hold the advancing flap in position. The skin is closed with running 7-0 silk (or chromic catgut) to maximize cosmesis. The resultant inner canthal suture line assumes a somewhat U-shaped configuration (Fig. 3–13H, I).

This procedure affords additional medial mobilization beyond that achieved by Y- to V-plasty and results in a less visible scar owing to conformity to Langer's lines (Figs. 3–14 and 3–15).

Blepharoptosis is corrected at the final stage of the first procedure or in a second operation. Usually, frontalis suspension is required because of the poor levator function present in these cases. In selected patients with less blepharoptosis and demonstrable levator function, a maximum levator resection may prove adequate. The

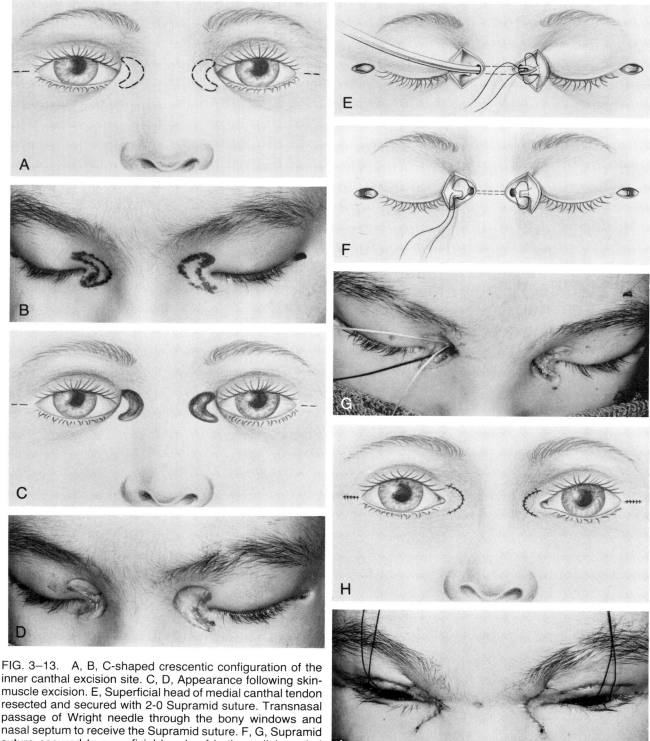

FIG. 3–13.   A, B, C-shaped crescentic configuration of the inner canthal excision site. C, D, Appearance following skin-muscle excision. E, Superficial head of medial canthal tendon resected and secured with 2-0 Supramid suture. Transnasal passage of Wright needle through the bony windows and nasal septum to receive the Supramid suture. F, G, Supramid suture secured to superficial heads of both medial canthal tendons through bony windows. H, I, Resultant U-shaped suture line at inner canthus and small suture line at outer canthus.

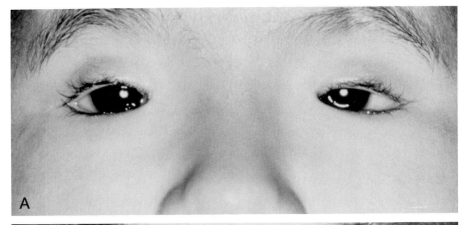

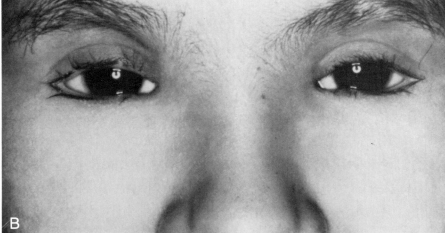

FIG. 3–14. C- to U-plasty. A, Preoperative appearance. B, Postoperative appearance demonstrating limited scar conforming to Langer's lines and significant improvement of this condition.

one case with bilateral levator aponeurosis dehiscence was corrected by dehiscence repair alone.

Rare cases with severe blepharophimosis may be helped by an enhanced lateral canthoplasty with conjunctival reattachment holding the outer canthus in a more open configuration. Cases with lower eyelid ectropion are amenable to retroauricular full-thickness skin grafting.

ANKYLOBLEPHARON

Ankyloblepharon is a partial fusion of the eyelids over a portion of their length, producing horizontal foreshortening of the palpebral aperture. This fusion occurs most commonly at the outer canthus (Fig. 3–16A), erroneously suggesting exotropia (pseudoexotropia). Occasionally, an inner canthal ankyloblepharon is noted, which may result in pseudoesotropia. Ankyloblepharon may be associated with other anomalies including anophthalmos, microphthalmos, and congenital phthysis bulbi.

The pathogenesis has been attributed to developmental arrest resulting in growth aberration at either canthus. Many cases have a hereditary component, usually dominant, although sporadic cases are seen.

The treatment of this condition involves incising the fused portion of the eyelid margin. The appropriate conjunctival and cutaneous surfaces are then joined to reapproximate normal anatomy (Fig. 3–16B).

ANKYLOBLEPHARON FILIFORME ADNATUM

Ankyloblepharon filiforme adnatum is a rare disorder in which fine attachments of extensile tissue fuse various portions of the upper and lower eyelids. This reduces the vertical palpebral fissure width and appreciably interferes with eyelid movement. The bands may be unilateral or bilateral, single or multiple, symmetrical or asymmetrical. These attachments arise at the gray line, posterior to the cilia and anterior to the meibomian gland orifices. They are comprised of a central vascularized connective tissue core surrounded by stratified squamous

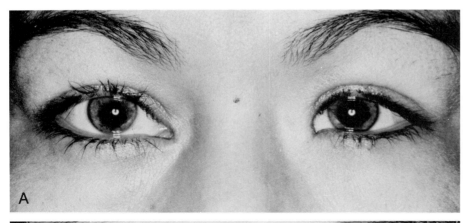

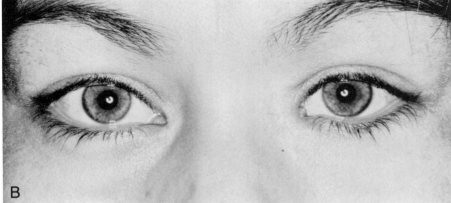

FIG. 3–15. Unilateral traumatic telecanthus (left eye). Unilateral C- to U-plasty. A, Preoperative appearance. B, Postoperative appearance.

epithelium. Associated findings may occasionally include cleft lip, cleft palate, adherent pinna, intraoral anomalies, ventricular septal defect, patent ductus arteriosus, syndactyly, hydrocephalus, meningomyelocele, imperforate anus, and the popliteal-pterygium syndrome.

The etiology of ankyloblepharon filiforme adnatum has been attributed to an interplay between a temporary arrest of epithelium and a rapid proliferation of mesenchyme, allowing the union of mesenchymal tissue along various points of the upper and lower eyelid margin. Subsequent eyelid movement stretches these attachments into formed bands. Although the condition is usually sporadic, autosomal dominant and recessive patterns have been reported.

Treatment involves simply severing the attachments. The resultant epithelial tags subsequently undergo rapid involution.

CONGENITAL ENTROPION AND EPIBLEPHARON

Congenital entropion of the lower eyelid is an uncommon, usually asymptomatic disorder manifested by an inward rolling of the eyelid margin, which causes the cilia to point inward toward the globe (Fig. 3–17). Confusion may result with the more common condition, epiblepharon, in which a horizontal redundant medial skin fold induces a vertical orientation of the cilia (Fig. 3–18). Both conditions may at times coexist and disproportionately occur in Orientals.

Improper development of the distal lower eyelid retractor, with attenuation or dehiscence near the tarsal plate, appears to be a common etiologic denominator in congenital lower eyelid entropion and epiblepharon. Secondary forms of congenital entropion can result from epicanthal folds, microphthalmos, and anophthalmos. These cases caused by mechanical factors.

The clinical course of congenital entropion is often asymptomatic with spontaneous resolution. Therefore, surgery should be reserved for persistent cases that threaten the cornea. When surgery is indicated, the recommended procedure is the tuck of the inferior aponeurosis as described by Jones and Reeh, detailed in Chapter 8.

Epiblepharon also improves and often resolves by age 3 as eyelid skin stretches. During this period, conservative treatment with lubricating ointment helps to spare the cornea. Surgery should be reserved for rare persistent cases. These may be corrected by either excising the

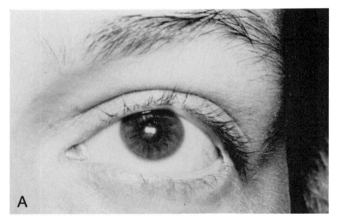

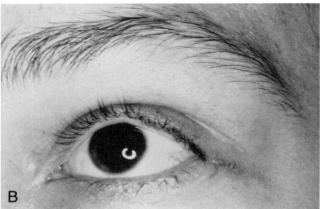

FIG. 3–16. Ankyloblepharon. A, Preoperative appearance. B, Postoperative appearance following lateral canthoplasty.

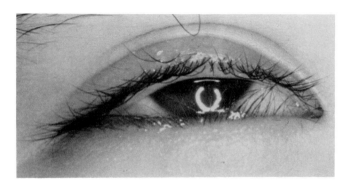

FIG. 3–17. Congenital entropion with inward rolling of eyelid margin and cilia pointing inward toward the globe.

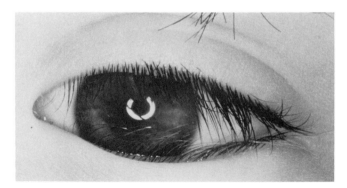

FIG. 3–18. Epiblepharon with redundant medial skin fold causing vertical orientation of the cilia.

skin and orbicularis oculi muscle comprising the redundant fold or by placing Quickert-Rathbun eyelid crease sutures.

Congenital entropion of the upper eyelid results from either congenital horizontal tarsal kink, as reported by Callahan, or cicatrization from inflammatory or infectious factors. Kink occurs from an anomalous fixed inward rotation of the distal tarsal margin causing the cilia to abrade the cornea. This may be corrected by resecting that portion of tarsus involved in the kink process. Congenital cicatricial entropion may be repaired by a Wies tarsal splitting procedure, as modified by Ballen for upper eyelid application (detailed in Chapter 6).

CONGENITAL ECTROPION

Primary congenital ectropion of the lower eyelid is a rare condition with occasional familial associations. Congenital ectropion is more commonly seen as a disorder secondary to microphthalmos, buphthalmos, euryblepharon, and tumors of the eyelid, or as part of the syndrome of blepharoptosis, blepharophimosis, epicanthus inversus, and telecanthus (Kohn-Romano syndrome) (Fig. 3–19). In the latter condition, ectropion results from vertical skin deficiency. Such cases are corrected using retroauricular full-thickness skin grafting to the lower eyelid. Rare cases of congenital ectropion due to excessive horizontal eyelid length are managed by horizontal eyelid shortening techniques such as the Bick procedures.

Congenital ectropion of the upper eyelid presents as total eversion. This disorder is postulated to arise from birth trauma that interferes with venous drainage. The resultant chemosis everts the eyelid and triggers orbicularis oculi muscle spasm. Orbicularis oculi muscle hypotonia has also been suggested as a cause. Conservative management involving lubricating ointments, a moisture

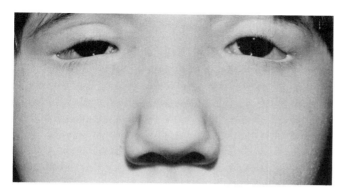

FIG. 3–19.   Congenital ectropion of the lateral portion of both lower eyelids in the syndrome of blepharoptosis, blepharophimosis, epicanthus inversus, and telecanthus (Kohn-Romano syndrome).

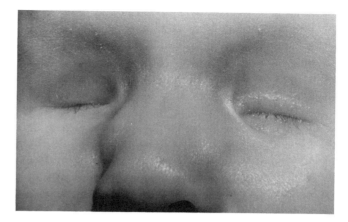

FIG. 3–21.   Bilateral congenital clinical anophthalmos with small, sunken eyelids.

chamber, and traction sutures placed at the eyelid margin often prove adequate. Persistent cases may additionally require excision of prolapsed conjunctiva.

MEDIAL CANTHAL TENDON ECTOPIA

Medial canthal tendon ectopia is a rare disorder in which the tendon and attached canthal structures are vertically displaced, particularly inferiorly (Fig. 3–20). In this disorder, the medial canthal tendon inserts at the junction of the medial orbital wall and the infraorbital rim, with the inferiorly displaced lacrimal sac subjacent. Nasal cleft deformities have been associated with this condition. The cause is considered to be a developmental arrest during the second month of embryonic life. Treatment consists of a medial canthal Z-plasty with supraplacement of the medial canthal tendon. Any concurrent lacrimal obstruction should also be corrected.

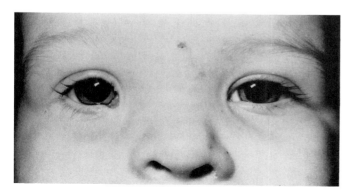

FIG. 3–20.   Medial canthal tendon vertical ectopia in a newborn.

CONGENITAL CLINICAL ANOPHTHALMOS

True anophthalmos is a rare disorder manifested by failure in the outgrowth of the primary optic vesicle. This results in total nonrepresentation of essential ocular structures derived from neuroectoderm. More commonly seen is microphthalmos, in which these tissues are variably represented. Clinical distinction between anophthalmos and microphthalmos is often indistinct and may be discernible only upon postmortem examination of serial sections of the orbit. Hence, the term congenital clinical anophthalmos is appropriate in describing both entities. Anophthalmos is embryologically subdivided into three categories.

Primary anophthalmos results from suppression of the optic vesicle during differentiation of the optic plate, following formation of the rudimentary forebrain. This results in absence of the optic nerve and neuroectoderm derivatives. Clinically, orbital and palpebral tissues are present, but underdeveloped, because they do not depend on the optic vesicle for differentiation.

Secondary (complete) anophthalmos results from an intrauterine insult during pregnancy that suppresses development of the entire forebrain. This causes numerous major abnormalities that are incompatible with life.

Degenerative anophthalmos results from absorption of the optic vesicle after its initial formation. The bony orbit, eyelids, lacrimal system, conjunctiva, extraocular muscles, cornea, and sclera do not depend on the optic vesicle for development. They may, therefore, be present with some degree of differentiation.

Congenital clinical anophthalmos most commonly presents as a small, amorphous, nodular mass near the orbital apex. The surrounding orbit is formed, but shallow with overlying small and sunken eyelids (Fig. 3–21).

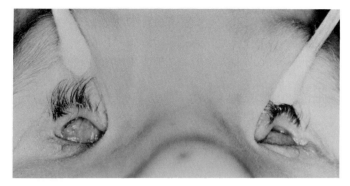

FIG. 3–22. Bilateral congenital clinical anophthalmos with palpebral fissures horizontally foreshortened.

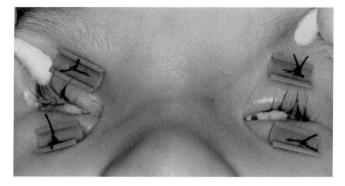

FIG. 3–23. Soft, malleable conformer secured with 4-0 silk mattress sutures, which have been tied over bolsters.

Commensurately, the palpebral aperture is horizontally foreshortened (Fig. 3–22). Cilia, meibomian glands, puncta, lacrimal tissue, and extraocular muscles are variably present. The optic nerve is usually absent, reducing optic foramen size.

Anophthalmos may be associated with eyelid colobomas, clefting disorders, polydactyly, cardiac malformations, mental retardation, craniofacial anomalies, and central nervous system defects. Most primary cases are sporadic, although dominant, recessive, and sex-linked cases have all been reported.

Surgery is best deferred until maximum benefit has been derived from mechanically stretching the fornices with progressively larger conformers beginning within the first several weeks of life. Conformers should be changed at 1- to 2-week intervals. Initially, even the smallest conformer may not fit or be self-retained. At this stage, soft malleable conformers may have to be trimmed to size and secured with 4-0 silk mattress sutures. These sutures are placed at the superior and inferior aspects of the conformer, penetrating the respective conjunctival fornix, engaging periosteum at the orbital rims, and emerging through the skin where they are tied over rubber bolsters to avoid skin excoriation (Fig. 3–23). After a short time, retention sutures will not be required. Pressure conformers may also prove useful in socket enlargement. In either system, vertical expansion exceeds horizontal expansion.

Eyelid and socket surgery rarely prove necessary for this condition. Early surgery promotes scar tissue formation, which significantly impedes any potential mechanical socket expansion. Therefore, all surgery should be delayed until this process has been completed.

Orbital volume may be reduced 50 to 60% in these cases. The ocular vestige should be left because it provides a better stimulus to orbital growth than would an enucleation sphere.

If the fornices remain insufficient, they may be aug-

mented by buccal mucous membrane grafting. These grafts are harvested from the lower lip internal to the vermilion border. A Castroviejo mucotome set at 0.3 mm thickness is optimal for this purpose. Thinner grafts may shred, while thicker grafts penetrate the fat layer of the lip and scar. Once harvested, the graft is sutured with 7-0 chromic catgut into a "bed" surgically opened in the fornices. This may be further supported by a stent or conformer (Fig. 3–24).

The palpebral fissure can be lengthened horizontally by a lateral canthotomy and canthoplasty. Major eyelid

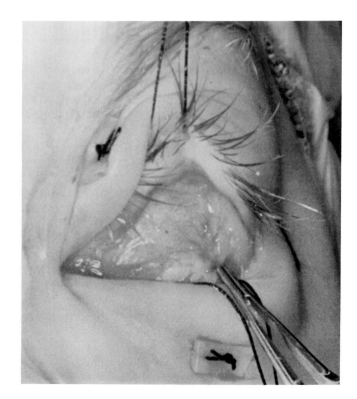

FIG. 3–24. Mucous membrane grafts sutured into fornices with 7-0 chromic catgut sutures.

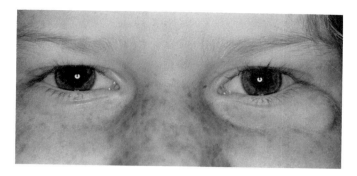

FIG. 3–25. Dermoid cyst in atypical location.

reconstruction is rarely indicated. Should it be required, Tenzel and Mustarde flaps are preferable to Hughes or Cutler-Beard flaps because they do not depend on the underdeveloped eyelids for donor tissues.

DERMOID CYSTS

Dermoid cysts are benign choristomas. During development, ectoderm and periosteum are in close apposition to bony suture lines. Pieces of ectoderm may become pinched off when suture lines close. As the skin develops, so does this ectodermal tissue, but in an ectopic location forming dermoid cysts (Fig. 3–25). They occur most commonly at the anterior aspect of the superior temporal orbit fixed to periosteum near the zygomaticofrontal suture (Fig. 3–26). They are less commonly seen in the deeper orbit in proximity to the sphenoid bone.

The peak incidence of orbital dermoids is from 3 to 10 years of age, while fewer may manifest in the third or fourth decades. In childhood, dermoids typically present as a painless, subcutaneous mass lesion of irregular configuration. They are firm and minimally mobile, although not usually attached to the overlying skin.

Superficial dermoids rarely present with radiologic evidence of bone erosion, while their deeper counterparts may demonstrate moderate fossa formation or erosion through orbital bone. Ultrasonographically, dermoids have smooth, well-defined contours with good sound transmission. They demonstrate internal echoes of variable amplitude because of the variable internal contents of these lesions. The degree of posterior extension can often be defined on B-scan ultrasonography. CT scans and tomographs may further demarcate these lesions, which may be highlighted by increased density of the surrounding bone.

Histopathologically, orbital dermoids are composed of epidermal tissue mixed with one or more dermal adnexal structures or skin appendages such as hair follicles, se-

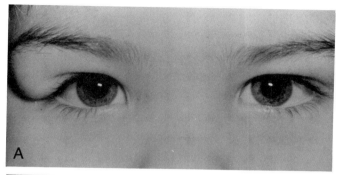

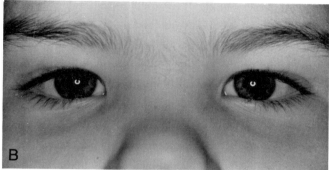

FIG. 3–26. A, Dermoid cyst in characteristic location. B, Appearance following surgical removal.

baceous glands, and sweat glands. Macroscopically, they have a prominent cystic structure lined by keratinizing epidermis, which may contain keratin, hair, or fat.

Superficial orbital dermoids can be readily removed through a skin incision made directly over the cyst. The dissection must carefully avoid disrupting the capsular lining, since release of the sebaceous material into the orbit will set up a moderate granulomatous inflammatory reaction. Diverticula, if present, should also be excised because they may provide a source for recurrence.

Deep orbital dermoids often necessitate a Kronlein lateral orbitotomy for removal. If they extend through the sphenoid bone toward the intracranial space, they are best removed in conjunction with a neurosurgical approach.

Some orbital dermoids present subconjunctivally (Fig. 3–27). The indications for surgical removal of such lesions are somewhat conservative because blepharoptosis, motility disturbances, and lacrimal gland obstruction may be encountered as postoperative sequelae. Indications for removal of subconjunctival dermoids include: direct obstruction of the visual axis, anisometropic amblyopia induced by pressure-astigmatic changes, or significant cosmetic disfigurement.

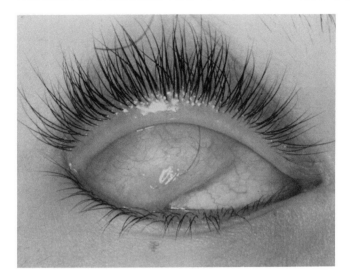

FIG. 3–27. Dermoid cyst with subconjunctival presentation and hair emerging through the surface.

ORBITAL TERATOMA

Orbital teratomas are rare, with fewer than 60 cases in the literature. They present in the newborn as unilateral, progressively expanding, polycystic tumors. Although usually confined to the orbit, bony erosion with intracranial extension can occur. Teratomas form mucin, which collects within and expands the cysts to enormous proportions. Marked enlargement of the eyelids and orbit may result (Fig. 3–28). The globe is normally developed, although the cornea and optic nerve may become compromised from marked proptosis. Clinical examination demonstrates a cystic, nonreducible mass that readily transilluminates. Some solid elements may also be present.

The evaluation of a suspected teratoma should include plain radiographs of the orbit and skull, CT scans of the orbit and anterior cranial areas, and ultrasonography. This should demonstrate a circumscribed cystic mass with calcifications variably present. The surrounding orbit may be considerably enlarged. These studies should characterize and localize the tumor to facilitate surgical planning.

The differential diagnosis of congenital orbital teratoma in a neonate should include rhabdomyosarcoma, undifferentiated sarcoma, lymphoma, lymphangioma, hemangioma, hematoma, neuroblastoma, neurofibroma, meningocele, encephalocele, inflammatory pseudotumor, dermoid cyst, microphthalmos with cyst, congenital cystic eyeball, and congenital glaucoma with buphthalmos.

Histopathologically, teratomas are composed of tissues

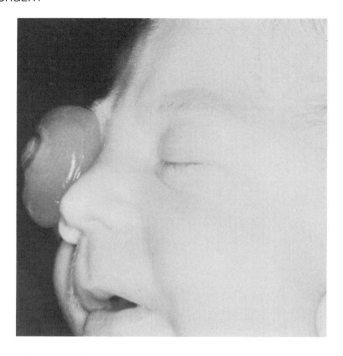

FIG. 3–28. Orbital teratoma with marked proptosis and enlargement of the eyelids (photograph courtesy of Arthur Grove, M.D. and W.B. Saunders, Publishers).

representing two or three germinal layers. Although they are principally composed of ectoderm, endodermal and mesodermal components are also represented. Differentiation may vary from an amorphous mass to complete fetal architecture. Malignant degeneration rarely occurs. The extensive fluid accumulation within these encapsulated cysts causes teratomas to be clinically destructive beyond their benign histologic structure.

The globe must be continuously protected during the preoperative assessment period. Prompt surgical removal of these tumors is essential, preserving the globe for vision or cosmesis if at all possible (Fig. 3–29). Sur-

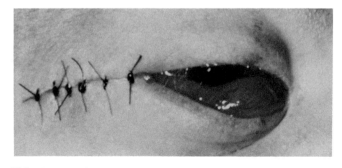

FIG. 3–29. Appearance immediately following surgical removal of orbital teratoma depicted in Fig. 3–28 (photograph courtesy of Arthur Grove, M.D. and W.B. Saunders, Publishers).

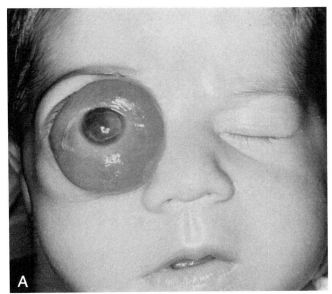

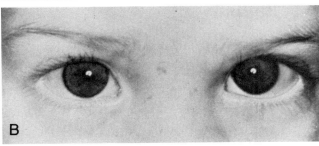

FIG. 3–30. A, Preoperative and, B, postoperative appearance of child with orbital teratoma. Vision was restored to 20/40 in the involved eye. (Photographs courtesy of Arthur Grove, M.D. and W.B. Saunders, Publishers.)

gery usually requires a lateral or anterolateral orbitotomy. Teratoma removal can sometimes be facilitated by coexistent needle aspiration of the fluid-filled encapsulated cysts to reduce tumor size. Although exenteration has been used in the past, many teratomas can be removed while retaining the globe, with useful vision resulting in some cases (Fig. 3–30).

BIBLIOGRAPHY

Barber, J., Barber, L., Guerry, D., and Geeraets, W.: Congenital orbital teratoma. Arch. Ophthalmol. 91:45, 1974.

Baylis, H., Bartlett, R., and Cies, W.: Reconstruction of the lower lid in congenital microphthalmos and anophthalmos. Ophthalmic Surg., 6:36, 1975.

Biglan, A. and Buerger, G.: Congenital horizontal tarsal kink. Am. J. Ophthalmol. 89:522, 1980.

Butler, M., Eisen, J., and Henry, J.: Cryptophthalmos with an orbital cyst and profound mental and motor retardation. J. Pediatr Ophthalmol. Strabismus 15:233, 1978.

Callahan, M. and Callahan, A.: Ophthalmic Plastic and Orbital Surgery. Birmingham, Aesculapius, 1979.

Carroll, R., Wilkins, R., Fredricks, S., and Small, R.: Congenital medial canthal tendon malposition. Ann. Ophthalmol. 10:665, 1978.

Chang, D., Dallow, R., and Walton, D.: Congenital orbital teratoma: Report of a case with visual preservation. J. Pediatr. Ophthalmol. Strabismus 17:88, 1980.

Codere, F., Brownstein, S., and Chen, M.: Cryptophthalmos syndrome with bilateral renal agenesis. Am. J. Ophthalmol. 91:737, 1981.

Cullen, J.: Orbital diploic dermoids. Br. J. Ophthalmol. 58:105, 1974.

Feldman, E., Bowen, S., and Morgan, S.: Euryblepharon: A case report with photographs documenting the condition from infancy to adulthood. J. Pediatr. Ophthalmol. Strabismus 17:307, 1980.

Geeraets, W.: Kohn-Romano syndrome. In Ocular Syndromes. Philadelphia, Lea & Febiger, 1976.

Gilbert, H., Smith, R., Barlow, M., and Mohr, D.: Congenital upper eyelid eversion and down's syndrome. Am. J. Ophthalmol. 75:469, 1973.

Golden, S. and Perman, K.: Bilateral clinical anophthalmia. South. Med. J. 73:1404, 1980.

Gupta, J. and Kumar, K.: Euryblepharon with ectropion. Am. J. Ophthalmol. 66:554, 1968.

Ide, C., Davis, W., and Black, S.: Orbital teratoma. Arch. Ophthalmol. 96:2093, 1978.

Johnson, C.: Epicanthus and epiblepharon. Arch. Ophthalmol. 96:1030, 1978.

Johnson, C.: Epiblepharon. Am. J. Ophthalmol. 66:1172, 1968.

Kazarian, E. and Goldstein, P.: Ankyloblepharon filiforme adnatum with hydrocephalus, meningomyelocele, and imperforate anus. Am. J. Ophthalmol. 84:355, 1977.

Keipert, J.: Euryblepharon. Br. J. Ophthalmol. 59:57, 1975.

Kennedy, R.: Growth retardation and volume determination of the anophthalmic orbit. Am. J. Ophthalmol. 76:294, 1973.

Kidwell, E. and Tenzel, R.: Repair of congenital colobomas of the lids. Arch. Ophthalmol. 97:1931, 1979.

Kohn, R. and Romano, P.: Blepharoptosis, blepharophimosis, epicanthus inversus, and telecanthus—a syndrome with no name. Am. J. Ophthalmol. 72:625, 1971.

Kohn, R.: Additional lacrimal findings in the syndrome of blepharoptosis, blepharophimosis, epicanthus inversus, and telecanthus. J. Pediatr. Ophthalmol. Strabismus 20:98, 1983.

Kohn, R.: Management of congenital and acquired telecanthus. In preparation.

Kohn, R.: Epicanthus. Chapter in Buyse, M., Birth Defects Encyclopedia, New York, Alan R. Liss, Inc., 1988.

Kohn, R.: Congenital Anomalies of the Eyelid and Socket. In Hornblass, A.: Oculoplastic, Orbital and Reconstructive Surgery, Baltimore, Williams and Wilkins, 1988.

Lemke, B. and Stasior, O.: Epiblepharon. Clin. Pediatr. 20:661, 1981.

McCarthy, G. and West, C.: Ablepharon macrostomia syndrome. Dev. Med. Child. Neurol. 19:659, 1977.

Patipa, M., Wilkins, R., and Guelznow, K.: Surgical management of congenital eyelid coloboma. Ophthalmic Surg. 13:212, 1982.

Pollard, Z. and Calhoun, J.: Deep orbital dermoid with draining sinus. Am. J. Ophthalmol. 79:310, 1975.

Quickert, M., Wilkes, D., and Dryden, R.: Nonincisional correction of epiblepharon and congenital entropion. Arch. Ophthalmol. 101:778, 1983.

Reeh, M., Beyer, C., and Shannon, G.: Practical Ophthalmic Plastic and Reconstructive Surgery. Philadelphia, Lea & Febiger, 1976.

Rodrigue, D.: Congenital ectropion. Can. J. Ophthalmol. 11:355, 1976.

Rosenman, Y., Ronen, S., Eidelman, A., and Schimmel, M.: Anky-loblepharon filiforme adnatum. Am. J. Dis. Child. 134:751, 1980.

Roy, E.: Kohn-Romano Syndrome. *In* Ocular Syndromes and Systemic Diseases. Orlando, Grune & Stratton, 1985.

Sassani, J. and Yanoff, M.: Anophthalmos in an infant with multiple congenital anomalies. Am. J. Ophthalmol. 83:43, 1977.

Soll, D.: Management of Complications in Ophthalmic Plastic Surgery. Birmingham, Aesculapius, 1976.

Stern, E., Campbell, C., and Faulkner, H.: Conservative management of congenital eversion of the eyelids. Am. J. Ophthalmol. 75:319, 1973.

Sugar, H.: The cryptophthalmos-syndactyly syndrome. Am. J. Ophthalmol. 66:897, 1968.

Waring, G. and Shields, J.: Partial unilateral cryptophthalmos with syndactyly, brachycephaly, and renal anomalies. Am. J. Ophthalmol. 79:437, 1975.

4

CRANIOFACIAL ABNORMALITIES

Andrew Choy, M.D.

The unfortunate patient with a craniofacial disfigurement may appear to the infrequent observer as a hopeless assortment of anomalies. Most of these patients are afflicted from birth. A few have acquired abnormalities resulting from trauma.

This chapter reviews some of the primary orbital, adnexal, and ocular problems of craniofacial patients. Throughout this chapter, emphasis is given to the importance of the development and preservation of vision. This emphasis is particularly vital in orbital translocation craniofacial surgery, where the eye is in the center of a maelstrom of major reconstruction and vision loss is a real threat.

An understanding of the bony abnormalities in the underlying craniofacial skeleton will help to explain the pathology and provide a framework to group these various craniofacial disorders into four general types: (1) teleorbitism (hypertelorism), (2) midfacial hypoplasia (craniofacial dysostosis, acrocephalosyndactyly), (3) hemifacial asymmetry, and (4) mandibulofacial dysostosis (Treacher Collins syndrome). Variations and subgroups are seen within each major category. Some patients may have a combination of the major disorders, and an occasional patient may defy classification. These four major categories, however, help to provide a basic understanding to us as physicians and to our fellow health professionals of the ophthalmologic problems experienced by craniofacial patients.

The pioneering craniofacial surgical efforts of Tessier and the subsequent refinements of others have led to the surgical subtotal translocation of the orbit in three dimensions. A horizontal translocation in a medial direction is used to correct teleorbitism (Fig. 4–1). A sagittal movement in an antero-posterior direction is used to advance the orbital roof (frontal bone) and the orbital floor (midface) in midfacial hypoplasia (Fig. 4–2). Vertical translocations in a superior and/or inferior direction are performed to correct orbital dystopia in hemifacial asymmetry (Fig. 4–3).

Tessier's extensive experience and careful observation have led to a craniofacial cleft classification that helps to explain some of these groups and their accompanying

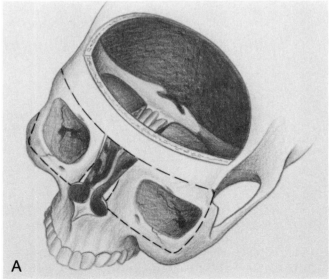 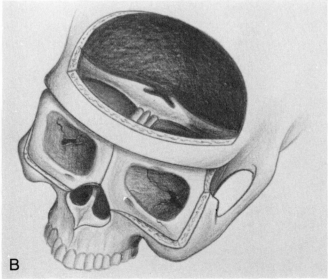

FIG. 4–1. A medial horizontal translocation of the orbit for teleorbitism. A, The osteotomy lines. B, After translocation of the orbits and bone grafting.

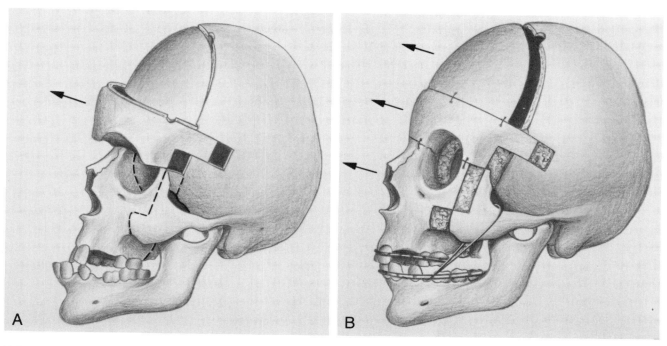

FIG. 4–2. An anteroposterior sagittal advancement of the orbital floor and orbital roof through a combined craniofacial route for midfacial hypoplasia. A, Lines of osteotomy with frontal bone advanced. B, Final position following advancement of all bony segments with bone grafts wedged into the resultant defects. Further stabilization is obtained by inter-maxillary wiring and the use of suspension wires to the zygomatic arches.

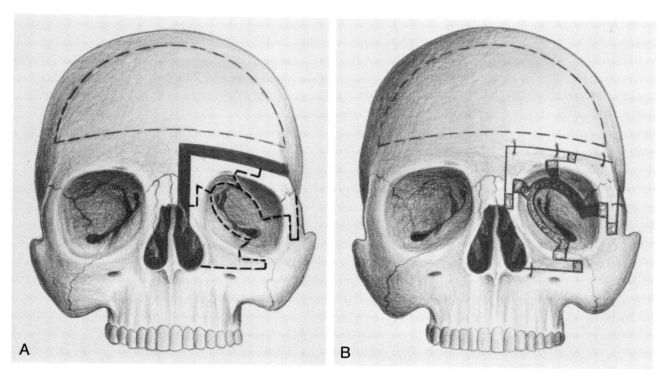

FIG. 4–3. Vertical type of translocation used for correction of orbital dystopia. A, Osteo-tomies and bony resection used in the expansion of the micro orbit. B, Bony defects are filled with bone grafts.

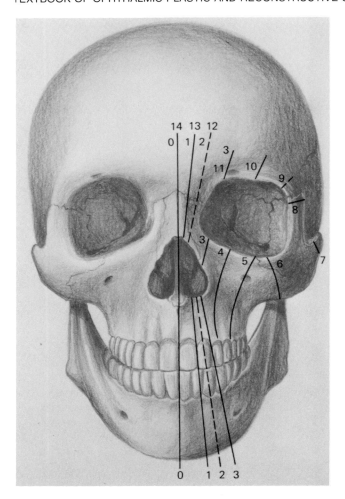

FIG. 4–4. Diagrammatic representation of bony facial clefts with the various locations around the orbit. (After Paul Tessier, M.D.)

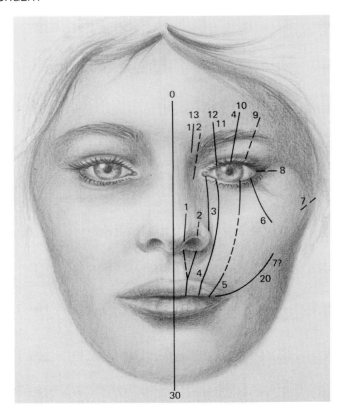

FIG. 4–5. Diagrammatic location of the corresponding soft tissue clefts. (After Paul Tessier, M.D.)

ophthalmologic problems. The bony abnormalities seen in Figure 4–4 and the accompanying soft tissue defects shown in Figure 4–5 are referred to throughout this discussion of the various craniofacial conditions.

In addition, premature closure or synostosis of the cranial sutures can lead to craniofacial malformations. Figure 4–6 illustrates the effect of premature synostosis of the coronal suture on one side of the calverium leading to an orbital dystopia frequently observed in hemifacial asymmetry patients.

TELEORBITISM (HYPERTELORISM)

Teleorbitism is associated with craniofacial skeletal defects in regions 1-13, 2-12, 3-11, and 4-10, as seen in Figures 4–4 and 4–5. Various disorders such as frontalnasal dysplasia, encephalocele, and median facial cleft

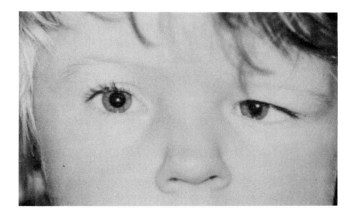

FIG. 4–6. Premature synostosis of the left-side coronal suture has led to plagiocephaly. There is a resultant orbital dystopia with hemifacial asymmetry. Esotropia and amblyopia accompany this patient's condition.

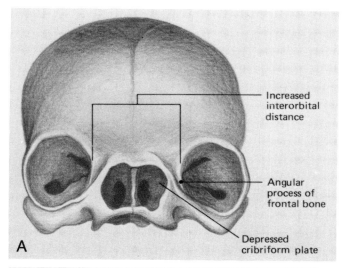

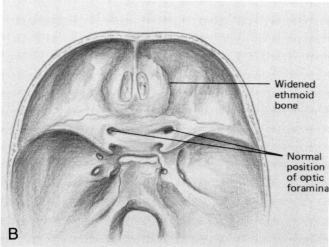

FIG. 4–7.   Infant skull with teleorbitism. A, Frontal view showing depressed cribriform plate and increased interorbital distance. B, Cranial view with widening of the ethmoid sinus complex. Note that optic foramina remain in normal position.

are associated with these defects. Figure 4–7 illustrates the typical increased interorbital distance with accompanying ethmoid sinus hyperplasia.

NASOLACRIMAL DRAINAGE DYSFUNCTION

Over 30 years ago, Urrets-Zavalia noted the frequency of lacrimal drainage system anomalies associated with the various craniofacial syndromes. The Tessier cleft classification strongly points to these bony defects as a major factor in compromising lacrimal drainage. The association of inferior bony clefts 1 through 4 and the superior extensions in Tessier Cleft numbers 11 through 13 in tele-

orbitism probably accounts for the increased incidence of nasolocrimal drainage disorders seen in this group of craniofacial patients (Figs. 4–4 and 4–8). These clefts are nasal to the overlying lacrimal puncta (Fig. 4–5). In a group of 31 teleorbitism patients, 16% had lacrimal drainage dysfunction before craniofacial reconstructive surgery.

The reconstructive craniofacial surgery also exposes a compromised lacrimal drainage system to the further potential of edema and possible secondary inflammation. The surgical technique involves extensive dissection around the lacrimal sac and nasolacrimal duct. These structures and surrounding area are frequently used as a pedicle in periorbital dissection (Fig. 4–9). This association is reflected in the same group of 31 teleorbitism

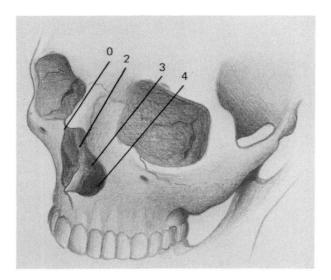

FIG. 4–8. Craniofacial bony clefts associated with nasolacrimal drainage disorders.

patients where the incidence of lacrimal drainage dysfunction rose to 32% following reconstructive surgery.

In cases with chronic dacryocystitis and an intact canalicular system, a dacryocystorhinostomy is necessary. Occasionally the canaliculi are also compromised, necessitating a conjunctivodacryocystorhinostomy.

BLEPHAROPTOSIS

Blepharoptosis appears frequently in teleorbitism patients. Prior to reconstructive surgery there was a 16% incidence of blepharoptosis. Following craniofacial surgery the incidence rose to involve approximately 35% of possible eyelids. Associated underaction of the superior rectus was demonstrable in nearly half of the patients.

This association of superior rectus underaction is not surprising, given the shared embryologic anlage between the levator palpebrae superioris and the superior rectus muscles. The levator is also the last extraocular muscle to develop. The frequent occurrence of superior rectus underaction in patients with craniofacial syndromes has been noted by other authors. The levator has been found to be divided at the time of surgical exposure in these patients. The superior Tessier clefts numbers 9, 10, or 11 could be associated with such findings (Fig. 4–5). While these factors may indicate a possible etiologic mechanism for preoperative blepharoptosis, Isaksson has noted that blepharoptosis may still occur despite normal musculature on electromyography (EMG) studies.

Postoperative blepharoptosis appears to have a more mechanical basis. Even with careful surgical techniques, the levator is a delicate structure prone to direct injury, damage to its nerve supply, edema, and/or hemorrhage into its fibers. The transverse ligament of Whitnall acts primarily as a check ligament because of its firm attachment to the lateral and medial orbital margins and to the periorbita along the superior orbital margin. This structure also limits excessive relaxation. Damage to Whitnall's ligament could conceivably produce blepharoptosis.

The upper and lower tarsi fuse medially and laterally into the medial and lateral canthal tendons (Fig. 4–10). The medial canthal tendon is repositioned by transnasal wiring after medial orbital translocation surgery (Fig. 4–11). This maneuver creates an additional horizontal pull that is transmitted as a vertical force on the eyelids.

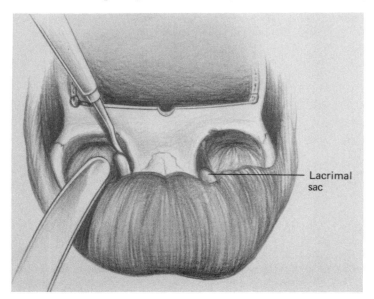

Lacrimal sac

FIG. 4–9. The lacrimal sac acts as a pedicle in the extensive periorbital dissection accompanying orbit translocation surgery.

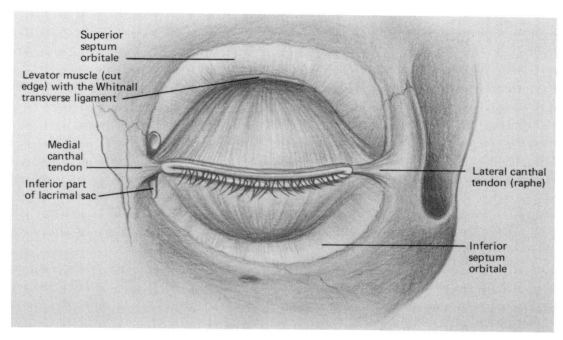

FIG. 4–10. The canthal tendon anatomy.

Therefore, the blepharoptosis seen in teleorbitism patients after reconstructive craniofacial surgery may result from pre-existing conditions, possible surgical trauma, and/or the development of new vertical vector forces on the eyelid.

STRABISMUS

The increased interorbital distance in hyperteloric patients changes the typical angulation of the bony orbits. This probably modifies the usual vector forces of the extraocular muscles because of the changed angle between the origin and the insertion of the rectus and oblique muscles on the globe. This change in the mechanical action of the extraocular muscles may account for the increased incidence of exodeviation reported in teleorbitism patients. In addition to showing a higher incidence of exodeviation, hyperteloric patients show a frequent incidence of V-pattern strabismus associated with underaction of the superior rectus or overaction of the yoke inferior oblique muscle.

As in other strabismus patients, the possibility of amblyopia also arises in congenital craniofacial anomaly patients. Vigorous amblyopia treatment by patching, penalization, a combination, or other means should be instituted whenever necessary to avoid the adverse long-term consequences of irreversible amblyopia. The usual careful regular monitoring of amblyopia therapy is recommended.

Patients with acquired teleorbitism such as that from trauma or fibrous dysplasia are usually older. They may have diplopia if their vision has been preserved bilaterally. Patching, Fresnel prisms, and/or botulinum toxin treatment may be necessary to eliminate double vision on at least a temporary basis. These therapies may also prevent secondary contracture and hypertrophy of an unopposed extraocular muscle, which may be observed in cranial nerve palsy after trauma or reconstructive surgery.

Correction of any horizontal deviation is accomplished by the standard horizontal rectus muscle surgery techniques. The strabismus surgeon, however, must be ready to modify the planned correction on the surgical table if absent or varied insertions of the extraocular muscles are encountered in craniofacial patients. Correction of the V-pattern deviation has proven more difficult. Maximal recession and/or extirpation of the inferior oblique muscles have not met with uniform success. Diamond has suggested lowering or raising the appropriate horizontal rectus muscle in conjunction with the horizontal strabismus correction to improve the results of correcting the V-pattern deviation. I have begun to combine this technique with extirpation of the inferior oblique, and my preliminary results have been encouraging. These results also point out the significance of mechanical factors upon the strabismus found in craniofacial patients.

The timing of corrective strabismus surgery in patients with teleorbitism and congenital strabismus has been a

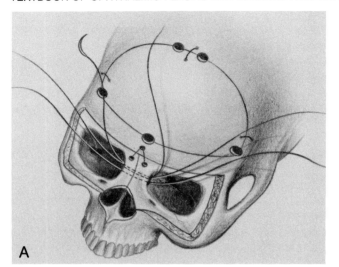

FIG. 4–11. Medial canthoplasties. A, Drill holes are made through the anterior lacrimal crests into which four stainless steel wires are passed. B, Transnasal wires are sutured to the medial canthal tendons. Two wires are then twisted on each side to anchor the medial canthal tendons. C, Excess soft tissue in the nasoglabellar area can be excised. A Z-plasty can be performed to lengthen the nose and aid in the redraping of the skin over the nasofrontal angle.

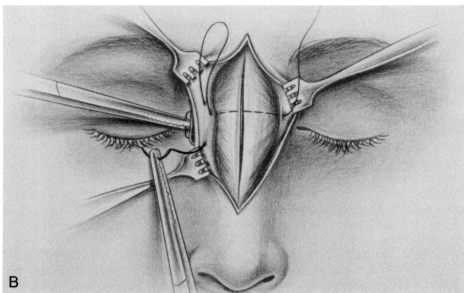

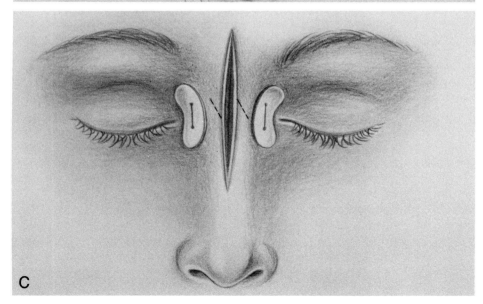

difficult decision. Despite great strides in craniofacial reconstructive surgery, the definitive procedure is usually not performed until the patients are older than the ideal age for the development of some binocularity in association with congenital strabismus.

Diamond and associates found surprising stability in ocular alignment after craniofacial surgery. They recommend early strabismus surgery to align the eyes before craniofacial reconstructive surgery. It should be noted that most patients in their study had a midfacial hypoplasia syndrome.

This is in contrast to our separate study involving 37 patients who underwent a medial horizontal translocation of the orbits for teleorbitism. Their preoperative orbital displacement ranged from 6 mm to 45 mm. Of these patients, 24 (65%) had a decrease in exodeviation after craniofacial reconstruction.

In patients with acquired teleorbitism, I recommend that corrective strabismus surgery be delayed for at least 6 months after hypertelorism correction. Major craniofacial neurosurgical and plastic-reconstructive procedures may cause temporary or permanent palsy of cranial nerves III, IV, and/or VI. A more accurate measurement of the angle of strabismus is obtained by allowing the patient to recover spontaneously as much function as possible, as in other cases of acquired cranial nerve injury.

MIDFACIAL HYPOPLASIA (CRANIOFACIAL DYSOSTOSIS, ACROCEPHALOSYNDACTYLY)

Various disease entities that exhibit midfacial hypoplasia include Crouzon's disease, Apert's syndrome. Saethre-Chotzen syndrome, and Carpenter's syndrome. Patients with a LeFort III facial fracture may also show some midfacial hypoplasia characteristics. Patients with midfacial hypoplasia, congenital or acquired, may have coexistent teleorbitism and orbital dystopia.

CORNEAL EXPOSURE

Globe proptosis or exorbitism is probably the most striking ophthalmologic finding in midfacial hypoplasia patients, particularly in patients with Crouzon's disease. The problem is attributed to diminished orbital volume with a shallow orbital floor (Fig. 4–12). Subluxation of the globe can occur in the more severe conditions. The retrusion of the eyelids behind the equator of the globe does not cause serious ocular damage if the globe is repositioned behind the eyelids immediately. Lateral tar-

sorrhaphies are often performed in recurrent cases to provide further protection against excessive corneal exposure.

The monoblock advancement technique has proved a more definitive procedure in increasing orbital volume to accommodate orbital contents. This technique has proven useful in infants and children with compromised orbital volume.

BLEPHAROPTOSIS

The preoperative finding of blepharoptosis is not surprising because several cases of an absent superior rectus muscle have been reported in patients with midfacial hypoplasia. In a series of 12 patients with midfacial hypoplasia, 25% had preoperative blepharoptosis. After reconstructive surgery, the incidence of blepharoptosis rose to 50%. This increase is probably of mechanical origin. It has also been postulated that the upper eyelid becomes stretched and the levator aponeurosis is elongated in its vertical dimension to protect the proptotic globe from corneal exposure. Persistent upper eyelid blepharoptosis after craniofacial surgery is presumed to be the result of redundant tissues and a lengthened levator aponeurosis (Fig. 4–13). This postoperative blepharoptosis tends to regress, and it is best to wait approximately 6 months after reconstructive surgery before proceeding with blepharoptosis repair.

LACRIMAL DRAINAGE DYSFUNCTION

Midfacial hypoplasia patients do not appear to have a higher incidence of nasolacrimal drainage dysfunction than the general population. This is in contrast to teleorbitism patients, who exhibit a higher than normal incidence of lacrimal dysfunction before reconstructive surgery.

We have observed an increase in obstruction and reduced tear drainage after reconstructive surgery for midfacial hypoplasia. The increase has not been dramatic, however. The probable causes of this postoperative finding include nasolacrimal drainage abnormality unrecognized before surgery or direct trauma from the surgical reconstruction. These findings are similar to those in previous reports.

STRABISMUS

An increased incidence of exotropia has been reported in midfacial hypoplasia patients. The frequency of V-

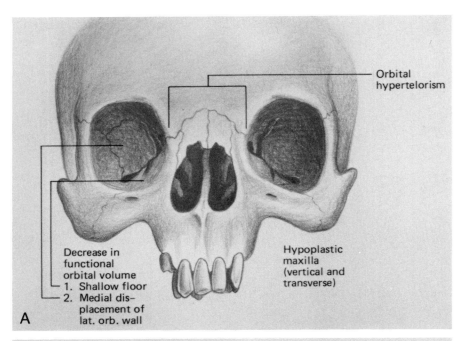

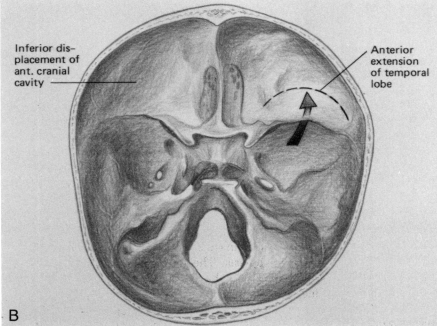

FIG. 4–12. Craniofacial dysostotic features in a skull. A, Frontal view shows maxillary hypoplasia, decrease in functional orbital volume, and teleorbitism. B, Cranial view shows anterior expansion of the middle cranial fossa plus inferior displacement of the anterior cranial vault.

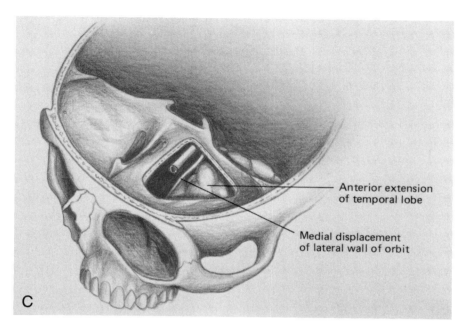

FIG. 4–12 Cont.   C, Oblique cutaway view shows the middle cranial fossa and temporal lobe medially displacing the lateral wall of the orbit, resulting in a loss of orbital volume.

pattern deviation is also increased. These findings are similar to those in teleorbitism patients. Mechanical effects of altered vector forces of the extraocular muscles probably contribute to the strabismus findings.

Unlike the teleorbitism group of craniofacial patients, the midfacial hypoplasia group shows less change in the amount of strabismus deviation after major craniofacial reconstructive surgery. In this group, there is also a tendency to delay definitive craniofacial reconstruction to a later age than in the teleorbitism group. These factors give rise to the present recommendation to proceed with corrective strabismus surgery in midfacial hypoplasia once the patient achieves visual equality, in an effort to preserve some degree of binocularity and prevent amblyopia.

Most children with congenital craniofacial disorders should be promptly referred by their family practitioner or pediatrician to major medical centers where a craniofacial team practices. Bertelsen has noted a previously increased incidence of optic nerve atropy and papilledema resulting from increased intracranial pressure. This occurred particularly in premature synostosis of the cranial sutures and in midfacial hypoplasia, such as Apert's syndrome and Crouzon's disease. Early craniofacial referral and treatment should avert the problem of optic atrophy and allow for development of binocular vision.

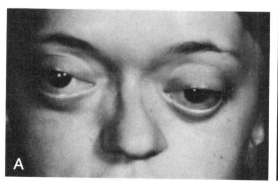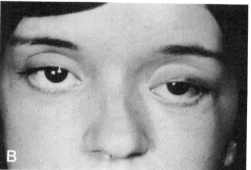

FIG. 4–13.   Residual blepharoptosis. A, Patient with Crouzon's disease and exophthalmos. B, Postoperative appearance following anterior advancement of orbital floor and orbital roof combined with an intracranial approach. Blepharoptosis persists bilaterally. (Courtesy of J. McCarthy, M.D.)

HEMIFACIAL ASYMMETRY

This group of craniofacial abnormalities is known by many designations, including first and second branchial arch syndrome, dysostosis otomandibularis, auriculo-branchiogenic dysplasia, oral-mandibular-auricular syndrome, hemifacial microsomia, otocraniocephalic syndromes, hemicraniofacial microsomia, and bilateral craniofacial microsomia. These congenital malformations are usually unilateral, but are occasionally bilateral, as the last term indicates. The bilateral forms must be distinguished from Treacher Collins syndrome (mandibulofacial dysostosis), which is transmitted as an autosomal dominant disease. The hemifacial asymmetry group of craniofacial disorders has probably more than one etiology responsible for the defect.

These deformities of the hemiface and cranium are characterized by varying degrees of hypoplasia of the skeletal and neuromuscular structures affecting the temporomandibular and pterygomandibular complexes. Similarities with the Treacher Collins syndrome include temporozygomatic defects and orbital deformities.

The orbital deformities with accompanying ocular defects are of interest to the ophthalmologist. A brief review of embryology shows that the maxillary process of the first branchial arch develops into the trigeminal nerve, mandible, and various parts of the external and inner ear. The facial nerve and posterior parts of the external ear are among the structures derived from the second branchial arch.

Jaw and ear deformities are most apparent in hemifacial asymmetry patients. There is, however, a close interlink with the structures derived from the first and second branchial arches and with the various bones of the cranium and skull. It is not surprising that associated deformities of the temporal bones and other cranial bones develop. Varying amounts of soft tissue hypoplasia such as microphthalmos, anophthalmos, cranial nerve palsy, and lateral facial clefts often accompany the skeletal deformities.

The extent of deformity varies within the hemifacial asymmetry group. It may range from extreme forms of dysplasia (Fig. 4–14) to micro forms that may show only slight facial asymmetry and minor auricular malformation.

Eyelid malposition and malformation, plus abnormalities of the width and/or length of the palpebral aperture, are often found in this group of patients. As in the other craniofacial disorders, correction of the overlying soft tissue deformities is best performed after completion of skeletal reconstructive surgery. The craniofacial surgery usually consists of translocation of the orbit in a superior and/or inferior direction to correct orbital dys-

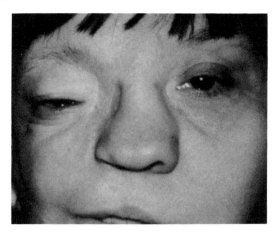

FIG. 4–14. Significant hemifacial asymmetry with microphthalmos, epibulbar dermoid, low-set ears, microtia, shortened mandibular rami, micrognathia, and anterior open bite.

topia, along with reconstruction of the lower face and jaw (Fig. 4–3).

A common finding in hemifacial asymmetry is dystopia of the involved lateral canthus that accompanies the antimongoloid palpebral aperture position. A lateral canthoplasty is usually the necessary repair. Staged reconstruction must be done when either the tendon or tarsus is lacking in the lower eyelid region. Grafting of tarsus, cartilage, or eye bank sclera is the first step. After several months, the vascular supply to the grafted tissue should be established, allowing a lateral canthoplasty to proceed as the second stage of the reconstruction.

Placement of the lateral canthal tendon superiorly upon the lateral orbital rim may correct an inferior displaced globe, corneal exposure, and/or lower eyelid ectropion. These hemifacial asymmetry patients, however, have a variety of problems that contribute to exposure keratitis and conjunctivitis, such as facial nerve paresis or palsy. Artificial tears and ointments may be adequate in mild cases. More severe cases may additionally require a moisture chamber at night. Such a chamber can be fashioned from an exposure bubble bandage or saran wrap. In some instances, a bandage soft contact lens may be helpful. Tarsorrhaphy may be required when exposure cannot be controlled by any other method. Additional therapeutic modalities used to combat exposure have included parotid gland duct transfers, orbicularis muscle transplantation, nerve redirection procedures, and implants of springs, silicone bands, or fascia lata in the eyelids. Such procedures have had limited success and should be applied only in selected cases.

Blepharoptosis is among the problems encountered in hemifacial asymmetry. Surgical repair of blepharoptosis is based upon the general principles reviewed in Chapter

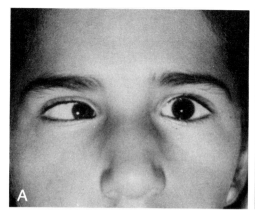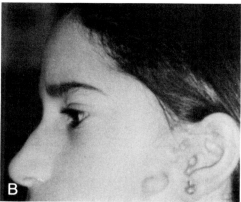

FIG. 4–15. Goldenhar's syndrome with bilateral Duane's syndrome. A, Restricted abduction of the left eye with widening of the palpebral fissure. The right eye adducts as the palpebral aperture narrows in this patient with bilateral Duane's syndrome. Note the hemifacial asymmetry. B, Lateral view of the more involved left side of the face with the characteristic preauricular skin tags found in Goldenhar's syndrome.

5. Such surgery should be deferred until the underlying skeletal foundation has been reconstructed.

A vertical strabismus is commonly encountered due to the frequency of orbital dystopia. Horizontal deviation may also occur separately or in conjunction with the vertical deviation. Goldenhar's syndrome (oculoauriculovertebral dysplasia) is a form of hemifacial asymmetry. Usually one or more epibulbar dermoids are present and may further compromise normal visual development. An increased incidence of Duane's syndrome is found in association with Goldenhar's syndrome (Fig. 4–15). Just as there is a tremendous spectrum of hemifacial asymmetry, a wide variety of vertical, horizontal, and oblique strabismus deviations can occur in these patients.

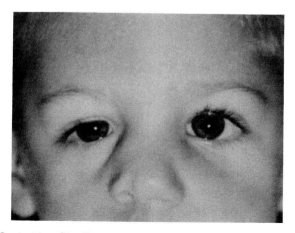

FIG. 4–16. Significant hemifacial asymmetry with mottled appearance of right retina. Consistent amblyopia prevention throughout life. At age 4, the patient has visual acuities of O.D.: 20/30, O.S.: 20/25.

Orbital malposition and accompanying strabismus predispose to amblyopia. In addition, intraocular abnormalities may further compromise the potential for normal visual development. Kushner, however, has reported surprising success in the development of vision in some eyes with compromised anatomy, and my personal experience has corroborated this. It has been achieved through persistent and consistent amblyopia therapy (Fig. 4–16).

MANDIBULOFACIAL DYSOSTOSIS (TREACHER COLLINS SYNDROME)

This well-known craniofacial anomaly is transmitted by an autosomal dominant gene with variable expression (Fig. 4–17). The result is a spectrum of findings with common characteristics. Franceschetti and Klein attempted to collate the mandibulofacial dystosis syndrome into five separate categories: complete, incomplete, unilateral, abortive, and atypical.

The complete form consists of all or most of the following: antimongoloid slant; notching or coloboma of the lateral portion of the lower eyelid (75% of cases), at times associated with deficient or absent eyelashes in the medial third of the lower eyelid (50% of cases); notching or coloboma of the lateral portion of the upper eyelid; hypoplasia of the facial bones (particularly the mandible and zygoma); deformities of the external, middle, and occasionally inner ear; macrostomia; high arched palate; abnormal dentition with malocclusion; blind dimples of the cheeks occurring on a line between the ears and the

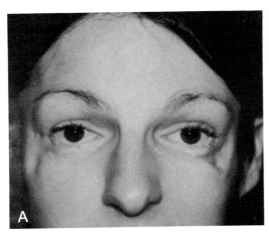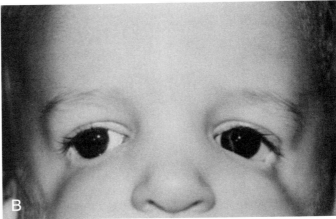

FIG. 4–17. Mandibulofacial dysostosis transmitted as an autosomal dominant with variable expression. A, Mother following several reconstructive procedures. B, Son with findings typical of this condition.

angle of the mouth; and atypical projections of the hairline toward or onto the cheeks.

A return of the Tessier cleft classification shows that the combination of Numbers 6, 7, and 8 clefts accounts for the complete expression of the syndrome (Figs. 4–4 and 4–5). The Number 6 cleft accounts for the eyelid coloboma. The zygomatic arch hypoplasia, external ear malformations, anterior displacement of the hairline, and mandibular deformities are derived from the Number 7 cleft. Defects of the lateral orbital rim are explained by the Number 8 cleft. The incomplete form of mandibulofacial dysostosis syndrome is presumably represented by the Number 6 cleft alone.

The deformities are less severe and less extensive in the incomplete form of the syndrome. Incomplete forms are characterized by antimongoloid palpebral apertures, eyelid colobomas, and underdevelopment of the malar bones and/or the mandible.

The abortive form of the syndrome has rarely been reported. These cases have only the eyelid abnormalities. The unilateral forms of mandibulofacial dysostosis are very rare and somewhat controversial because this disease is considered a bilateral craniofacial anomaly.

The atypical form involves the incomplete group of the syndrome, in which one or more of the principal characteristics of the full Treacher Collins syndrome are missing. In addition, atypical cases contain abnormalities such as microphthalmos that do not belong in the complete or fully developed forms of mandibulofacial dysostosis. Additional atypical features include orbital hypoplasia, cataract, corectopia, exotropia, esotropia, V-pattern strabismus, distichiasis, and lacrimal drainage abnormalities.

The treatment depends on the extent of deformity. A series of reconstructive surgical procedures is usually necessary. Augmentation of the malar region and reconstruction of the eyelid and ear should begin in early childhood. Other reconstructive procedures such as chin advancement and rhinoplasty are deferred until teenage or adult years.

The importance of rebuilding and augmenting the underdeveloped zygomaticomaxillary area before eyelid reconstruction has been emphasized. If this is not done, the eyelid repair frequently fails, particularly in cases where the lower eyelid height is insufficient for normal eyelid closure.

Most reconstructive surgeons currently favor the use of onlay bone grafts to reconstruct the lateral orbital wall, orbital rim, zygoma, zygomatic arch, and anterior maxillary wall (Fig. 4–18). The principal sources for onlay grafts are autogenous rib and iliac bone. This is endochondral bone, which has shown a tendency to reabsorb when implanted in the craniofacial region, diminishing the long-term reconstructive result. Zins and Whitaker have demonstrated greater volume maintenance with autogenous membranous onlay bone grafts to the craniofacial skeleton. This bone is harvested from the cranium and provides hope for maintaining volume in reconstructing the hypoplastic zygomaticomaxillary areas in patients with mandibulofacial dysotosis.

After repair of the skeletal foundation, attention should be directed toward the eyelid deformities and antimongoloid palpebral apertures. Repair of eyelid notching or coloboma was covered in Chapter 3. Correction of the antimongoloid obliquity has proven an even greater challenge. This repair is carried out at the same time as the repair of the lower eyelid deletion deformity and involves vertical repositioning of the lateral canthal tendon along

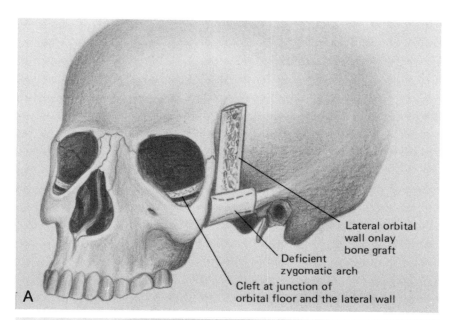

Lateral orbital
wall onlay
bone graft

Deficient
zygomatic arch

Cleft at junction of
orbital floor and the lateral wall

A

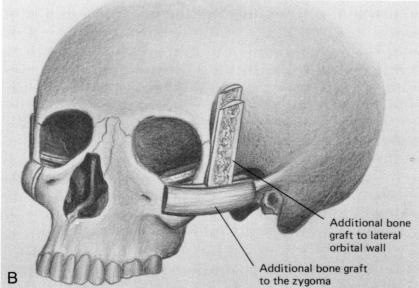

Additional bone
graft to lateral
orbital wall

Additional bone graft
to the zygoma

B

FIG. 4–18. Onlay bone graft reconstruction. A, Autogenous grafts have been added to the cleft at the junction of the orbital floor and the lateral orbital wall, along the deficient lateral wall, and the zygomatic arch. B, Additional bone grafts are layered along the lateral wall and the zygoma. The grafts are secured with wires. Distribution and size of the onlay bone grafts depend on individual pathology. Further grafting may be necessary over the zygomatic arch or the anterior wall of the maxilla.

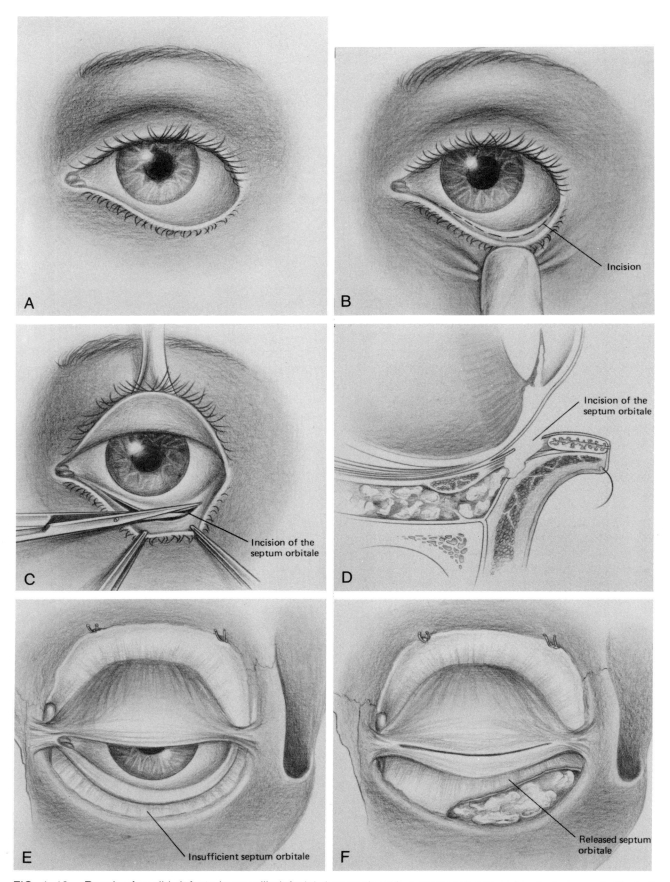

FIG. 4–19. Repair of eyelid defects in mandibulofacial dysostosis with a tarsoconjunctival flap technique. A, Typical antimongoloid slant of the palpebral aperture and deficiency of the lateral portion of the lower eyelid. B, C, D, Technique of septum orbitale release. The incision provides enough laxity to increase the vertical dimension of the septum. Periorbita can also be incised along the orbital floor to further release the orbital septum. E, A deficient or short orbital septum. F, Following release of the orbital septum.

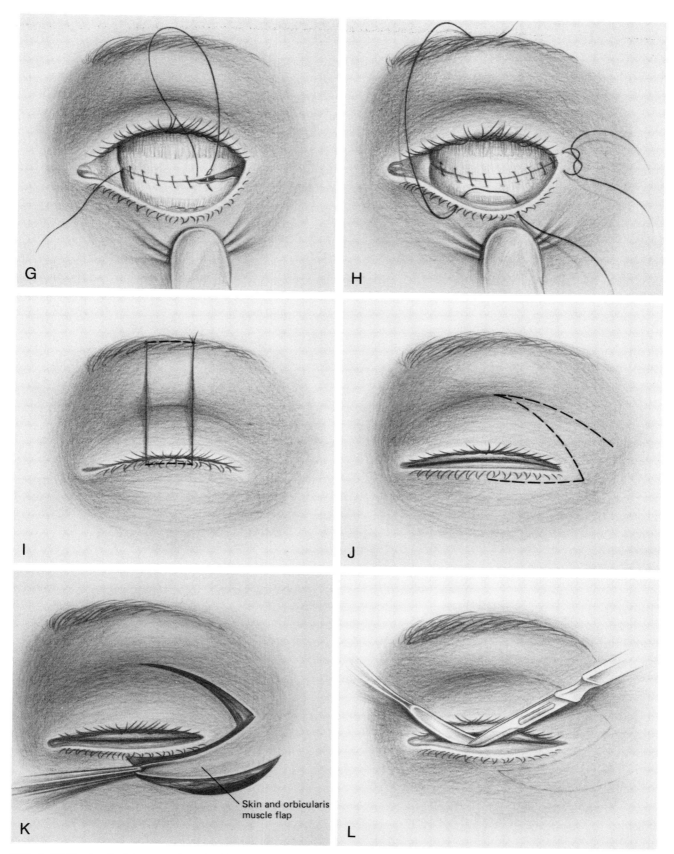

FIG. 4–19 Cont.   G, A tarsoconjunctival flap from the upper eyelid has been released and is sutured to the tarsoconjunctiva of the lower eyelid. H, A traction mattress suture is placed after the suture line is closed. I, The mattress suture is tied. J, Outline of skin-muscle transposition flap. K, Additional skin and muscle is added to the lateral portion of the lower eyelid by transposition of a full-thickness skin and orbicularis oculi muscle flap into the lower eyelid incision. L, The tarsoconjunctival flap is sectioned at a later date at a position suitable to restore the vertical height of the lower eyelid and correct the antimongoloid slant. (From Smith, B., and Converse, J. (eds.): Plastic and Reconstructive Surgery of the Eye and Adnexa. St. Louis, C.V. Mosby, 1967.)

with Z-plasty of the lateral canthal angle (Fig. 2–29A through D). A method using tarsoconjunctival transfer has also been used and is illustrated in Figure 4–19.

The abnormalities found along the medial aspect of the lower eyelid in patients with mandibulofacial dysostosis often lead to lacrimal drainage obstruction. Epiphora may result from punctal aplasia, canalicular aplasia or hypoplasia, or maldevelopment of the nasolacrimal duct. Lacrimal reconstruction in this disorder follows the guidelines covered in Chapter 13.

As in patients with other craniofacial anomalies, the threat of amblyopia is also present in patients with mandibulofacial dysostosis under age 8 years. Amblyopia must be treated with the best available methods. Because of the frequent orbital abnormalities in this syndrome, a V-pattern strabismus is often observed. An elevation in adduction of both eyes gives the appearance of inferior oblique overaction. This may prove functionally troublesome in downgaze (reading position). As in most strabismus associated with the other craniofacial syndromes, mechanical factors have a major influence on the observed deviation.

BIBLIOGRAPHY

Aleksic, S., Budzilovich, G., Choy, A., Ruben, R., Randt, C., Finegold, M., McCarthy, J., Converse, J., and Feigin, I.: Congenital ophthalmoplegia in oculo-auriculo-vertebral dysplasia. A clinicopathologic study and review of the literatue. Neurology 26:638, 1976.

Berry, G.: Note on a congenital defect (? coloboma) of the lower lid. Royal London Ophthalmol. Hosp. Report 12:255, 1889.

Bertelsen, T.: Premature synostosis of the cranial sutures. Acta Ophthalmol. 51 (suppl), 9-175, 1958.

Caronni, E.: Embryogenesis and Classification of Branchial Auricular Dysplasia. In: Trans. Fifth Internatl. Congr. Plast. Reconstr. Surg., Melbourne, Australia, Butterworths, 1971.

Choy, A., Margolis, S., and Breinin, G.: Ophthalmologic Complications of Craniofacial Surgery. In Converse, J, McCarthy, J., and Wood-Smith, D.: Symposium on the Diagnosis and Treatment of Craniofacial Anomalies, St. Louis, C.V. Mosby, 1979.

Choy, A., Margosis, S., Breinin, G., and McCarthy J.: Analysis of Preoperative and Postoperative Extraocular Muscle Function in Surgical Translocation of Bony Orbit: A Preliminary Report. In Converse, J., McCarthy, J., and Wood-Smith, D.: Symposium on Diagnosis and Treatment of Craniofacial Anomalies, St. Louis, C.V., Mosby, 1979.

Converse, J., Wood-Smith, D., McCarthy, J., and Coccaro, P.: Craniofacial Surgery. Clin. Plast. Surg. 1:499, 1974.

Converse, J., McCarthy, J., Wood-Smith, D., and Coccaro, P.: Principles of Craniofacial Surgery. In Converse, J.: Reconstructive Plastic Surgery, Vol. IV, Philadelphia, W.B. Saunders, 1977.

Converse, J, McCarthy, J. Wood-Smith, D., and Coccaro, P.: Craniofacial Microsomia. In Converse, J.: Reconstructive Plastic Surgery, Vol. IV, Philadelphia, W.B. Saunders, 1977.

Cuttone, J., Brazis, P., Miller, M., and Folk, E.: Absence of the superior rectus muscle in Apert's syndrome. J. Pediatr. Ophthalmol. Strabismus 16:349, 1979.

Diamond, G., Katowitz, J., Whitaker, L, Quinn, G., and Schaffer, D.: Variations in extraocular muscle number and structure in craniofacial dysostosis. Am. J. Ophthalmol. 90:416, 1980.

Diamond, G., Katowitz, J., Whitaker, L, Quinn, G., and Schaffer, D.: Ocular alignment after craniofacial reconstruction. Am. J. Ophthalamol. 90:248, 1980.

Diamond, G.: Surgical Treatment of Overaction in Adduction in Patients with Craniostenosis. Presented at the Eleventh Annual Meeting of the American Association of Pediatric Ophthalmology and Strabismus, Dorado, Puerto Rico, 1985.

Duke-Elder, S.: Congenital Deformities. Part 2, System of Ophthalmology, London, Henry Kimpton Publishing, 1963.

Edgerton, M., Udvarhelyi, G., and Knox, D.: The surgical correction ocular hypertelorism. Ann. Surg. 172:473, 1970.

Enlow, D.: Handbook of Facial Growth, Philadelphia, W.B. Saunders, 1982.

Franceschetti, J. and Klein, D.: The mandibulofacial dysostosis: a new hereditary syndrome. Acta Ophthalmol. 27:144, 1949.

Gorln, R. and Findborg, J.: Syndromes of the head and neck. New York, McGraw-Hill, 1984.

Isakowitz, J.: Eine Seltene Erblicke Anomalie der Lidspalte (Atypisches Lidkolobom?). Klin. Monatsbl. Augenheilkd. 78:509, 1927.

Isaksson, I.: Studies on congenital genuine blepharoptosis. Acta Ophthalmol. 72 (suppl.), 1962.

Kushner, B.: Functional amblyopia associated with organic ocular disease. Am. J. Ophthalmol. 90:39, 1981.

Longacre, J., deStefano, G., and Homstrand, K.: The early versus the late reconstruction of congenital hypoplasia of the facial skeleton and skull. Plast. Reconstr. Surg. 27:489, 1961.

Margolis, S., Aleksic, S., Charles, N., McCarthy, J., Greco, A., and Budzilovich, G.: Retinal and optic nerve findings in Goldenhar-Gorlin syndrome. Ophthalmology 91:1327, 1984.

Marino, H. and Appiani, E.: Disostosis mandibolofacial. Prensa Med. Argent. 51:3083, 1954.

Morax, S.: Oculomotor Disorders in Craniofacial Malformations. In Caronni, E.: Craniofacial Surgery, Boston, Little Brown, 1985.

Morax, S.: Changing of the Eye Position After Craniofacial Surgery. In Caronni, E.: Craniofacial Surgery, Boston, Little Brown, 1985.

Munro, I.: Orbito-cranial facial surgery: the team approach. Plast. Reconstr. Surg. 55:170, 1975.

Murray, J. and Swanson, L.: Mid-face osteotomy and advancement for craniosynostosis. Plast. Reconstr. Surg. 41:229, 1968.

O'Connor, G. and Conway, M.: Treacher Collins syndrome (dysostosis mandibulo-facialis). Plast. Reconstr. Surg. 5:419, 1950.

Ortiz-Monasterio, F., DelCampo, A., and Carrillo, A.: Advancement of the orbits and the midface in one piece, combined with frontal repositioning, for the correction of Crouzon's deformities. Plast. Reconstr. Surg. 61:507, 1978.

Pruzansky, S.: Findings of Hemifacial Microsomia. Presented at the First International Symposium of Craniofacial Anomalies, New York University Medical Center, 1971.

Pruzansky, S., Miller, M., and Kammer, J.: Ocular Defects in Craniofacial Syndrome. In Goldberg, M.: Genetic and Metabolic Eye Disease, Boston, Little Brown, 1974.

Schachter, M.: Atrésie Congénitale des paupières inférieures, facies de "clown" et malformations squélétiques multiples chez un petit oligophrène: malformations identiques chez le père. Ann. Pédiatr. 169:345, 1947.

Scobee, R.: The fascia of the orbit. Am. J. Ophthalmol. 31:152.

Serson Neto, D.: Disostose mandibulo-facial. O Hospital 51:333, 1957.

Snyder, C.: Bilateral facial agenesia (Treacher Collins Syndrome). Am. J. Surg. 92:81, 1956.

Stark, R. and Saunders, D.: The first branchial syndrome: the oral-mandibular-auricular syndrome. Plast. Reconstr. Surg. 29:229, 1962.

Stenstrom, S. and Sundmark, E.: Contribution of the treatment of the eyelid deformities in dysostosis mandibulo-facialis. Plast. Reconstr. Surg. 38:567, 1966.

Straith, C. and Lewis, J.: Associated congenital defects of the ears, eyelids, and malar bones (Treacher Collins Syndrome). Plast. Reconstr. Surg. 4:209, 1949.

Tessier, P.: Anatomical classification of facial, craniofacial, and latero-facial clefts. J. Maxillofac. Surg. 4:69, 1976.

Tessier, P., Guiot, G., Delbet, J., and Pastoriza, J.: Osteotomis cranio-naso-orbito-faciales hypertelorism. Chir. Plast. 12:103, 1967.

Tessier, P.: Relationship of craniostenoses to craniofacial dysostoses and to faciostenoses: a study with therapeutic implications. Plast. Reconstr. Surg. 48:224, 1971.

Tessier, P.: The definitive plastic surgical treatment of the severe facial deformities of craniofacial dysostosis, Crouzon's and Apert's diseases. Plast. Reconstr. Surg. 48:419, 1971.

Urrets-Zavalia, A.: The peristomodeal malformations. Arch. Ophthalmol. 55:526, 1956.

Walsh, F. and Hoyt, W.: Clinical Neuro-ophthalmology, 3rd Edition, Vol. I, Baltimore, Williams and Wilkins, 1969.

Weinstock, F. and Hardesty, H.: Absence of superior recti in craniofacial dysostosis. Arch. Ophthalmol. 74:152, 1965.

Whitaker, L., Katowitz, J., and Randall, P.: The nasolacrimal apparatus in congenital facial anomalies. J. Maxillofac. Surg. 2:59, 1974.

Whitaker, L. and Katowitz, J.: Nasolacrimal Apparatus in Craniofacial Deformity. In Converse, J., McCarthy, J., and Wood-Smith, D.: Symposium on Diagnosis and Treatment of Craniofacial Anomalies, St. Louis, C.V. Mosby, 1979.

Wood-Smith, D., Epstein, F., and Morello, D.: Transcranial decompression of the optic nerve in the osseous canal in Crouzon's disease. Clin. Plast. Surg. 3:631, 1976.

Zins, J. and Whitaker, L.: Membranous versus Endochondral bone: implications for craniofacial reconstruction. Plast. Reconstr. Surg. 72:778, 1983.

5

BLEPHAROPTOSIS

The most common disorder in ophthalmic plastic surgical practice is blepharoptosis. A thorough preoperative evaluation is the most important step in the treatment of this disorder because it defines the type and extent of blepharoptosis, which dictates the choice of operation and degree of correction.

EVALUATION

In addition to obtaining a *complete medical history*, it is important that the examiner explore certain specific questions in detail. Ascertaining the *age of onset* clarifies whether blepharoptosis is congenital or acquired. A review of old photographs may help to avoid historical ambiguity. Assessment of *diurnal variance* and *progression* is essential. Diurnal variation suggests myasthenia gravis and unremitting motility disturbance suggests progressive external ophthalmoplegia.

A history of *previous ocular surgery* or *trauma* helps to define a myogenic or neurogenic etiology. *Contributing ocular, neurologic, and systemic diseases* should be explored, as well as such symptoms as *fatigue, dysphagia, jaw winking, and anhydrosis*. Contributing *medications* should be ruled out (reserpine, vincristine). Determination of *family history* discloses an occasional genetically transmitted case.

During a complete ophthalmic examination the *best corrected visual acuity* should be recorded. The *position of the eyelid margin* is observed in relation to the pupil and/or limbus. This is evaluated in primary position, with the frontalis muscle immobilized. In primary position, the upper eyelid margin normally rests 1.5 mm below the superior limbus. The *vertical width of the palpebral fissure* is measured with a small ruler, noting the interval between upper and lower eyelid margins. This should be recorded and photographed in primary position (Fig. 5–1A), as well as in upgaze (Fig. 5–1B) and downgaze (Fig. 5–1C). Involutional blepharoptosis generally demonstrates a link between vertical extraocular muscle movement and eyelid movement. In congenital blepharoptosis, this linkage is reduced and the patient often demonstrates relative lid lag in upgaze and downgaze.

Evaluating additional gaze positions may also contribute in suspected cases of Marcus Gunn jaw-winking syndrome (Fig. 5–2) or misdirected third nerve regeneration.

It is essential to quantify *levator palpebrae superiorus muscle action* while immobilizing the frontalis muscle. This may be determined by placing the ruler at the upper eyelid margin. The interval of excursion is measured as the eyelid moves from extreme downgaze to extreme upgaze. Normal levator action is approximately 14 to 16 mm. An inability to reposition an everted upper eyelid while looking up is an additional indication of poor levator function (Fig. 5–3).

The *height of the eyelid creases* above the eyelid margin should be determined. A high or absent fold suggests either dehiscence of the levator aponeurosis (if levator action is good) (Fig. 5–4) or severe blepharoptosis (if levator action is poor) (Fig. 5–1). The eyelid crease is normally absent in the Oriental eyelid. Any secondary eyelid fold should be recorded (Fig. 5–5). Abnormalities of the eyelid margin *contour* and *eyelashes* should also be documented.

In extraocular muscle evaluation, one must pay particular attention to *superior rectus function and the presence or absence of Bell's phenomenon* (Fig. 5–6). Limitation of either may dictate a more conservative therapeutic approach. Pain on extraocular movement might suggest a cavernous sinus or orbital apex disorder, pseudotumor, or myositis. *Anomalies* such as Marcus Gunn jaw-winking syndrome and misdirected third nerve regeneration should be ruled out.

Visual field examination delineates the extent of functional limitation. The *dominant eye* should be identified in patients with bilateral blepharoptosis. In unilateral surgery on the nondominant eye, an over-correction will likely result; on the dominant eye, accentuation of the blepharoptosis on the unoperated side will probably result (Hering's law).

Shirmer testing and evaluation of *corneal sensitivity* will identify any predisposition to corneal desiccation. Positive findings dictate a more conservative surgical approach. *Orbicularis oculi muscle strength* should be as-

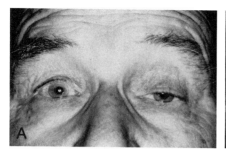
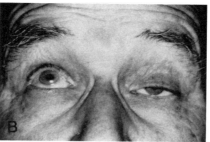
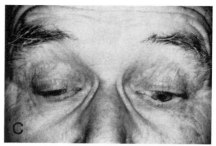

FIG. 5–1. Acquired blepharoptosis photographed in, A, primary position, B, upgaze (note diminished superior rectus function), and C, downgaze.

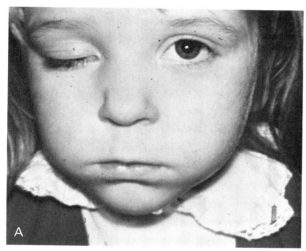
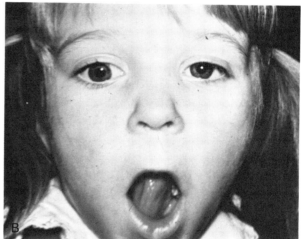

FIG. 5–2. Six-year-old girl with blepharoptosis associated with the Marcus Gunn phenomenon. Note that blepharoptosis is, A, present when the mouth is closed and, B, absent when the mouth is opened.

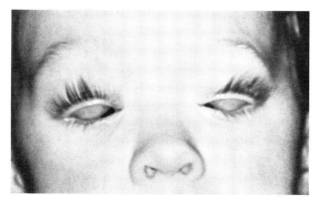

FIG. 5–3. Positive Iliff sign. Levator function is so poor that the infant's eyelids remain everted even after the patient has looked upward. (Courtesy Arthur J. Schaefer, M.D.)

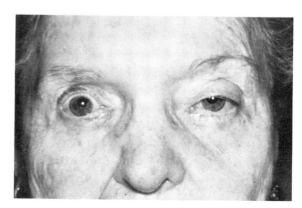

FIG. 5–4. Blepharoptosis associated with a high or absent eyelid fold suggests levator aponeurosis dehiscence if associated with good levator action.

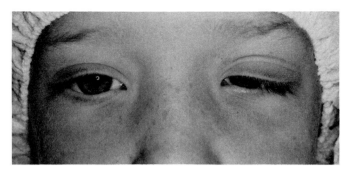

FIG. 5–5. Left upper eyelid congenital blepharoptosis with a secondary eyelid crease.

sessed. Preoperative *lagophthalmos* likewise dictates conservatism unless it could be corrected.

Pupillary changes may suggest dysfunction of cranial nerve III or Horner's syndrome. Except in cases with a narrow anterior chamber angle, the pupils can be dilated with phenylephrine (a dose of 2½% causes fewer cardiovascular effects than higher doses); this serves as a *phenylephrine test*. Any resultant additional eyelid elevation is a manifestation of Müller's muscle and sympathetic nerve function.

Examination of the periorbital area discloses whether dermatochalasis (Fig. 5–7) or epicanthal folds contribute to blepharoptosis. Inflammation may disclose other causes such as blepharitis, cellulitis, or myositis.

Additional diagnostic support may come from the following: testing with hydroxyamphetamine hydrochloride (Paredrine) in suspected Horner's syndrome; testing with edrophonium chloride (Tensilon) in suspected myasthenia gravis; radiologic studies, including CT scanning and possibly MRI, in cases with suspected orbital or neurologic disorders; and ultrasonography in suspected intraorbital foreign body, tumor, or Graves' disease. Consultation with a neurologist may be beneficial in the diagnosis and treatment of neurogenic blepharoptosis; likewise, consultation with a specialist in internal medicine may be helpful in cases possibly caused by Graves' disease or corticosteroids.

CLASSIFICATION

To understand and treat blepharoptosis correctly, the clinician must have a thorough working knowledge of its classification. We are indebted to Crowell Beard, M.D., whose devotion to this subject has resulted in this comprehensive collation:

A. Congenital
1. Simple blepharoptosis
2. Blepharoptosis with superior rectus paresis
3. Blepharoptosis with double elevator palsy
4. Blepharoptosis with levator aponeurosis dehiscence
5. The syndrome of blepharoptosis, blepharophimosis, epicanthus inversus, and telecanthus (Kohn-Romano syndrome)
6. Synkinetic blepharoptosis
   a. Marcus Gunn jaw-winking syndrome
   b. Misdirected cranial nerve III regeneration
   c. Duane's syndrome
7. Congenital Horner's syndrome
8. Congenital cranial nerve III palsy
9. Birth trauma (myogenic origin)
B. Acquired
1. Neurogenic
   a. Cranial nerve III palsy
      1. Diabetes

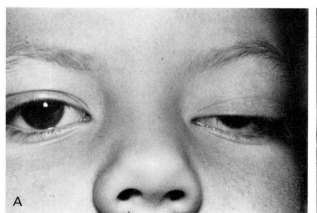
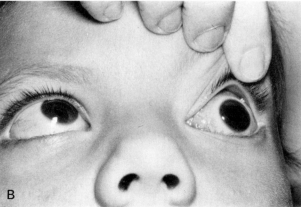

FIG. 5–6. A, Three-year-old girl with congenital blepharoptosis and, B, associated paresis of left superior rectus muscle. The extraocular muscle anomaly was corrected first, followed by correction of the ptotic eyelid.

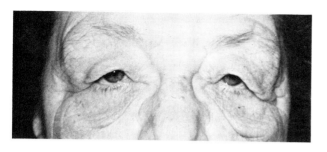

FIG. 5–7. A 75-year-old woman who complained of difficulty in seeing, upper visual field restrictions, and fatigue at the end of the day from dermatochalasis.

    2. Vascular
    3. Traumatic
    4. Tumor
    5. Inflammatory
  b. Acquired Horner's syndrome
  c. Ophthalmoplegic migraine
  d. Multiple sclerosis
2. Myogenic
  a. Involutional
  b. Late acquired hereditary blepharoptosis
  c. Chronic progressive external ophthalmoplegia
  d. Myotonic dystrophy
  e. Myasthenia gravis
  f. Corticosteroid-induced blepharoptosis
  g. Blepharoptosis of pregnancy
  h. Graves' disease
3. Traumatic
  a. Laceration
  b. Enucleation
  c. Orbitotomy
  d. Intraocular surgery
  e. Motility surgery
  f. Eyelid surgery or radiation
  g. Intraorbital foreign body
  h. Orbital roof fracture
  i. Orbital hematoma
4. Mechanical
  a. Tumor
  b. Infiltrate
  c. Inflammation
  d. Blepharochalasis
  e. Cicatricial
  f. Prosthesis-induced
C. Pseudoptosis

CONGENITAL BLEPHAROPTOSIS

For blepharoptosis to be classified as congenital, its onset must occur at birth. Old photographs may be nec-essary to distinguish a congenital case from an early ac-quired one. This distinction is more than academic; it may influence the choice of surgical procedure and the amount of surgical correction. Congenital blepharoptosis represents 60 to 80% of all blepharoptosis cases. It is subdivided into the nine categories listed previously and described in the following paragraphs.

Simple Blepharoptosis. Simple blepharoptosis (Fig. 5–5) represents 75% of the congenital cases and results from a dystrophic process isolated to the levator palpebrae superiorus muscle. Of these cases, 75% are unilateral and 25% are bilateral. The levator is relatively nonelastic, frequently resulting in lid lag on downgaze and dimin-ished blink reflex. Poor levator function is common, re-sulting in a high or absent eyelid crease and an inability to reinvert the everted eyelid (Fig. 5–3). Superior rectus muscle function is normal in this group. The condition remains stable over time.

Blepharoptosis with Superior Rectus Paresis. This group represents 16% of all congenital cases and, with the ex-ception of poor superior rectus muscle function (Fig. 5–6), is identical to the preceding category. Vertical ex-traocular muscle surgery, if indicated, should precede the eyelid correction.

Blepharoptosis with Double Elevator Palsy. This cate-gory is identical to congenital simple blepharoptosis with the addition of paresis of the superior rectus and inferior oblique muscles. Preservation of Bell's phenomenon in these rare cases suggests a supranuclear etiology. Vertical extraocular muscle surgery, if indicated, should precede blepharoptosis correction.

Blepharoptosis with Levator Aponeurosis Dehiscence. Congenital blepharoptosis with dehiscence of the levator aponeurosis is uncommon (Fig. 5–8). This disorder is characterized by mild to moderate blepharoptosis, good levator function, a high or absent eyelid crease, and ab-sence of lid lag. The upper eyelid is somewhat thin.

Syndrome of Blepharoptosis, Blepharophimosis, Epi-canthus Inversus, and Telecanthus (Kohn-Romano Syn-drome). This condition is reviewed in detail in Chapter 3.

Synkinetic Blepharoptosis. The *Marcus Gunn jaw-wink-ing* syndrome results from misdirection of the external pterygoid portion of cranial nerve V (trigeminal) fibers into the distribution of cranial nerve III (oculomotor) fibers. This disorder represents 4 to 6% of the congenital group.

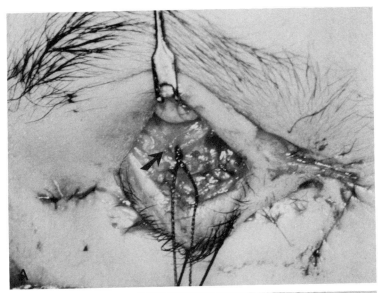

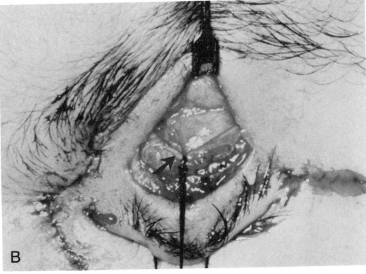

FIG. 5–8. Congenital blepharoptosis caused by dehiscence of the levator aponeurosis (arrow). A, Right upper eyelid. B, Left upper eyelid.

Jaw winking is usually an isolated finding and rarely has familial or hereditary associations. Patients present with varying degrees of blepharoptosis and jaw winking. The wink is a rapid and transient elevation of the ptotic eyelid (Fig. 5–2), in some cases to a level higher than the normal contralateral eyelid. This anomaly is triggered by jaw movement, swallowing, or sucking. The winking movement is made more obvious by having the patient chew gum. Superior rectus paresis is a frequently associated feature. The condition is usually unilateral and found more commonly on the left side than the right. Without surgery, the jaw winking remains stable over time; it may be expressed to a lesser degree as patients learn to assume facial positions that lessen this anomalous movement.

Misdirected cranial nerve III is a rare cause of con-genital blepharoptosis. In such cases, the third cranial nerve malfunctions because of an adverse gestational factor. It may regenerate in an untoward manner, establishing atypical reinnervations. This may result in bizarre eyelid movement associated with extraocular muscle movement.

A patient with *Duane's syndrome* may show pseudop-tosis on adduction. Because true blepharoptosis is not present, no treatment is required.

Congenital Horner's Syndrome. Congenital Horner's syndrome results from intrauterine malformation or birth trauma along the sympathetic chain, often at the level of the brachial plexus. The patient presents with mild blepharoptosis with good levator function associated with ipsilateral miosis, anhydrosis, and apparent enophthalmos. Hypopigmentation of the ipsilateral iris distinguishes congenital Horner's syndrome from its more common acquired form. Evaluation with a Paredrine test distinguishes preganglionic from postganglionic lesions.

Congenital Cranial Nerve III Palsy. Congenital blepharoptosis rarely results from cranial nerve III palsy. Such cases are caused by intrauterine disease or birth trauma. Before any eyelid surgery, it is imperative to evaluate completely and surgically treat any concomitant extraocular muscle imbalance. Such vertical motility surgery often influences blepharoptosis by producing palpebral fissure changes. Once this stabilizes, the blepharoptosis may be corrected.

The choice of operation should follow the ordinary guidelines for congenital blepharoptosis. Diminution of superior rectus function or Bell's phenomenon resulting from cranial nerve III dysfunction may necessitate less surgical correction or a nonsurgical approach (crutch glasses). Ignoring such factors might significantly increase the risk of maintaining corneal exposure postoperatively.

It is important to recognize that children with this condition probably have strabismic amblyopia. If the blepharoptosis is complete, deprivation amblyopia may also supervene. Long-term patching of the dominant eye may be required.

Birth Trauma. Birth trauma may rarely cause injury to the levator palpebrae superiorus muscle or its aponeurosis. Evaluation and treatment should follow the guidelines for congenital blepharoptosis.

ACQUIRED BLEPHAROPTOSIS

For blepharoptosis to be classified as acquired, its onset must occur after birth. Although the history usually accurately distinguishes congenital from acquired cases, photographic corroboration may sometimes be useful. Acquired blepharoptosis represents 20 to 40% of all blepharoptosis cases. It is subdivided into four general categories: neurogenic, myogenic, traumatic, and mechanical.

NEUROGENIC BLEPHAROPTOSIS

Acquired neurogenic blepharoptosis may result from a myriad of central and peripheral foci. Central lesions can be both supranuclear and nuclear. Supranuclear locations may involve the frontal, parietal, or temporal cortices, as well as the angular gyrus, tegmentum, or

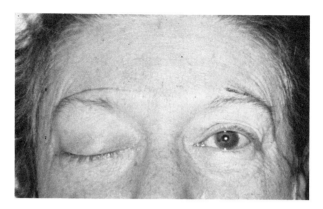

FIG. 5–9. A 70-year-old woman with total oculomotor nerve paralysis from metastatic lung carcinoma.

pineal body. Nuclear lesions arise in the floor of the cerebral aqueduct in the midbrain, often presenting as blepharoptosis in association with loss of accommodation and pupillary changes.

Peripheral (infranuclear) lesions may arise anywhere along the course of the third cranial nerve from the brain stem, through the cavernous sinus, through the supraorbital fissure, to its innervation into the muscular portion of the intraorbital levator complex. Likewise, patients may present with blepharoptosis in association with loss of accommodation and a dilated pupil (cavernous sinus foci may cause miosis). Associated exotropia is more characteristic of a peripheral focus.

Cranial Nerve III Palsy. Acquired third nerve dysfunction may result from diabetes, trauma, aneurysm or other vascular disorders, tumor (primary or metastatic) (Fig. 5–9), inflammation, infections (measles, influenza, encephalitis, meningitis, diphtheria, poliomyelitis, botulism, and syphilis), and neurotoxic conditions (heavy metal poisoning).

This form of blepharoptosis is often accompanied by a motility disturbance placing the globe in a down-and-out position. Gradual resolution is common; patients with incomplete resolution often demonstrate evolution of paralysis into paresis. Therefore, 6 to 12 months should be allowed before treatment is considered. Blepharoptosis surgery should be considered when further improvement ceases for 3 months. The choice of operation and the extent of correction follows the guidelines for acquired blepharoptosis.

Diminution of superior rectus function or Bell's phenomenon resulting from cranial nerve III dysfunction may necessitate less surgical correction or a nonsurgical approach (crutch glasses). Ignoring such factors might significantly increase the risk of maintaining corneal exposure postoperatively.

One must recognize that successful blepharoptosis repair might unmask diplopia caused by motility dysfunction from the underlying third nerve palsy; therefore, motility surgery and/or prism glasses should be implemented first.

Acquired Horner's Syndrome. Horner's syndrome is the most frequent cause of acquired neurogenic ptosis. It results from dysfunction along the sympathetic chain caused by tumor, aneurysm, inflammation, or trauma (usually surgical). Acquired Horner's syndrome is characterized by mild blepharoptosis, miosis, anhydrosis, and apparent enophthalmos. The lower eyelid may be somewhat elevated. Cluster headaches may infrequently coexist (Horton's headache/histamine cephalalgia). Diagnostically, Paredrine helps to differentiate preganglionic from postganglionic lesions.

Some mild cases require no surgery. Those that do respond to either the Fasanella-Servat procedure or to Müller's muscle resection as advocated by Putterman.

Ophthalmoplegic Migraine. This rare cause of acquired blepharoptosis may result from the expansion of an intracranial aneurysm, sphenoid sinus mucocele, or pyocele into the orbit. It is characterized by ophthalmoplegia associated with headache. The paralysis is usually transient. Although the diagnosis is often one of exclusion, when this condition is suspected, a complete workup is indicated. Treatment is directed at the underlying cause. Any residual blepharoptosis should be managed according to the usual guidelines for acquired blepharoptosis.

Multiple Sclerosis. Demyelinating diseases are rare causes of blepharoptosis. When present, the blepharoptosis assumes variable presentations and is prone to exacerbation. This may be associated with optic neuritis, internuclear ophthalmoplegia, skew deviation, and nystagmus. Surgical treatment should be directed toward correcting residual blepharoptosis that has stabilized.

MYOGENIC BLEPHAROPTOSIS

This is the most common category of acquired blepharoptosis, and is dominated by the involutional group.

Involutional Blepharoptosis. Most cases of involutional blepharoptosis are caused by stretching of the levator palpebrae superiorus and/or Müller's muscle. A minor contribution may be diminution of eyelid support from orbital fat atrophy, causing enophthalmos in the aging orbit. Dehiscence or disinsertion of the levator aponeu-

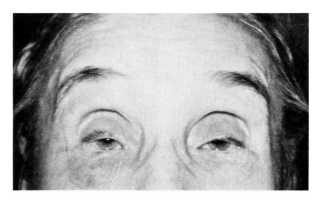

FIG. 5–10. An 82-year-old woman with bilateral involutional blepharoptosis, worse on the left side. Note absence of eyelid crease.

rosis is another category that has become recognized increasingly over the last 10 years; this is the cause of the frequently encountered, and incompletely understood, aphakic blepharoptosis.

Involutional cases with an intact levator aponeurosis are characterized by mild to moderate blepharoptosis with moderate to good levator function and a normally placed eyelid crease.

Involutional cases with levator dehiscence or disinsertion are characterized by mild to moderate blepharoptosis, good levator function, a high or absent eyelid crease, and abnormal lid lag (Fig. 5–10). The upper eyelid is thin, sometimes allowing visualization of iris coloration through the closed eyelids. Almost all cases of aphakic blepharoptosis result from either levator dehiscence or disinsertion.

Late Acquired Hereditary Blepharoptosis. Blepharoptosis in this group starts in the fourth or fifth decade. It is similar to the involutional group, with an additional hereditary component. Correction follows acquired blepharoptosis guidelines.

Chronic Progressive External Ophthalmoplegia. This is a rare progressive muscular dystrophy affecting the extraocular muscles, including the levator palpebrae superiorus (Fig. 5–11). At times a small neurogenic component may be superimposed. Both sexes are equally affected and 50% of cases are familial.

Progressive external ophthalmoplegia (PEO) characteristically begins in childhood or adolescence with gradually increasing blepharoptosis. Other extraocular muscles are involved later. The eyes often become fixed in slight infraduction. Diplopia is uncommon because of the superimposed eyelid droop. Other muscle groups may become involved. The orbicularis oculi muscle may later be affected, resulting in an inability to open and close

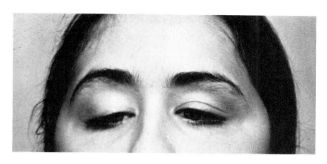

FIG. 5–11. A 28-year-old woman with blepharoptosis from progressive external ophthalmoplegia. A conservative frontalis suspension procedure was performed.

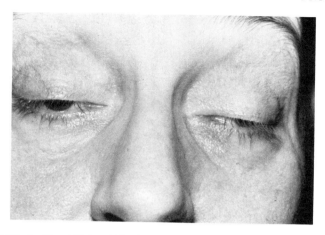

FIG. 5–12. Bilateral blepharoptosis from myasthenia gravis. Within 2 minutes of receiving 1 ml of edrophonium (Tensilon) intravenously, the blepharoptosis transiently disappeared.

the eyelids properly. Pupillary and accommodative functions are normal. Features occasionally associated with PEO include pigmentary retinopathy, endocrine dysfunction, and cardiomyopathy.

A subcategory of this condition is termed oculopharyngeal muscular dystrophy. This disorder occurs in older individuals, frequently on a familial basis in French Canadians. These patients may have dysphagia from weakness of the pharyngeal and facial muscles.

Because superior rectus function and Bell's phenomenon are usually compromised, surgery is contraindicated in all but the mildest cases of progressive external ophthalmoplegia. When blepharoptosis surgery is performed, the goal should be minimal elevation. Most patients instead require crutch glasses, which affords eyelid elevation while the patient is awake and corneal protection while the patient sleeps.

Myotonic Dystrophy. The mild blepharoptosis of myotonic dystrophy has a somewhat random incidence, but has been associated with young aphakic individuals. Paresis of the orbicularis oculi muscle and decreased Bell's phenomenon may coexist. Surgery, when indicated, should be conservative.

Myasthenia Gravis. Myasthenia gravis is caused by a relative acetylcholine deficiency at the myoneural junction. It rarely occurs in childhood, and appears most commonly in young women and older men (Figs. 5–12 and 5–13). Myasthenia may cause variable blepharoptosis and diplopia, with a diurnal and fatigue-related component. Patients occasionally present with thymic hyperplasia.

The diagnosis is suggested by the presence of Cogan's eyelid twitch sign, which is elicited when the eye moves from infraduction to primary position. The ptotic eyelid demonstrates one or more upward twitches. Horizontal eye movement may likewise induce mild flutter in the ptotic eyelid.

The definitive diagnosis may rest with a Tensilon test. The return of function after Tensilon administration is sometimes subtle. In such cases Tensilon tonography, performed by administering Tensilon while a tonographic tonometer is in contact with the cornea, may be useful. A subtle return of extraocular muscle function may be noted by a sudden shift of the tonographic recorder. In Tensilon testing, atropine sulfate and an Ambu bag should be readily available as a precaution. In a different test the presence of acetylcholine receptor antibodies may add further specificity to the diagnosis.

Many cases of myasthenia gravis are cured completely with medication alone, usually pyridostigmine bromide (Mestinon). Cases that are not completely helped by medication may require surgery. As for all blepharoptosis categories, the selection of surgery and the amount of

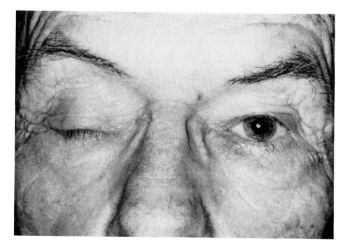

FIG. 5–13. Unilateral blepharoptosis from myasthenia gravis.

correction are based on the severity of blepharoptosis and the amount of levator function.

Corticosteroid-induced Blepharoptosis. The long-term use of oral or parenteral corticosteroids may result in mild blepharoptosis, often reversible on discontinuation of the drug.

Blepharoptosis of Pregnancy. Blepharoptosis may occur either during or immediately after pregnancy. Its characteristics are similar to those of the involutional group, and it tends to stabilize with time.

Graves' Disease. Blepharoptosis is an uncommon finding in Graves' disease. Because of occasional concurrence between this disease and myasthenia gravis, Tensilon testing should be considered. The ptotic eyelid in Graves' disease usually results from aponeurotic dehiscence, and surgical correction should repair this defect.

TRAUMATIC BLEPHAROPTOSIS

A multitude of traumatic events may produce blepharoptosis. Eyelid lacerations, particularly those horizontally configured, may damage the levator complex (Fig. 5–14). Contour abnormalities or blepharoptosis may be immediate, from partial or complete levator transection, or delayed, from cicatricial tethering. Their correction rests with repair of the levator palpebrae superiorus muscle or aponeurosis through an external approach and/or removal of cicatricial bands. When the anatomy is distorted, a severed and retracted levator can often be found by following the medial and lateral horns superiorly. In adults, local anesthesia may help facilitate surgery by allowing the patient to move his eyelid, thereby identifying the severed levator by its movement.

Blepharoptosis may be the sequela of various surgical procedures. After enucleation, the upper eyelid may droop from a rare injury to the third nerve or levator complex. Blepharoptosis repair should be performed with the prosthesis in place to best quantify the result. Modification of the prosthesis may still by required post-operatively. Blepharoptosis may likewise follow orbitotomy, particularly in the removal of dermoids. Anterior segment surgery, especially cataract extraction, frequently antedates mild blepharoptosis. This results from levator dehiscence or disinsertion; its cause is unknown. Surgery on the superior oblique or superior rectus muscle occasionally causes blepharoptosis by cicatricial tethering (Fig. 5–15). Eyelid surgery for other disorders, periorbital radiation, intraorbital foreign body, orbital roof fracture, and orbital hematoma are other rare causes of traumatic blepharoptosis.

MECHANICAL BLEPHAROPTOSIS

Mechanical blepharoptosis may result from structural changes within the eyelid, orbit, or socket. Causal factors may include: tumors (hemangioma [Fig. 5–16A], neurofibroma, rhabdomyosarcoma, plexiform neuroma [Fig. 5–16B], lacrimal gland tumors, granuloma, and dermoid); infiltrates (amyloid, lymphoma, and leukemia); inflammation (blepharitis, cellulitis, and myositis); blepharochalasis, cicatricial processes in the upper eyelid (trachoma, Stevens-Johnson syndrome, and ocular pemphigoid); or a poorly fitting enucleation prosthesis. Resolution of the causal factor usually eliminates the induced blepharoptosis; any residual deformity should be corrected surgically.

PSEUDOPTOSIS

Dermatochalasis with severe hooding and associated upper visual field loss is the most common presentation

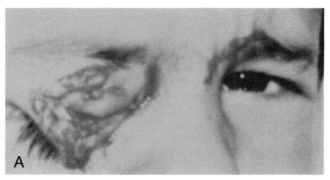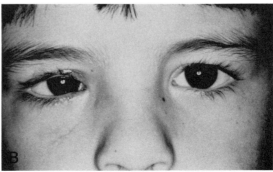

FIG. 5–14.   A, Traumatic blepharoptosis from a dog bite with transection of the levator aponeurosis. B, Appearance 6 weeks after surgical repair.

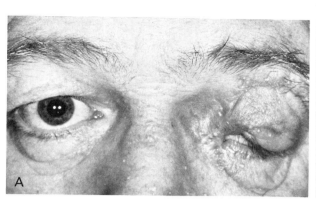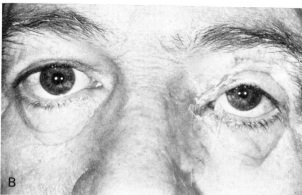

FIG. 5–15. A, Hasty closure of an eyelid wound in an emergency room by an inexperienced physician resulted in blepharoptosis with cicatricial tethering. B, Later reconstructive surgery resulted in a normally functioning eyelid. (Photograph courtesy of Charles Beyer-Machule, M.D.)

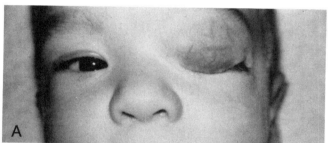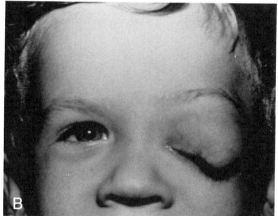

FIG. 5–16. Mechanical blepharoptosis from, A, capillary hemangioma and, B, plexiform neuroma.

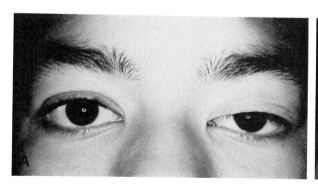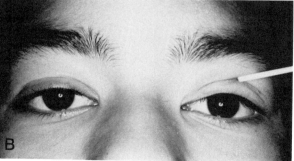

FIG. 5–17. A, Pseudoptosis of the left upper eyelid caused by unilateral dermatochalasis with severe hooding. B, The apparent blepharoptosis disappears when the hood is retracted.

of pseudoptosis (Figs. 5–7 and 5–17). Other causes may include: enophthalmos after enucleation or blowout fracture, hypotropia, contralateral mild exophthalmos or eyelid retraction, congenital clinical anophthalmos (microphthalmos), phthysis bulbi, blepharospasm, and protective blepharoptosis (uveitis, foreign body, corneal abrasion, conjunctivitis). Most pseudoptosis cases resolve after treatment of the cause. Additional blepharoptosis surgery may be necessary in selected cases.

BLEPHAROPTOSIS SURGERY

Surgical correction may be considered when accurate, stable and reproducible measurements are obtained. Earlier surgery is indicated when the blepharoptosis is so severe that vision is compromised and deprivation amblyopia is threatened. This circumstance is uncommon. The choice of operation and size of correction are based on the etiology of the blepharoptosis and the preoperative measurements. Preoperative photographs and measurements should be available at surgery.

In all blepharoptosis surgery, the goal is to achieve optimal eyelid *height, crease (fold), contour, and symmetry.* Symmetry should be both static and dynamic. Postoperative lid lag in vertical gaze positions is inversely proportional to the amount of preoperative levator function.

CONGENITAL BLEPHAROPTOSIS

In congenital cases, frontalis suspension should be performed when levator function is 3 mm or less. If the condition is bilateral (even though less severe on the contralateral side), frontalis suspension should be performed bilaterally. If the condition is unilateral, the surgeon may perform the suspension either bilaterally (to maximize symmetry) or unilaterally (to avoid surgery on a normal eyelid) (Fig. 5–18). In the latter circumstance, if asymmetry in vertical gaze proves bothersome postoperatively, suspension of the second eyelid can be performed later.

In treating the Marcus Gunn syndrome and anomalous cranial nerve III reinnervation, it is imperative to distinguish the ptotic element from the anomalous element. If the anomaly is mild, blepharoptosis should be treated according to normal guidelines for congenital blepharoptosis. If the anomaly is significant, complete levator transection on the involved side must be performed to disassociate this linkage.

In such situations, Beard recommends bilateral levator transection followed by bilateral frontalis suspension to ensure symmetry. Callahan has modified this somewhat, recommending ipsilateral levator transection followed by bilateral frontalis suspension, leaving the contralateral normal levator alone. This achieves symmetry while leaving the normal eyelid relatively undisturbed. A third and more conservative approach is ipsilateral levator transection followed by ipsilateral frontalis suspension, leaving the contralateral eyelid completely undisturbed. This achieves symmetry in primary position, with asymmetry in upgaze and downgaze. Parents of some patients request the latter approach to avoid disturbing the normal eyelid. If asymmetry in vertical gaze proves bothersome postoperatively, it can be corrected by later contralateral frontalis suspension with or without levator transection.

In congenital cases, levator resection should be performed when levator function is greater than 3 mm. This can be accomplished from either the conjunctival or cutaneous approach (Fig. 5–19).

The quantity of levator aponeurosis resected is a manifestation of the degree of blepharoptosis and the amount of preoperative levator function. More levator must be resected in congenital cases than in comparable acquired cases.

A useful starting point is to quantify the droop as mild (1 to 2 mm), moderate (3 mm), or severe (4 mm or more). Levator action is also quantified as excellent (greater than 10 mm), good (7 to 10 mm), fair (4 to 6 mm), or poor (3 mm or less). The severity of blepharoptosis usually correlates with the extent of levator action. These figures translate into small, medium, and large levator resections. In surgical terms, this approximately quantifies levator resections into 14 mm (small), 18 mm (medium), and 22 mm (large). Selected cases may benefit from resections of 23 mm or more. Levator resections of 10 mm or less in congenital blepharoptosis usually bring no improvement whatsoever.

At surgery, these approximates are used as a starting reference point. During the procedure, if the eyelid appears too low or high, the amount of resection can be increased or decreased respectively. Likewise, if a contour abnormality develops during surgery, the medial and lateral sutures can be repositioned accordingly.

The rare congenital case with an aponeurotic dehiscence is best corrected by aponeurotic dehiscence repair techniques alone. Most such cases resolve with repositioning the levator aponeurosis to the upper tarsal border. In most dehiscence cases, any appreciable levator resection results in significant overcorrection with upper eyelid retraction. Occasionally, a small levator resection (or advancement lower on the tarsal plate) or recession may also be necessary to achieve optimal results.

Mild cases (1 to 2 mm) of congenital blepharoptosis or cases of congenital Horner's syndrome may be managed

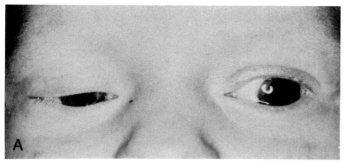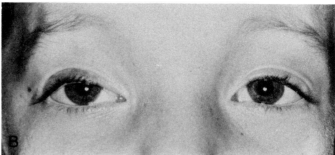

FIG. 5–18. A, Severe unilateral congenital blepharoptosis. Surgery was performed unilaterally at the parents' request. B, Appearance following a unilateral frontalis suspension.

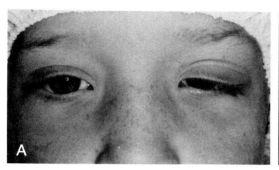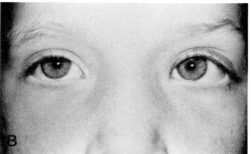

FIG. 5–19. Congenital blepharoptosis. A, Preoperative appearance. B, Postoperative appearance after external levator resection.

with either the Fasanella-Servat procedure or Müller's muscle resection as advocated by Putterman.

ACQUIRED BLEPHAROPTOSIS

Mild cases of acquired blepharoptosis with good levator function and cases of acquired Horner's syndrome should be managed with either a Fasanella-Servat procedure (Fig. 5–20) or Müller's muscle resection.

Moderate cases (the most common group) require aponeurosis surgery (resection or aponeurosis repair) (Fig. 5–21).

Most patients have an aponeurotic defect (dehiscence, disinsertion, rarefaction, attenuation) and respond to aponeurotic repair alone. They typically require repositioning of the levator aponeurosis at the upper tarsal border. In a typical case of dehiscence, any appreciable levator resection results in significant overcorrection with upper eyelid retraction. Occasionally, a small le-

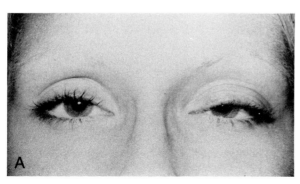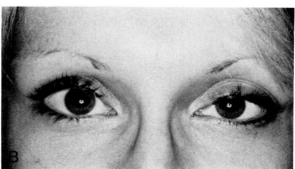

FIG. 5–20. Acquired blepharoptosis. A, Preoperative appearance. B, Postoperative appearance after the Fasanella-Servat procedure.

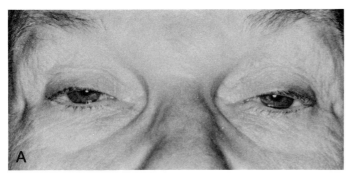 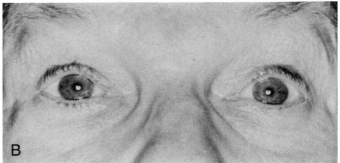

FIG. 5–21. Acquired blepharoptosis. A, Preoperative appearance. B, Postoperative appearance after repair of levator aponeurosis dehiscence.

vator resection (or advancement lower on the tarsal plate) or recession may also be necessary to achieve optimal results.

The remainder of moderate blepharoptosis cases require levator resection. In this group, levator resection is beneficial when levator function is greater than 2 mm. This can be accomplished from either the conjunctival or cutaneous approach. The latter is often preferable because it affords better surgical exposure and allows larger surgical resection.

Quantification of levator aponeurosis to be resected is a manifestation of the degree of blepharoptosis and the amount of preoperative levator function. Less levator must be resected in acquired cases than in comparable congenital cases.

A useful starting point is to quantify the droop as mild (1 to 2 mm), moderate (3 mm), or severe (4 mm or more). Levator action is also quantified as excellent (13 mm or greater), good (8 to 12 mm), fair (3 to 7 mm), or poor (2 mm or less). The severity of blepharoptosis usually correlates with the extent of levator action. These figures translate into small, medium, and large levator resections. In surgical terms this quantifies levator resections approximately into 10 mm (small), 14 mm (medium), and 18 mm (large). Selected cases may benefit from still greater levator resection.

At surgery, these approximates are used as a starting reference point. During the procedure, if the eyelid appears too low or high, the amount of resection can be increased or decreased respectively. Likewise, if a contour abnormality develops during surgery, the medial and lateral sutures can be repositioned accordingly.

Frontalis suspension in acquired blepharoptosis is necessary in rare severe cases (droop of 4 mm or more) with poor levator function (2 mm or less) (Figs. 5–22 and 5–23).

Anesthesia. In children, blepharoptosis surgery requires general anesthesia. In adults, it is preferable to proceed under local anesthesia. This not only lessens the anesthetic risk, but allows the adult patient to demonstrate the degree of correction and the eyelid contour as the operation progresses. This information feedback yields better results and lessens the chance of reoperation.

Although epinephrine is commonly used as part of the local anesthetic for oculoplastic procedures, I do not recommend its use in blepharoptosis surgery. Although it enhances hemostasis, it also exerts an effect on Müller's muscle, causing variable accentuation of eyelid lift during the operation. This misleading information may cause the surgeon to lessen the extent of the surgical correction, resulting in undercorrection.

Nerve blocks (supraorbital, supratrochlear, infratrochlear) are also not recommended in blepharoptosis correction. The anesthetic from any of these blocks may diffuse deeper into the orbit. This can block the action of the third nerve in and around the area of the ciliary ganglion, causing variable diminution of eyelid lift during the operation. This misleading information may cause the surgeon to increase the extent of the surgical correction, resulting in overcorrection.

The order of discussion of operations in the following text ranges from those for minimal blepharoptosis with good levator function to those for severe blepharoptosis with poor or absent levator function.

MODIFIED FASANELLA-SERVAT PROCEDURE (TARSOMYECTOMY)

This procedure is ideal for patients with minimal blepharoptosis and good levator action. After topical and local infiltration anesthesia (general anesthesia in children), the upper eyelid is everted over a Desmarres retractor. Three double-armed 4-0 silk sutures are placed horizontally at the superior aspect of this folded eyelid. These sutures should enter just below the upper fornix

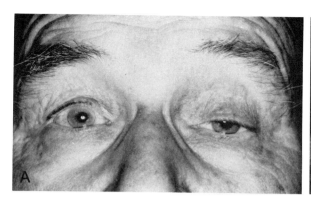
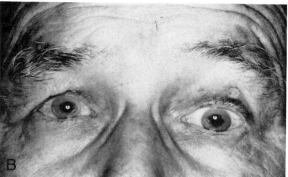

FIG. 5–22. Acquired severe unilateral blepharoptosis. A, Preoperative appearance. B, Postoperative appearance after frontalis suspension.

and exit through tarsus. They hold the levator aponeurosis in position as the tarsal complex (tarsus, Müller's muscle, conjunctiva) is resected (Fig. 5–24A).

Two curved mosquito hemostats (or a Putterman clamp) are placed symmetrically on the everted tarsus. The amount of tarsal complex within the hemostats can be titrated somewhat, depending on the amount of correction desired. The maximum "tarsectomy" is 3 mm. To avoid a postoperative peak, excessive tarsus should not be incorporated centrally. After removing the hemostats, a full-thickness excision is made with a #64 Beaver blade or Stevens scissors directly over the hemostat crush line, avoiding the 4-0 silk sutures (Fig. 5–24B). With a conformer protecting the globe, hemostasis should be obtained with electrocautery.

A double-armed 6-0 chromic catgut suture enters from the cutaneous surface of the lateral eyelid and emerges at the lateral end of the tarsectomy. It is then run in a mattress fashion incorporating conjunctiva, Müller's muscle, and tarsus in each pass (Fig. 5–24C). Each bite should be as close to the cut edges as possible to minimize later suture contact with the cornea. When the suture reaches the medial end of the tarsectomy, it is then passed in a running fashion laterally, joining conjunctival edge to conjunctival edge (Fig. 5–24D). These suture passes should be buried as much as possible to minimize postoperative corneal erosion. When the suture again reaches the lateral end of the tarsectomy, it is externalized next to its entrance site, tied, and then cut (Fig. 5–24E). The three 4-0 silk sutures are removed and the eyelid is placed in its normal position.

Antibiotic ointment is applied to the suture line and the cornea, and no dressing is required. This ointment should be used several times a day postoperatively to

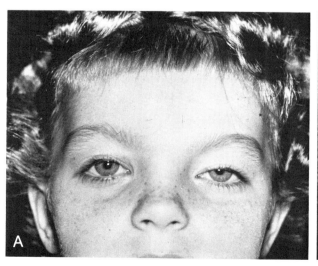
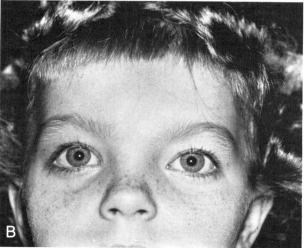

FIG. 5–23. Congenital blepharoptosis. A, Preoperative appearance with only 3 mm of levator function in each eyelid. B, Postoperative appearance 1 year after frontalis suspension with preserved fascia lata using the Crawford technique.

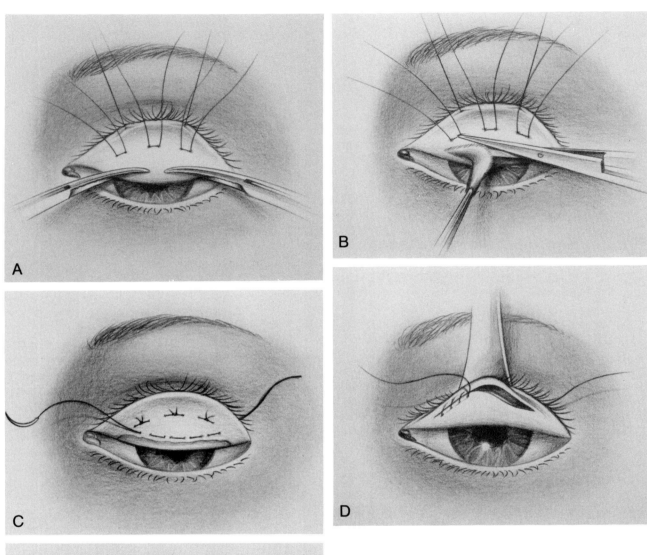

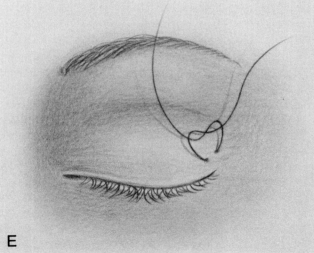

FIG. 5–24.   Modified Fasanella-Servat procedure. A, Three double-armed 4-0 silk sutures are placed in the everted eyelid to fixate levator aponeurosis, tarsus, Müller's muscle, and conjunctiva. Two curved mosquito hemostats (or a Putterman clamp) are placed symmetrically on the everted tarsus. B, A full-thickness tarsectomy is performed with Stevens scissors in the bed demarcated by the hemostat crush line. C, A double-armed 6-0 chromic catgut suture is placed in mattress fashion incorporating conjunctiva, Müller's muscle, and tarsus in each pass. D, The same suture is continued laterally to reunite conjunctiva. E, The suture is externalized laterally, where it is tied and cut. The three fixation sutures are removed.

minimize suture-induced corneal erosion. Should this develop, more frequent installation of Lacri-Lube ointment, semi-pressure patching, or the use of a bandage soft contact lens may help.

MÜLLER'S MUSCLE-CONJUNCTIVAL RESECTION

This procedure is applicable in children and adults with either Horner's syndrome or minimal blepharoptosis, with good levator action and a positive phenylephrine test. After topical and local infiltration anesthesia (general anesthesia in a child), the upper eyelid is everted on a Desmarres retractor. A 6-0 silk marking suture is placed 7 to 9 mm above the superior tarsal border. A toothed forceps is used to separate Müller's muscle and conjunctiva from their deeper attachment to the levator aponeurosis. This should be performed in the interval between the superior tarsal border and the marking suture.

A Putterman clamp is positioned with one blade next to the superior tarsal border and the other blade next to the marking suture. As the Desmarres retractor is withdrawn, this clamp is closed, incorporating Müller's muscle and conjunctiva within its grasp. The clamp and skin are now pulled in opposite directions to ensure that the levator aponeurosis has not been unintentionally included.

A 7-0 chromic catgut horizontal mattress suture is run from a temporal-to-nasal direction 1.5 mm distal to the clamp. Each bite is 2 mm apart, engaging conjunctiva and tarsus on one side and Müller's muscle and conjunctiva on the other side. When the nasal extent has been reached, a #64 Beaver blade is used to excise the contents of the clamp, carefully avoiding the suture. The suture is then passed temporally in a running fashion, joining conjunctival edges. The suture should be tied within the lateral extent of the wound. All suture bites should be buried as effectively as possible. The marking suture is removed and the eyelid is placed in its normal position.

Antibiotic ointment is applied to the suture line and the cornea, and no dressing is required. This ointment should be used several times a day postoperatively to minimize suture-induced corneal erosion. Should this develop, more frequent installation of Lacri-Lube ointment, semi-pressure patching, or the use of a bandage soft contact lens may again prove helpful.

EXTERNAL LEVATOR RESECTION

The area of the intended eyelid crease is designated with a marking pen. This should be in conformity with the contralateral eyelid. If both eyelids are involved, the crease should be placed approximately 6 mm above the eyelid margin. This should taper somewhat inferiorly both medially and laterally. Subjacent to this, local anesthesia should be infiltrated (general anesthesia in children). A 4-0 silk-modified Frost traction suture may be placed in the central portion of the upper eyelid margin.

According to the marked lines, a skin incision should be made with a #64 Beaver blade (Fig. 5–25A). This incision should be carried to the anterior tarsal surface with blunt and sharp dissection with Stevens scissors. This is facilitated by placing the scissors at a 45-degree angle. A flatter dissection may damage the eyelash follicles near the eyelid margin. A steeper dissection may pass through the orbital septum and distal levator aponeurosis while searching for the tarsus. Once the tarsus is identified, its upper portion is cleaned of epitarsal tissue.

The Stevens scissors are next used to separate preseptal orbicularis from the orbital septum (Fig. 5–25B). With the orbital septum identified, it is opened approximately 5 mm above the superior tarsal border (Fig. 5–25C). Any opening lower than this may pass directly through the fusion of septum with levator aponeurosis. The optimal place to open the septum is sometimes demonstrable as a furrowing caused by the lower end of the subjacent preaponeurotic fat pad. Once the orbital septum is opened, the lower end of the preaponeurotic fat pad ("friendly fat") will be visible (Fig. 5–25D). Directly below this is the levator aponeurosis. Voluntary eyelid movement by the patient under local anesthesia will further facilitate its identification. If an aponeurotic dehiscence is present, it is demonstrable at this point and its repair should proceed as described in the section on dehiscence repair.

If there is no dehiscence, the eyelid is everted and openings are made at the medial and lateral junctions of levator aponeurosis with tarsus (Figs. 5–25E and F). A Berke clamp is placed through these openings, incorporating levator aponeurosis, Müller's muscle, and conjunctiva as one complex (Fig. 5–25G and H). This complex is disinserted from the tarsus (Fig. 5–25I).

The conjunctiva is separated from the Berke clamp (Figs. 5–25J and K) and resutured to the upper tarsal border with running 7-0 chromic catgut (Figs. 5–25L and M). Blunt dissection now separates Müller's muscle from the clamped levator up to the height of Whitnall's ligament (Figs. 5–25N and O). Whitnall's ligament should never be cut so as to maintain the pulley effect of the levator muscle and aponeurosis. The levator aponeurosis may be further dissected medially and laterally, depending upon the anticipated size of resection (Fig. 5–25P). This freed segment should encompass the cen-

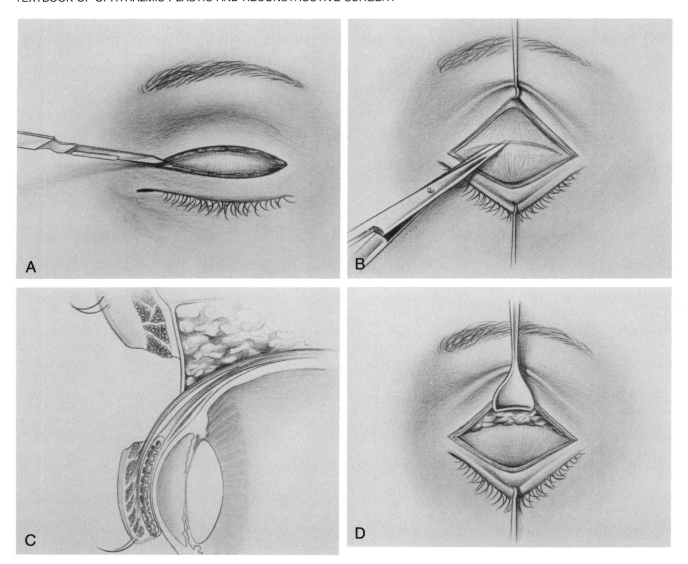

FIG. 5–25. External levator resection. A, At the position of the desired eyelid fold, an incision is made with a #64 Beaver blade. B, Preseptal orbicularis is separated from the orbital septum with Stevens scissors. C, Lateral view demonstrating the fusion of orbital septum with levator aponeurosis for a variable distance above the upper tarsal border. D, Orbital septum opened, revealing the lower end of the preaponeurotic fat pad and the subjacent levator aponeurosis.

tral two-thirds of the aponeurosis. The horns are cut only when necessary for a large resection. To ensure that the levator has been adequately separated from the septum, pull down on the clamp while touching the superior orbital rim. Any appreciable transmitted tug suggests inadequate separation. Damage to deeper structures (trochlea-medially, lacrimal gland-laterally) can be avoided by always keeping the scissors tips visible.

Three double-armed 5-0 Vicryl sutures should be placed horizontally (2 to 3 mm below the upper tarsal border (Fig. 5–25Q). (This position is chosen to allow for later recession up the tarsus in case of an overcorrection and to avoid ectropion from too low an insertion). Tarsal sutures should be lamellar, not full-thickness, to spare the cornea postoperatively. The central suture should be passed through the levator aponeurosis at the position determined by the preoperative measurements (Fig. 5–25R). This suture should be temporarily tied with a slip knot (Fig. 2–25S) and the eyelid height is observed. This is most accurate with the surgical lights turned off

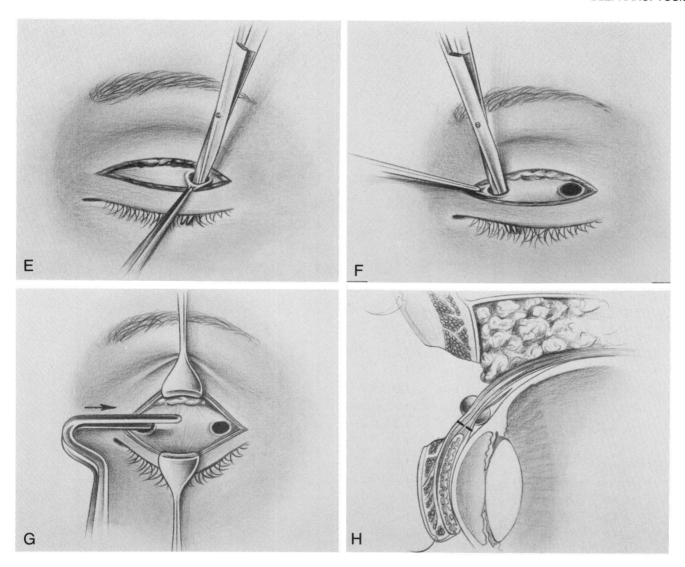

FIG. 5–25 Cont. E, Lateral opening made at the levator-tarsal junction. F, Medial opening made at the levator-tarsal junction. G, Berke clamp placed through these openings, incorporating levator aponeurosis, Müller's muscle, and conjunctiva as one complex. H, Lateral view of the structures contained within the Berke clamp.

to reduce any artifact from photophobia-induced eyelid squeezing. If the eyelid is too low, the suture is repositioned higher (greater resection) upon the aponeurosis. If the eyelid is too high, it is repositioned lower (lesser resection) upon the aponeurosis.

Once proper height is achieved, the medial and lateral sutures are placed at comparable positions in the medial and lateral portions of the aponeurosis respectively. These sutures are tied with slip knots and the contour is assessed. The medial and lateral sutures can be repositioned upon the aponeurosis until optimal contour is achieved. When the desired eyelid height and contour are attained, these sutures are tied permanently and cut.

The distal fringe of redundant levator aponeurosis is excised (Fig. 5–25T). A small fringe of aponeurosis should be left. This allows additional levator for recession in case of postoperative overcorrection. It also plays a role in the formation of the eyelid crease. The crease is achieved by closing the skin with running 7-0 silk sutures (or chromic catgut in children). If appreciable dermatochalasis coexists, the skin may be trimmed before closure (Fig. 5–25U). In joining skin edges, each pass should engage subjacent portions of the aponeurotic fringe (Fig. 5–25V). This imbrication of aponeurosis into the posterior aspect of the skin correctly simulates the anatomic levator contribution to the eyelid crease.

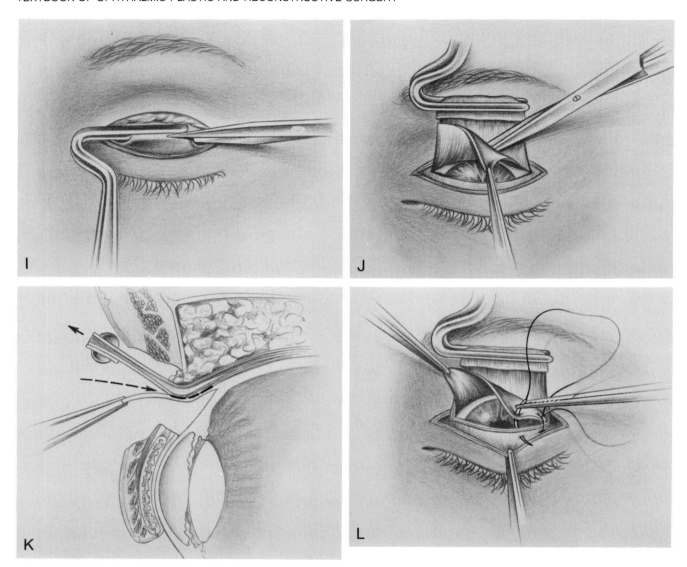

FIG. 5–25 Cont.   I, Levator complex disinserted from the upper tarsal border. J, Conjunctiva separated from levator complex within the clamp. K, Lateral view demonstrating the separation of conjunctiva from the structures within the clamp. L, Conjunctiva resutured to the upper tarsal border with 7-0 chromic catgut.

A second 4-0 silk modified Frost suture is placed in the lower eyelid central margin. The two modified Frost sutures are interlaced and secured to the cheek and brow respectively with tincture of benzoin and Steri-strips (Fig. 5–25W). This avoids corneal exposure in the immediate postoperative period. The lower eyelid modified Frost suture is removed on the first postoperative day. The upper eyelid modified Frost suture may be removed on the second postoperative day if there is no apparent overcorrection. If overcorrection remains a possibility, this suture should be left taped in place longer. It can then be used as a handle for downward traction, if necessary, to treat mild overcorrection. The 7-0 silk skin-

levator imbrication sutures should be removed on the tenth postoperative day to allow for eyelid crease formation.

LEVATOR APONEUROSIS DEHISCENCE REPAIR

Whether anticipated preoperatively or discovered at surgery, the repair of an aponeurotic dehiscence begins in a manner identical to external levator resection surgery (Fig. 5–26A through C). Once the aponeurosis is

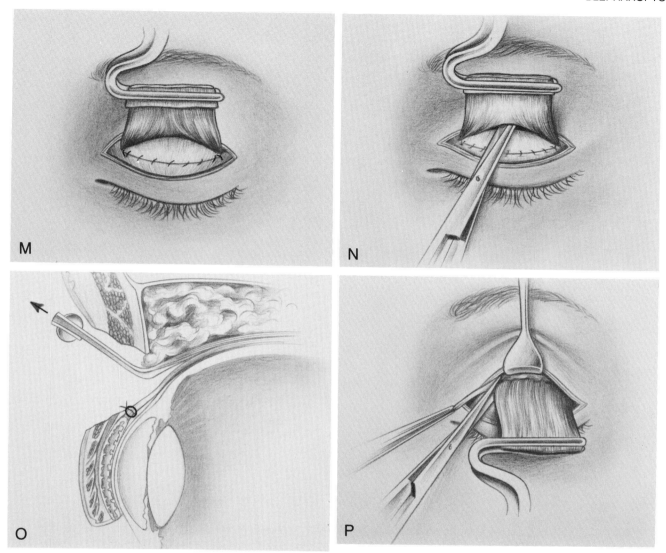

FIG. 5–25 Cont.   M, Conjunctiva resutured to the upper tarsal border with 7-0 chromic catgut. N, Levator aponeurosis separated from Müller's muscle to the height of Whitnall's ligament. O, Lateral view demonstrating the resutured conjunctiva and the upward dissection of levator aponeurosis. P, The levator aponeurosis may be further dissected medially and laterally. Levator horns should be cut only when necessary for large resections.

located, the surgery differs somewhat from external levator resection (Fig. 5–26D).

Three types of dehiscence have been identified: rarefaction, dehiscence, and disinsertion. In rarefaction, the aponeurosis is thin, but normally positioned and without full thickness defects, and the consistency of the aponeurosis is usually extremely friable and attenuated. A dehiscence is a circumscribed aponeurotic defect with the surrounding aponeurosis intact. Disinsertion is a normal-appearing aponeurosis with its leading edge separated from tarsus and positioned superior to the upper tarsal border. In a disinsertion, the exact position of the

leading edge of the aponeurosis may vary from just above the tarsus to behind the fat pad. It will sometimes appear to have a rolled edge.

If the dehiscence represents an intraaponeurotic separation (Fig. 5–26E), the aponeurosis is reconstituted with three double-armed 5-0 Vicryl sutures in a mattress fashion.

If the dehiscence represents a disinsertion from tarsus, these two structures should be rejoined as follows: Three double-armed 5-0 Vicryl sutures should be placed horizontally at the upper tarsal border. The central suture should be passed through the distal fringe of levator

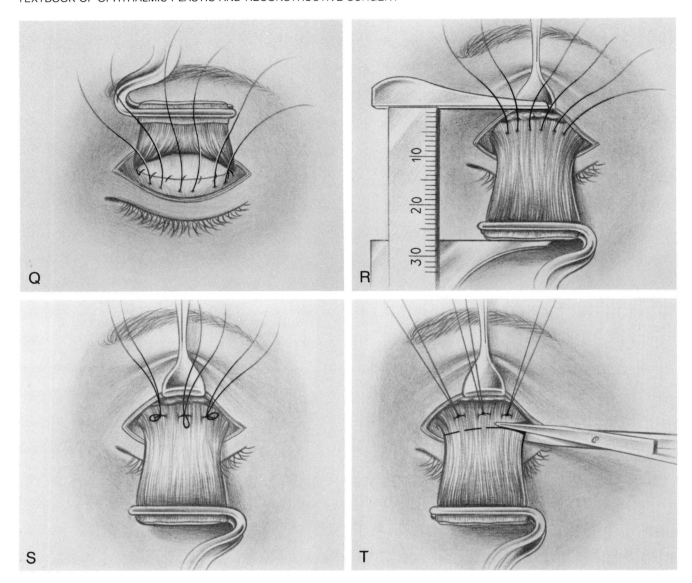

FIG. 5–25 Cont. Q, Three double-armed 5-0 Vicryl sutures placed 2 to 3 mm below the upper tarsal border. R, The Vicryl sutures passed through levator aponeurosis at the position suggested by the preoperative measurements. S, Vicryl sutures temporarily tied with slip knots. T, Once proper height is achieved, the sutures are tied permanently. The distal fringe of redundant levator aponeurosis is then excised.

aponeurosis. Enough aponeurosis should be engaged, though, to avoid a recurrent dehiscence. This suture should be temporarily tied with a slip knot and the eyelid height should be observed. This is most accurate with the surgical lights off to reduce any artifact from photophobia-induced eyelid squeezing. If the eyelid is too low, the sutures are repositioned higher (greater resection) on the aponeurosis or slightly lower on the tarsus. No significant levator resection should ever be per-

formed in the presence of an aponeurotic dehiscence because it carries a risk of severe upper eyelid retraction. If the eyelid is too high, the aponeurosis is secured to the tarsus, using pedicle tarsal flaps or a spacer (see Chapter 6).

Once proper height is achieved, the medial and lateral sutures are placed at comparable positions in the medial and lateral portions of the aponeurosis, respectively. These sutures are tied with slip knots and the contour

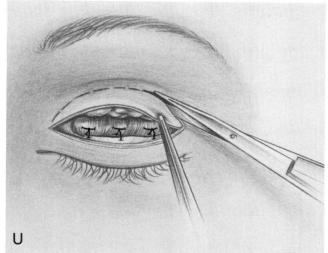

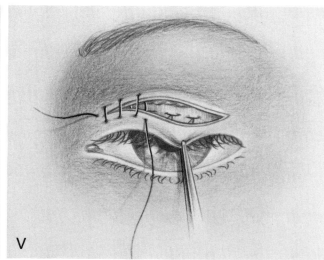

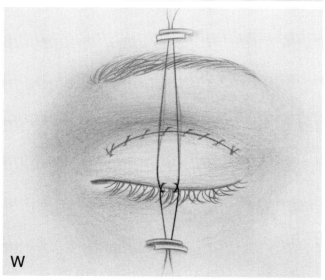

FIG. 5–25 Cont. U, Excess skin may be trimmed before closure. V, The skin closure incorporates the aponeurotic fringe to create a postoperative eyelid crease. W, Two modified Frost sutures may be interlaced at the close of surgery to avoid corneal exposure in the immediate postoperative period.

is assessed. The medial and lateral sutures can be partially adjusted to achieve optimal contour. Once the eyelid height and contour are satisfactory, these sutures are tied permanently and cut (Fig. 5–26F).

The skin is closed with running 7-0 silk sutures (or chromic catgut in children). In joining skin edges, each pass should engage subjacent portions of the aponeurosis fringe (Figs. 5–26G and H). This imbrication of aponeurosis into the posterior aspect of the skin simulates the anatomically correct eyelid fold. If appreciable dermatochalasis coexists, the skin may be trimmed before closure. A postoperative dressing and/or modified Frost sutures are optional (Fig. 5–26I).

INTERNAL LEVATOR RESECTION

After topical and infiltrative anesthesia (general anesthesia in children), a 4-0 silk-modified Frost suture may be placed in the upper eyelid margin and tied long. This eyelid is everted over a Desmarres retractor. Stevens scissors are used to make a horizontal tarsotomy 1.5 mm below the upper tarsal margin (Fig. 5–27A). This should enter the pretarsal (postaponeurotic) space, exposing the levator aponeurosis. Within this space, the scissors are directed horizontally, undermining the levator aponeurosis (Fig. 5–27B). The scissors are withdrawn and replaced with a Berke ptosis clamp (Fig. 5–27C). The clamp should engage a small segment of attached tarsus, levator aponeurosis, and orbital septum. Discard the tarsal fragment. The distal end of the levator complex is severed by sharp dissection.

Removal of the Desmarres clamp facilitates separation of the orbital septum from the levator complex. The septum is further separated from the levator aponeurosis by blunt dissection (Fig. 5–27D). Downward tension on

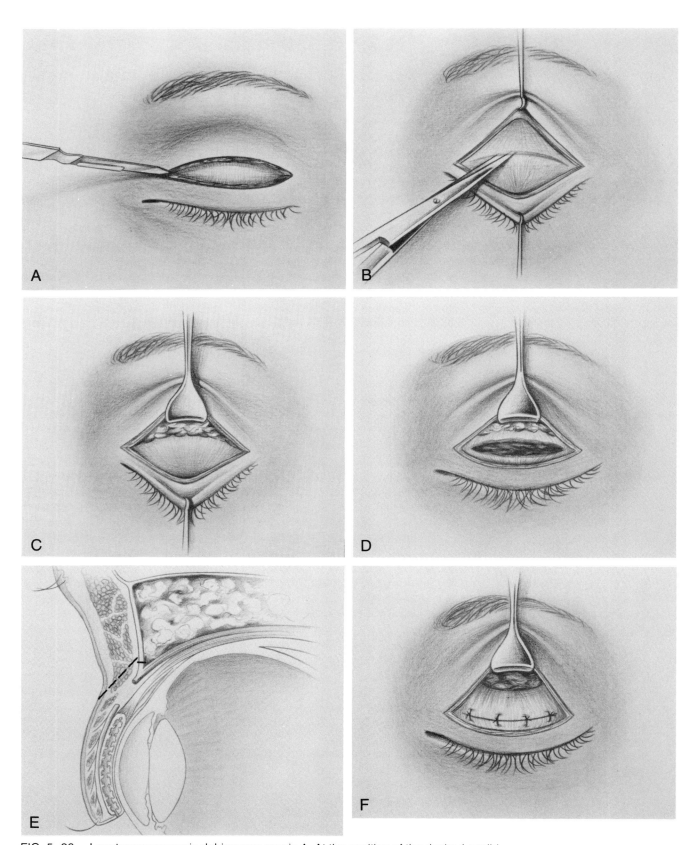

FIG. 5–26.   Levator aponeurosis dehiscence repair. A, At the position of the desired eyelid fold, an incision is made with a #64 Beaver blade. B, Preseptal orbicularis is separated from the orbital septum with Stevens scissors. C, Orbital septum opened, revealing the lower end of the preaponeurotic fat pad and the subjacent levator aponeurosis. D, Levator aponeurosis is isolated and found to be in a dehiscence configuration. E, Lateral view showing site of incisions to expose the levator aponeurosis and an intra-aponeurotic separation. F, Once proper eyelid height and contour are achieved, the sutures closing the levator dehiscence are tied permanently and cut.

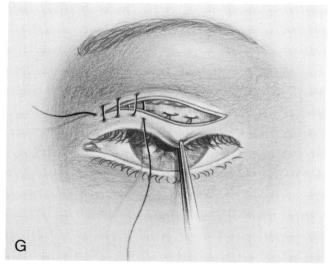

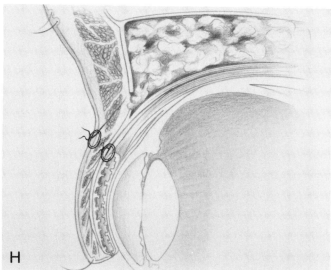

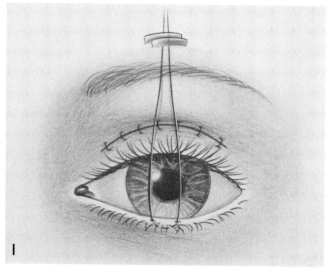

FIG. 5–26 Cont.   G, The skin closure incorporates the aponeurotic fringe to create a postoperative eyelid crease. H,
Lateral view demonstrating closure of an aponeurotic dehiscence and closure of overlying skin. The skin closure should
incorporate deeper bites to augment the eyelid crease. I,
Placement of a modified Frost suture in the lower eyelid margin is optional.

the Berke clamp identifies the medial and lateral horns
of the levator (Fig. 5–27E). If necessary, the horns
should be severed (Fig. 5–27F) to an extent dictated by
the anticipated size of levator resection. Care should be
taken to avoid the superior oblique tendon and lacrimal
gland in the process. Conjunctiva and Müller's muscle
should be separated from the undersurface of the exposed levator aponeurosis (Fig. 5–27G).

The amount of levator to be resected is measured from
the clamp (Fig. 5–27H). Three double-armed 5-0 Vicryl
sutures are placed through medial, central, and lateral
levator positions at this point. The central suture is then
passed through tarsus, emerging on the skin surface at
the position of the desired eyelid crease. The suture
should be temporarily tied with a slip knot and the eyelid
height should be observed. This is most accurate with
the surgical lights off to reduce any artifact from pho-

tophobia induced eyelid squeezing. If the eyelid is too
low, the suture is repositioned higher (greater resection)
upon the aponeurosis. If the eyelid is too high, it is
repositioned lower (lesser resection) upon the aponeurosis.

Once proper height is achieved, the medial and lateral
sutures are placed at comparable positions on the aponeurosis and tarsus, emerging through the skin (Fig.
5–27I). These sutures are tied with slip knots and the
contour is assessed. The medial and lateral sutures can
be repositioned upon the aponeurosis until optimal contour is achieved. Once the eyelid height and contour are
satisfactory, these sutures are tied permanently and cut
(Fig. 5–27, J through L).

The distal fringe of redundant levator aponeurosis is
excised (Fig. 5–27I). A small fringe of aponeurosis should
be left. This allows additional levator for recession in

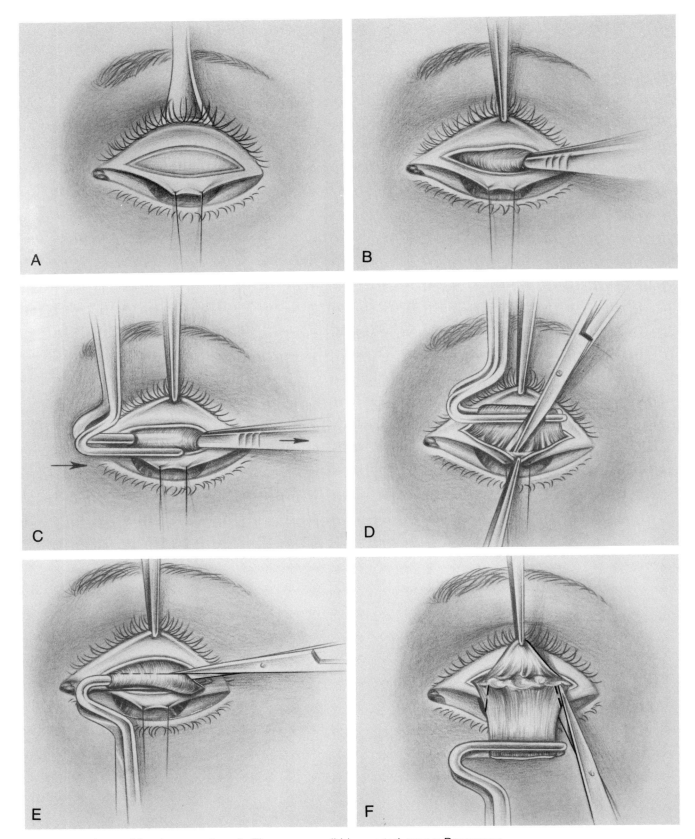

FIG. 5–27.   Internal levator resection. A, The upper eyelid is everted over a Desmarres retractor and Stevens scissors are used to make a horizontal tarsotomy 1.5 mm below the upper tarsal margin. B, The pretarsal (postaponeurotic) space is entered, undermining the levator aponeurosis. C, A Berke ptosis clamp replaces the Stevens scissors. D, The septum and levator aponeurosis are further separated by blunt dissection. E, Levator horns are identified by downward traction. F, The horns are optionally severed to facilitate large resections.

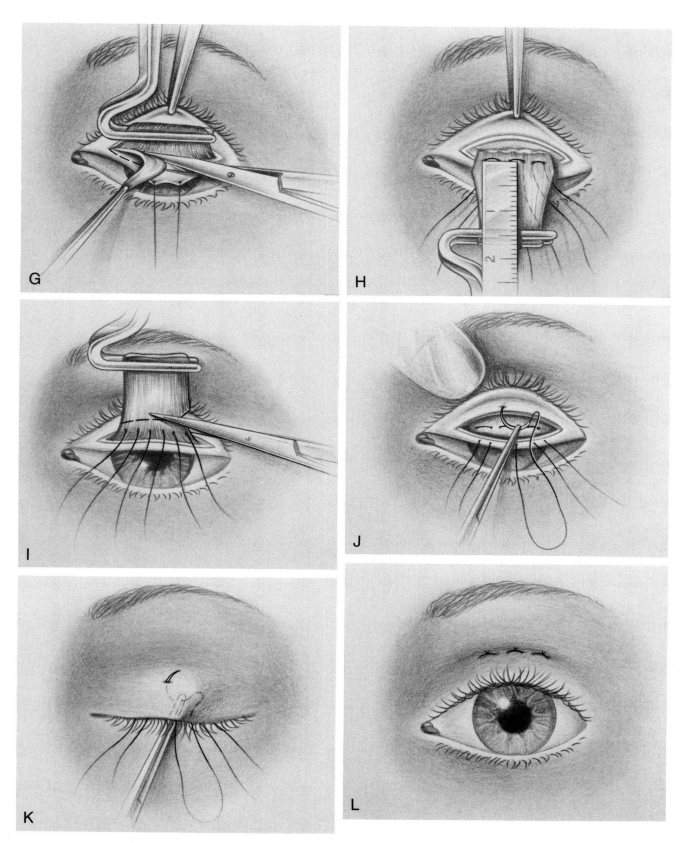

FIG. 5–27 Cont.   G, Conjunctiva and Müller's muscle are separated from levator aponeurosis. H, The amount of levator for resection is measured from the clamp. I, Once proper
height is achieved, all three sutures are positioned and the distal fringe of aponeurosis is
excised. J, K, and L, The Vicryl sutures are externalized, tied, and cut. Conjunctiva is closed
with running 7-0 chromic catgut.

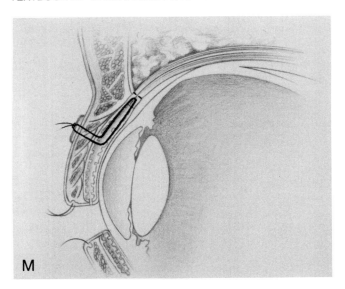

FIG. 5–27 Cont.   M, Lateral view of suture placement at the close of the procedure.

case of postoperative overcorrection. The conjunctiva is closed with a running 7-0 chromic catgut suture, with effort directed toward burying the suture to minimize postoperative corneal erosion (Figs. 5–27M).

A second 4-0 silk-modified Frost suture is placed in the lower eyelid central margin and tied long. The two modified Frost sutures are interlaced and secured to the cheek and brow respectively with tincture of benzoin and Steri-strips. This avoids corneal exposure in the immediate postoperative period. The lower eyelid modified Frost suture is removed on the first postoperative day. The upper eyelid modified Frost suture may be removed on the second postoperative day if there is no apparent overcorrection. If overcorrection remains a possibility, this suture should be left taped in place longer. It can then be used as a handle for downward traction, if necessary, to treat mild overcorrection.

Most ophthalmic plastic surgeons choose external levator resection over the conjunctival approach for the following reasons: (1) the anatomy is clearer, (2) larger levator resections can be accomplished, (3) aponeurotic dehiscence can be better visualized and treated, and (4) excision of redundant skin can be accomplished through the same incision. In reoperation, external levator resection is clearly preferable for these reasons.

FRONTALIS SUSPENSION

The frontalis muscle is a secondary eyelid elevator, used ineffectively by patients trying to raise a severely ptotic eyelid. Frontalis suspension accentuates this proc-

ess, affording more efficient transfer of frontalis muscle contraction into eyelid lift.

Indications for frontalis suspension include (1) severe blepharoptosis (either myogenic or neurogenic) with poor levator function (3 mm or less in congenital cases, 2 mm or less in acquired cases), (2) incomplete success of prior maximal levator resection, (3) incomplete success of prior frontalis suspension, (4) temporary eyelid fixation to avoid deprivation amblyopia in a neonate or infant, (5) severe trauma in levator or third nerve injury, (6) selected cases of myasthenia gravis, and (7) severe myotonia. In (8) third nerve palsy and (9) progressive external ophthalmoplegia, frontalis suspension, if performed, must be conservative to avoid corneal exposure. In (10) Marcus-Gunn jaw winking and (11) anomalous third nerve reinervation, a distinction must be made between the ptotic element and the anomalous reinervation element. In cases with severe blepharoptosis and significant synkinesis, frontalis suspension should be combined with levator transection.

Materials used for frontalis suspension may be divided into biologic (absorbable) and synthetic (nonabsorbable) categories. The absorbable materials leave behind dense fibrous tissue to function as a permanent suspensory material. Although many substances have been used, autogenous fascia lata and homogenous (preserved) fascia lata have proven distinctly the best tolerated and easiest to work with. Synthetic materials are used for temporary eyelid elevation, but otherwise are not recommended because of frequently encountered problems such as rounding of the suspensory material, extrusion, infection, or recurrent blepharoptosis. The most common material used within this category is Supramid Extra. Additionally, silk, silcone, silastic, nylon, gold wire, and tantelum wire have been used.

The characteristics desired in frontalis suspension materials include accessibility, low infection rate, low rejection rate, ease of handling, permanence, tensile strength, decreased tendency toward recurrent blepharoptosis, and avoidance of a second operative site. It would appear that fascia lata, either preserved (obtainable from the University of Toronto Fascia Bank) or autogenous, suits these criteria. Preserved fascia lata is preferable in children to avoid traumatizing the developing leg.

Harvesting Fascia Lata. To harvest autogenous fascia lata, one can use a Masson fascia lata stripper, or a Mustarde fascia lata stripper (Fig. 5–28). The Crawford fascia lata stripper is equally effective but somewhat more complicated to use.

Frontalis suspension with a fascial sling should proceed under general anesthesia. The fascial element is removed

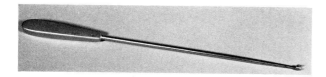

FIG. 5–28. The Mustarde fascial splitter, with curved end and knife-sharp leading edge.

from the area between the lateral knee (head of the fibula) and the anterior superior iliac crest (Fig. 5–29A). Internally rotating the leg facilitates this process.

After careful preparation, the 4 cm-long incision is placed 5 to 6 cm above the lateral knee (Fig. 5–29B). Deeper dissection brings the glistening fascia lata into view. Metzenbaum scissors help to separate fascia from overlying fat. Two parallel incisions are made in the fascia 6 to 8 mm apart and in the same direction as the fascial fibers (Fig. 5–29C). The fascia lata stripper engages the fascia and is advanced to the desired length while applying countertraction with a hemostat (Fig. 5–29D). The cutting blade of the stripper severs the fascia. A piece of fascia lata 7.5 to 10 cm long is then removed (Fig. 5–29E). The fascia lata does not require closure and the leg incision is closed in two layers with 4-0 Vicryl and 5-0 silk. Once removed, the fascia is cleaned of fat and subcutaneous tissue and subdivided into multiple strips 3 mm wide by 10 cm long. The fascia is then placed in an antibiotic solution until it is used.

Frontalis Suspension—General Principles. The techniques that I recommend are the Crawford double triangle and the modified Tillett and Tillett single rhomboid. In either technique, horizontal incisions are made 2 mm above the eyelid margin down to the level of the anterior tarsal surface. Each incision is 2 to 3 mm long. Comparable brow incisions should be placed at the upper edge of the brow hairline, and extended deep to the level of frontal bone periosteum. This makes the fascia less perceptible postoperatively.

In the eyelid, the fascia is passed in the epitarsal space anterior to the orbital septum. To avoid lid lag in the brow, the periosteum should not be engaged. Either a Wright or a Crawford needle is well suited for fascia lata passage. It is important that posterior penetration be avoided to minimize postoperative infection and extrusion. If posterior penetration occurs, the fascial strip should be reformatted.

Once placed, the fascia should be pulled taut and tied with a square knot (rather than a surgeon's knot) with tension based on the desired postoperative eyelid position. Slippage of this knot is avoided by securing it with a Mersilene suture. It is hard to overcorrect and very easy to undercorrect frontalis suspension, therefore effort should be made to optimize elevation. Excess fascia should be excised, leaving behind a fringe that can be used in cases of overcorrection. In most cases, the ideal postoperative eyelid height is 1 to 2 mm above the pupillary border with the brow relaxed. The brow incisions are closed with 7-0 silk (or chromic catgut in children). Postoperatively, upward tension upon the sling from frontalis muscle contraction elevates the eyelid and provides an eyelid crease.

Crawford Technique. Three eyelid and three brow incisions are evenly placed. The central brow incision is highest, located above the hairline. The medial and lateral brow incisions should be farther apart than the medial and lateral eyelid incisions (Fig. 5–30A).

A Wright needle is introduced into the nasal eyelid incision and extended temporally emerging through the central eyelid incision. The fascia is placed through the eyelet opening and becomes properly positioned in the epitarsal space as the Wright needle is withdrawn (Fig. 5–30B). In a similar fashion, the nasal brow incision is used to engage and properly position both of these fascial strands. This provides the nasal fascial triangle. A second piece of fascia is similarly positioned to form the temporal fascial triangle. Each fascial triangle is tied with one square knot at its apex (Fig. 5–30C). Tension applied to each triangle dictates eyelid height and contour. The square knots are reinforced with a 4-0 Mersilene suture. One end of each fascial knot is cut, leaving a small fringe, while the other end is tunneled subcutaneously to the higher central brow incision using a Wright needle (Fig. 5–30D). These ends are united with one square knot, adding some further eyelid lift, if desired, in the process. This knot linking the two triangles is reinforced with a 4-0 Mersilene suture. The remaining fascial ends are cut, again leaving a small fringe. Skin is closed with interrupted 7-0 silk sutures (or chromic catgut in children.)

Management in the immediate postoperative period includes placement of a modified Frost traction suture in the lower eyelid margin to prevent postoperative corneal exposure (Fig. 5–30E). Additionally, lubricating drops and ointment may be used to minimize corneal desiccation in the early postoperative period. This can usually be rapidly tapered and eliminated. Oral antibiotics lessen the incidence of infection from placement of suspensory materials. The silk sutures may be removed on the sixth postoperative day.

Modified Tillett and Tillett Techniques. Two eyelid and three brow incisions are evenly placed. The medial and lateral brow incisions should be farther apart than the medial and lateral eyelid incisions (Fig. 5–31A). A

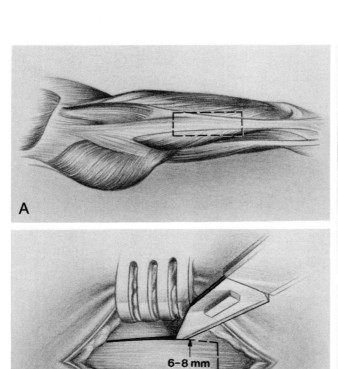

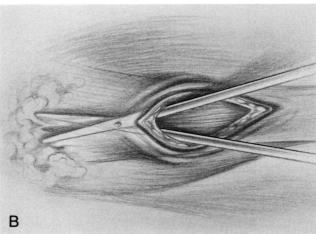

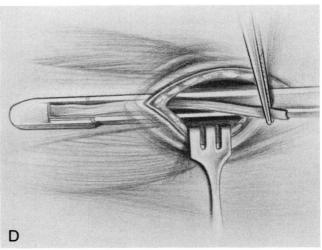

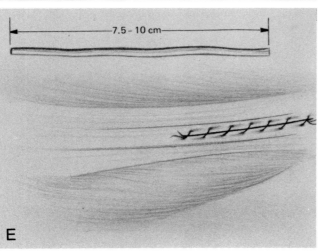

FIG. 5–29. Harvesting fascia lata. A, Fascia is removed from the area between the lateral knee (head of the fibula) and the anterior superior iliac crest. B, A 4 cm incision is placed 5 to 6 cm above the lateral knee. C, Two parallel incisions are made 6 to 8 mm apart in the direction of the fascial fibers. D, The fascial stripper is advanced while countertraction is applied to the fascia. E, A piece of fascia 7.5 × 10 cm long is removed and further subdivided. The leg incision is closed in two layers.

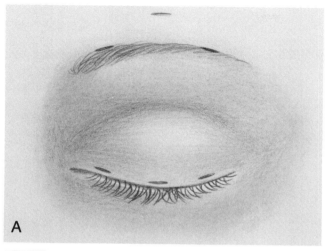

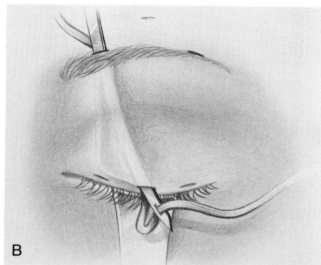

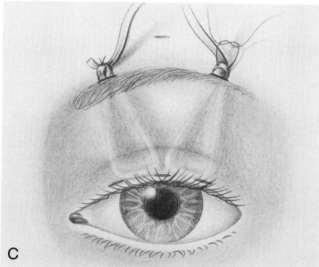

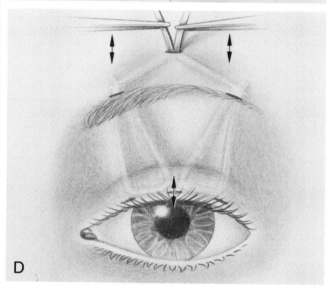

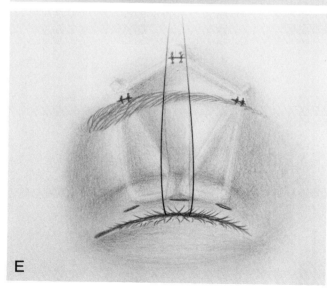

FIG. 5–30. Crawford technique. A, Placement of all six incision sites. B, Wright needle passing from the nasal brow incision through the central eyelid incision. Fascia is placed through the eyelet opening and becomes properly positioned as the Wright needle is withdrawn. C, After all fascial elements are passed, each triangle is tied with one square knot at its apex. The knots are reinforced with 4-0 Mersilene sutures. D, One end of each fascial knot is tunneled to the central brow incision. These ends are united with one square knot and a 4-0 Mersilene suture. E, Following skin closure, a modified Frost suture minimizes corneal exposure in the early postoperative period.

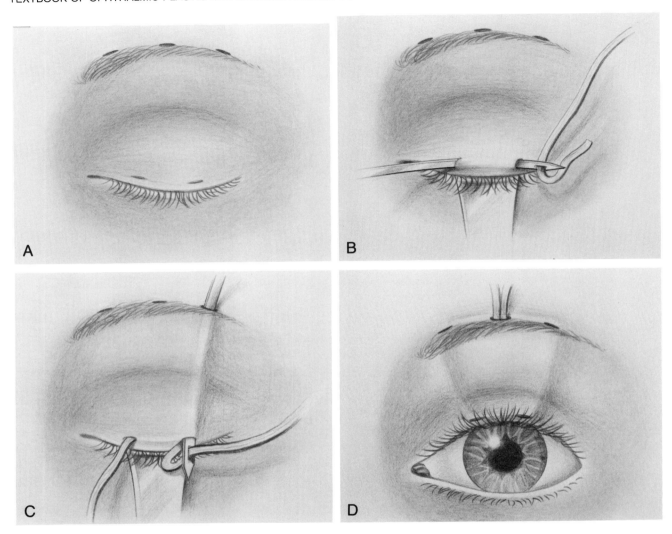

FIG. 5–31. Modified Tillett and Tillett technique. A, Placement of all five incision sites. B, A Wright needle extends from the nasal eyelid incision to the temporal eyelid incision, where it initially engages fascia. C, The temporal brow incision is used to engage and position the temporal fascial strand. D, The fascial rhomboid is completed and joined with one square knot and a 4-0 Mersilene suture.

Wright needle is introduced into the nasal eyelid incision and extended temporally, emerging through the temporal eyelid incision (Fig. 5–31B). The fascia (instead of the silicone used in the original Tillett and Tillett description) is placed through the eyelet opening and becomes positioned in the epitarsal space as the Wright needle is withdrawn. In a similar manner, the nasal and temporal brow incisions are used to engage and properly position the nasal and temporal fascial strands (Fig. 5–31C). The Wright needle is introduced through the central brow incision, making nasal and temporal passes to gather the nasal and temporal fascial strands. This fascial rhomboid is closed with one square knot (Fig.

5–31D). Tension on this knot dictates eyelid height and contour. The square knot is reinforced with a 4-0 Mersilene suture and the fascia is cut, leaving a small fringe. Skin is closed with interrupted 7-0 silk sutures (or chromic catgut in children).

Management in the immediate postoperative period includes placement of a modified Frost traction suture in the lower eyelid margin to prevent postoperative corneal exposure. Additionally, lubricating drops and ointment may be used to minimize corneal desiccation in the early postoperative period. Use of these can usually be rapidly tapered and eliminated. Oral antibiotics lessen the incidence of infection from placement of suspensory

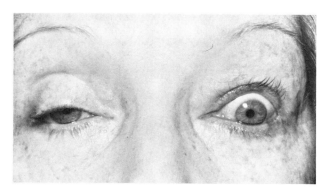

FIG. 5–32. Too large a levator resection resulted in a gross overcorrection in this patient.

materials. The silk sutures may be removed on the sixth postoperative day.

Features to be expected with frontalis suspension include blepharoptosis on upgaze, lid lag on downgaze, mild lagophthalmos, and arching of the brow with lid lifting.

COMPLICATIONS IN BLEPHAROPTOSIS SURGERY

Undercorrections, overcorrections (Fig. 5–32), and contour abnormalities are the most frequent postoperative complications. Additional surgery should be considered if minor adjustment techniques prove inadequate. Candidates for reoperation should be evaluated in the same manner as for the initial procedure. In general, the choice of reoperation and the degree of correction are determined by the severity of residual blepharoptosis and the amount of resultant levator function. This is further influenced by the previous surgery performed. The earlier a reoperation is performed, the less scar tissue is encountered. This decision, however, should not be made too early because many cases improve appreciably once edema subsides after the first postoperative 2 weeks. Many potential reoperations can therefore be avoided.

Undercorrection after the Fasanella-Servat procedure or levator aponeurosis surgery may require external levator resection. Additional tarsomyectomy is rarely indicated because it would further deplete tarsus. Aponeurosis revision should be from an anterior incision to optimize surgical exposure and access to the levator aponeurosis. Undercorrection after maximum levator resection may require frontalis suspension. Undercorrection, overcorrection, or contour abnormality in the first 6 weeks after frontalis suspension should be managed in minor surgery by opening the brow incision over the

knot (or knots) and adjusting the tension of the suspensory element. Undercorrection can occur later from migration or extrusion of alloplastic material. In this situation, the alloplastic element should be removed and a fascia lata sling procedure should follow.

Overcorrection after the Fasanella-Servat procedure is rare and may benefit from removal of the chromic catgut suture. Persistent overcorrection may require external levator recession, possibly implementing techniques used in treating eyelid retraction. Overcorrection in the first 2 weeks after levator aponeurosis surgery can be helped by daily everting the upper eyelid over a Desmarres retractor and/or applying intermittent downward force on the 4-0 silk-modified Frost suture. These maneuvers stretch and slightly weaken the tarsal-levator junction. In the conjunctival approach, early suture removal drops the eyelid further. Cases that involve levator resection should have additional room to adjust the tarsal-levator relationship. The sutures can be repositioned higher on the tarsal plate or lower on the aponeurosis fringe. Larger overcorrections require application of eyelid retraction techniques. Contour abnormalities are adjusted by segmentally altering the tarsal-levator relationship or by segmentally excising an ellipse of tarsus.

Although uncommon, permanent loss of eyelashes may result from carrying levator aponeurosis surgery too close to the eyelid margin or from a postoperative infection. Eyelash grafts are relatively ineffective and are not recommended.

Mild lid lag and lagophthalmos are common and proportional to the amount of surgery performed. They may be particularly noticeable following frontalis suspension or large levator resection. Resultant exposure tends to improve over time. This may be helped with lubricating ointment and drops, a moisture chamber, and/or a humidifier. Severe lid lag or lagophthalmos may require further surgery to diminish the surgical effect.

Corneal irritation, staining, the erosion occasionally occur after surgery involving a conjunctival suture line, particularly the Fasanella-Servat procedure. Most patients improve with more frequent use of lubricating or antibiotic ointments. Those with persistent problems may benefit from temporary use of a bandage soft contact lens. By the second or third postoperative week, the chromic catgut suture is usually soft enough to pose no further problem. Conjunctival suture removal is rarely required.

Entropion after blepharoptosis correction is rare, and results from excessive tarsectomy in the Fasanella-Servat procedure or conjunctival levator resection. A Wies procedure is effective in resolving any maintained postoperative entropion.

Ectropion may occur after levator resection from su-

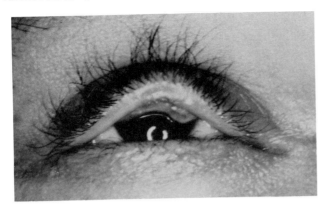

FIG. 5–33. Conjunctival prolapse several days after external levator resection.

turing the levator aponeurosis too low on tarsus. It usually resolves over time. Should it persist, surgical repositioning of the aponeurosis higher on the tarsus is indicated.

Superior rectus and superior oblique dysfunction occur rarely after posterior dissection in large levator resection. Any persistent extraocular muscle dysfunction should be evaluated and treated on a case-by-case basis.

A deficient eyelid crease may follow levator resection if imbrication sutures joining distal levator aponeurosis to skin are not placed. This can be corrected simply by placing several Pang sutures (full-thickness mattress sutures placed and tied at the position of desired eyelid fold), or more elaborately by opening the wound and placing supratarsal fixation sutures.

Conjunctiva may prolapse from early postoperative edema (Fig. 5–33). This usually resolves with time. Any persistent prolapse may be repositioned in the fornix with mattress sutures or simply excised.

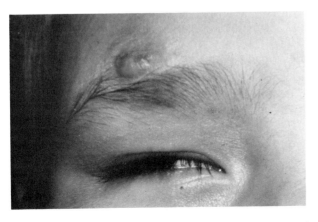

FIG. 5–34. Supramid suture infection and scar, which developed within 3 weeks of frontalis suspension with this alloplastic material. The infection could not be controlled with medication, necessitating removal of this material.

With the exception of frontalis suspension, infection is exceedingly rare after blepharoptosis surgery. Autogenous fascia lata is least prone to infection, followed in order by homogenous fascia lata (eyebank fascia), heterogenous fascia lata (bovine fascia), and alloplastic materials. These materials may occasionally induce a serum accumulation. This responds to heat and minimal surgical drainage with retention of the sling material. If infection occurs, as evidenced by a purulent discharge, the suspensory element must be removed. This will also require appropriate culture and sensitivity studies, topical and systemic antibiotics, heat, and drainage in case of abscess. Later replacement of the suspensory material with fascia lata is required unless the original sling was present long enough to develop a fibrous tract sufficient to support the eyelid. Up to 10% of alloplastic suspensory materials require removal because of infection or extrusion (Fig. 5–34).

Scarring is usually minimal in blepharoptosis surgery. Anterior approaches conceal the scar in the eyelid crease, while in posterior approaches the conjunctival scar is not directly accessible. In frontalis suspension, the brow incisions may remain perceptible. They are least obvious when placed at the superior aspect of the brow hairline. Frontalis suspension may predispose to granuloma formation. This may require removal of the granuloma and sometimes of the supensory material.

BIBLIOGRAPHY

Anderson, R. and Beard, C.: The levator aponeurosis. Arch. Ophthalmol. 95:1437–1441, 1977.

Anderson, R. and Dixon, R.: The role of Whitnall's ligament in ptosis surgery. Arch. Ophathalmol. 97:705–707, 1979.

Anderson, R. and Dixon, R.: Aponeurotic ptosis surgery. Arch Ophthalmol. 97:1123–1228, 1979.

Anderson, R. and Gordy, D.: Aponeurotic defects in congenital ptosis. Am. J. Ophthalmol. 86:1493–1499, 1979.

Baylis, H. and Shorr, N.: Anterior tarsectomy reoperation for upper eyelid blepharoptosis or Contour Abnormalities. Am. J. Ophthalmol. 84:67–71, 1977.

Beard, C.: Blepharoptosis repair by modified Fasanella-Servat operation. Am. J. Ophthalmol. 69:850, 1970.

Beard, C.: Blepharoptosis. In Soll, D.B. (ed): Management of Complications in Ophthalmic Plastic Surgery, Birmingham, Aesculapius, 1976.

Beard, C.: Ptosis, 3rd Ed., St. Louis, C.V. Mosby, 1981.

Beard, C. and Sullivan, J.: Ptosis. In Beyer Machule, C., and von Noorden, G.: Atlas of Ophthalmic Surgery. New York, Thieme-Stratton, 1985.

Berke, R.: Results of resection of the levator muscle through a skin incision in congenital ptosis. Arch. Ophthalmol. 61:177, 1959.

Berke, R.: Surgical treatment of traumatic blepharoptosis. Am. J. Ophthalmol. 72:691, 1971.

Beyer, C. and Carroll, J.: Moderately severe cicatricial entropion. Arch. Ophthalmol. 89:33, 1973.

Beyer, C. and Johnson, C.: Anterior levator resection: problems and management. Trans. Am. Acad. Ophthalmol. Otolaryngol. 70:687–695, 1975.

Bosniak, S. and Smith, B.: Advances in ophthalmic plastic and reconstructive Surgery. New York, Pergamon Press, 1982.

Callahan, A.: Correction of unilateral blepharoptosis with bilateral eyelid suspension. Am. J. Ophthalmol. 74:321–326, 1972.

Callahan, M.: Surgically mismanaged ptosis associated with double elevator palsy. Arch. Ophthalmol. 99:108, 1981.

Cogan, D.: Myesthenia gravis: a review of the disease and a description of lid twitch as a characteristic sign. Arch. Ophthalmol. 74:217–221, 1965.

Crawford, J.: Repair of ptosis using frontalis muscle and fascia lata. Trans. Am. Acad. Ophthalmol. Otolaryngol. 60:672–678, 1956.

Crawford, J.: Repair of ptosis using frontalis muscle and fascia lata: a 20 year review. Ophthalmic Surg. 8:31, 1977.

Dortzbach, R.: Superior tarsal muscle resection to correct blepharoptosis. Ophthalmology 86:1883, 1979.

Fasanella, R. and Servat, J.: Levator resection for minimal ptosis: another simplified operation. Arch. Ophthalmol. 65:493–496, 1961.

Fasanella, R.: Surgery for minimal ptosis: the Fasanella-Servat operation. Trans. Ophthalmol. Soc. U.K. 93:425, 1973.

Friedenwald, J. and Guyton, J.: A simple ptosis operation: utilization of the frontalis by means of a single rhomboid-shaped suture. Am. J. Ophthalmol. 31:411, 1948.

Frost, A.: Supporting suture in ptosis operations. Am. J. Ophthalmol. 17:633, 1934.

Frueh, B.: The mechanistic classification of ptosis. Ophthalmology 87:1019–1021, 1980.

Geeraets, W.: Ocular Syndromes (Kohn-Romano Syndrome). Philadelphia, Lea & Febiger, 1976, p. 256.

Johnson, C.: Selection of operation, operative techniques, complications. Arch. Ophthalmol. 66:793, 1961.

Jones, L.: The anatomy of the upper eyelid and its relation to ptosis surgery. Am. J. Ophthalmol. 57:943, 1964.

Jones, L., Quickert, M., and Wobig, J.: The cure of ptosis by aponeurotic repair. Arch. Ophthalmol. 93:629–634, 1975.

Kearns, T.: External ophthalmoplegia, pigmentary degeneration of the retina, and cardiomyopathy: a newly recognized syndrome. Trans. Am. Ophthalmol. Soc. 63:559-625, 1965.

Kohn, R. and Romano, P.: Blepharoptosis, blepharophimosis, epicanthus inversus, and telecanthus—a syndrome with no name. Am. J. Ophthalmol. 72:625, 1971.

Kohn, R.: Additional lacrimal findings in the syndrome of blepharoptosis, blepharophimosis, epicanthus inversus, and telecanthus. J. Pediatr. Ophthalmol. Strabismus 20:98, 1983.

Kohn, R.: Management of congenital and acquired telecanthus. Submitted for publication.

Kohn, R., Romano, P.: Kohn-Romano Syndrome. *In* Roy, F.H.: Ocular Syndromes and Systemic Disease, Grune and Stratton, 1985, p. 170.

Kohn, R.: Epicanthus. *Chapter in* Buyse, M., Birth Defects Encyclopedia, New York, Alan R. Liss, Inc., 1988.

Kohn, R.: Congenital Anomalies of the Eyelid and Socket. *In* Hornblass, A.: Oculoplastic, Orbital and Reconstructive Surgery, Williams and Wilkins, 1988.

Older, J.: Levator aponeurosis disinsertion in the young adult. Arch. Ophthalmol. 96:1857, 1978.

Pang, H.: Surgical formation of upper lid fold. Arch. Ophthalmol. 65:783, 1961.

Paris, G. and Quickert, M.: Disinsertion of the aponeurosis of the levator palpebrae superiorus muscle after cataract extraction. Am. J. Ophthalmol. 81:337–340, 1976.

Putterman, A. and Urist, M.: Transconjunctival isolation and transcutaneous resection of the levator palpebrae superiorus muscle. Am. J. Ophthalmol. 77:90, 1974.

Putterman, A. and Urist, M.: Müller's muscle—conjunctiva resection. Arch. Ophthalmol. 93:619, 1975.

Putterman, A. and Urist, M.: Reconstruction of the upper eyelid crease and fold. Arch. Ophthalmol. 94:1941, 1976.

Putterman, A. and Urist, M.: Müller's muscle—conjunctival resection ptosis procedure. Ophthalmic Surg. 9:27, 1978.

Reeh, M.: Congenital blepharoptosis. Am. J. Ophthalmol. 69:431, 1970.

Reeh, M., Beyer, C., and Shannon, G.: Practical Ophthalmic Plastic and Reconstructive Surgery. Philadelphia, Lea & Febiger, 1976.

Riley, F. and Moyer, N.: Oculosympathetic paresis associated with cluster headaches. Am. J. Ophthalmol. 72:763–768, 1971.

Small, R.: Supratarsal fixation in ophthalamic plastic surgery. Ophthalmic Surg. 9:73–85, 1978.

Smith, B., McCord, C., and Baylis, H.: Surgical treatment of blepharoptosis. Am. J. Ophthalmol. 68:92, 1969.

Tillett, C. and Tillett, G.: Silicone sling in the correction of ptosis. Am. J. Ophthalmol. 62:521, 1966.

6

THYROID OPHTHALMOPATHY AND EYELID RETRACTION

Thyroid ophthalmopathy (Graves' disease) is a multisystem disorder that is the most common cause of unilateral and bilateral exophthalmos in adults. Women are affected approximately eight times more often than men, with onset typically in the third to fifth decade (Fig. 6–1). Genetic predisposition may exist in some cases. Thyroid dysfunction is designated as Graves' disease when it includes one or more of the following characteristics: hyperthyroidism associated with diffuse hyperplasia of the thyroid gland, infiltrative ophthalmopathy, and infiltrative dermopathy (localized pretibial myxedema).

CLINICAL MANIFESTATIONS

Clinical manifestations of Graves' disease can be unilateral or bilateral and may include exophthalmos (40 to 70%), limitation of extraocular movement, diplopia corresponding to this limitation, upper and/or lower eyelid retraction (Dalrymple's sign), pseudo-retraction (from proptosis), upper lid lag on downgaze, restriction of downward traction on the upper eyelid (Grove's sign), eyelid edema, conjunctival chemosis, epibulbar vascular congestion overlying the insertion of the rectus muscles, and increased orbital resistance to retrodisplacement.

Extraocular muscle contracture and fibrosis most commonly and severely affects the inferior rectus (Fig. 6–2A and B), followed by the medial rectus. In equivocal cases, forced duction testing may demonstrate resistance on moving the globe away from the suspected restricted muscle. Increased intraocular pressure may also be de-

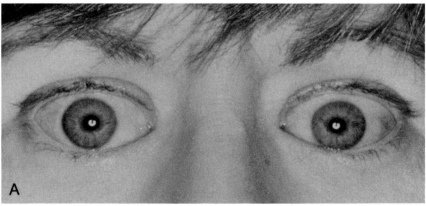
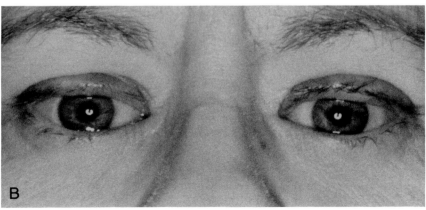

FIG. 6–1. A, Preoperative appearance of 46-year-old woman with bilateral upper eyelid retraction secondary to Graves' disease. B, Postoperative appearance 4 years after bilateral recession of the levator aponeurosis with two pedicle tarsal rotation flaps. (From Kohn, R.: Treatment of eyelid retraction with two pedicle tarsal rotation flaps. Am. J. Ophthalmol., 95:539–544, 1983.)

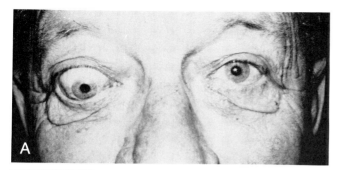

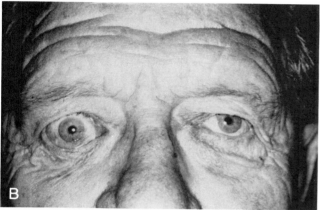

FIG. 6–2. Graves' disease demonstrating contracture and fibrosis of the right inferior rectus muscle in A, primary position and, B, attempted upgaze.

tected when the patient is looking away from the position of the restricted muscle.

Vision may be jeopardized from optic neuropathy in an orbital apex crowded with enlarged extraocular muscles (2.5%). This often occurs in a setting of mild to moderate proptosis (incomplete spontaneous decompression). Patients present with painless and slowly progressive loss of vision associated with a central scotoma. Diminution of color vision, afferent pupillary defect, and diminished visual evoked response (VER) may also be elicited. These changes sometimes occur rapidly, within a 1- to 2-week interval. Congested orbits may occasionally present with papilledema or optic atrophy. Severe proptosis (complete spontaneous decompression) may likewise compromise vision, in this case from increased intraocular pressure (uncommon) or corneal exposure, which may lead to corneal ulceration.

PATHOPHYSIOLOGY

Although the exact etiology is unknown, the ocular changes in Graves' disease are thought to result from an autoimmune mechanism. Immune complexes may reach the orbit through the superior cervical lymphatic channels, which drain both the thyroid gland and the orbit. These complexes may then bind to extraocular muscles, orbital fat, and/or the lacrimal gland, resulting in an inflammatory reaction composed of lymphocytes, plasma cells, mast cells, and hyaluronic acid. The later is hyperosmotic, drawing fluid into the orbit. This infiltration stimulates fibroblasts in the extraocular muscles to produce acid mucopolysaccharides. The result is progressive fibrosis. Extraocular muscle infiltration in Graves' disease is therefore a restrictive myopathy resulting from inflammation and edema, leading to muscle degeneration and fibrosis.

Inflammation and edema of the extraocular muscles and orbital fat, along with the resultant venous engorgement, result in increased intraorbital pressure. These infiltrated structures deep within the orbit are minimally compressible. Therefore, orbital pressure is transmitted anteriorly, causing exophthalmos. The eyelids, orbital septum, extraocular muscles, and optic nerve check the forward movement of the globe.

Upper eyelid retraction may result from enhanced adrenergic stimulation and enhanced superior rectus and levator muscle contraction in an attempt to overcome a restricted inferior rectus muscle. Initial infiltration of the levator muscle by glycoprotein and mucopolysaccharide, followed later by fibrosis, may also contribute to the retraction. Lower eyelid retraction is caused by enhanced adrenergic stimulation and fibrotic contraction of the lower eyelid retractors.

RELATIONSHIP OF OPHTHALMOPATHY TO THYROID FUNCTION

Although most patients with Graves' disease demonstrate hyperthyroidism, some never develop a hyperthyroid state and instead have euthyroid or hypothyroid Graves' disease throughout. The onset and clinical course of Graves' disease does not necessarily parallel that of the thyroid disease. Ophthalmopathy may precede, follow, or concur with the period of clinical thyroid dysfunction. This disease is usually self-limited and resolves within months or a few years of its onset. Occasional patients may worsen clinically after treatment changes their hyperthyroid state to a euthyroid level.

EVALUATION

The diagnosis of Graves' disease is based on the clinical presentation, supported by ultrasonographic and CT scan findings. Axial views on CT scans may demonstrate en-

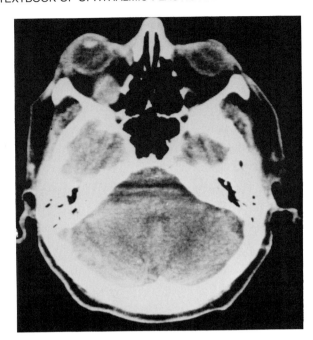

FIG. 6–3. CT scan in axial view, demonstrating enlarged right inferior rectus muscle with sparing of the tendinous insertion caused by Graves' disease. Such muscle enlargement should be distinguished from a tumor on the basis of clinical findings, CT direct coronal views, and/or ultrasonography.

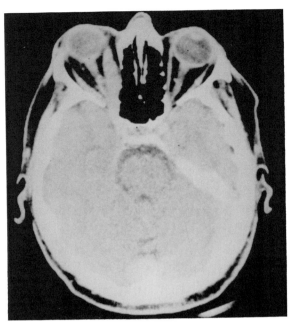

FIG. 6–4. CT scan in axial view, demonstrating enlarged right medial rectus muscle from Graves' ophthalmopathy.

larged extraocular muscles with sparing of tendinous insertions (Figs. 6–3 and 6–4). Direct coronal views on CT scans may yield a graphic view of this process, while additionally disclosing optic nerve compression from crowding at the orbital apex. Ultrasound may demonstrate one or more enlarged extraocular muscles, possibly associated with accentuation of orbital walls and irregular retrobulbar fat pads.

Radionuclide scans may show increased uptake of technetium-labeled compounds by the extraocular muscles. In suspected cases, coexistent myasthenia gravis may be ruled out on the basis of Tensilon testing and acetylcholine receptor antibody assays. The increased association of Graves' disease with collagen vascular diseases should not be overlooked. An endocrinologic consultation is recommended.

The initial laboratory work-up should include triiodothyronine (T_3) and thyroxine (T_4) determinations. If these are elevated, the diagnosis is confirmed. If they are normal or low, the T_3 suppression test (Werner) and thyrotropin releasing hormone (TRH) test should be performed. The TRH test has the highest specificity for Graves' disease. These thyroid function tests are more useful in support of the diagnosis and as a guide in medical management of endocrine dysfunction than they are

in establishing the diagnosis of Graves' disease, which is based on clinical findings.

MANAGEMENT OF THE ACTIVE PHASE OF GRAVES' DISEASE

The natural history of Graves' disease shows steady clinical deterioration over several months, followed by stability, then slow subsidence over months to years. Eventual remission is characteristic, although few patients return to a completely normal clinical state. Therefore, treatment in the active phase of Graves' disease should be conservative. Any coexistant endocrine abnormality should be treated. If possible, definitive surgical procedures should be performed 6 to 12 months after clinical stabilization to lessen the chance that the ophthalmopathy will progress after such surgery.

Mild cases of corneal exposure from proptosis or eyelid retraction may be managed with lubricating ointments and tears, along with nocturnal use of a humidifier and moisture chamber. Intractable exposure may predispose to corneal erosion or ulceration. This should be treated with a short course of prednisone. Optic neuropathy may result from swollen extraocular muscles compressing the optic nerve in the confined space of the orbital apex. This should also be treated with a short course of prednisone. To be effective, 80 to 100 mg/day of prednisone is given over a 2-week period, followed by incremental tapering over an additional week. Less gastric irritation develops if the drug is taken in conjunction with antacids or milk.

A less efficacious alternative to steroids is irradiation (1500 to 3000 rads) in 10 fractions over a 2-week period. This carries the short-term risk of tissue swelling further compromising an already crowded orbital apex. A long-term risk may be tissue shrinkage enhancing orbital fibrosis.

Steroids and irradiation are temporizing modalities that rarely prove curative. They may help to recompensate the optic nerve or cornea so that definitive surgery can be delayed until the disease is in the inactive phase. If steroids do not adequately resolve the optic neuropathy or corneal compromise, orbital decompression should be performed immediately.

Diplopia, particularly in the vertical plane, may result from extraocular muscle involvement. Motility surgery should not be performed while the disease is active; otherwise further muscle fibrosis may spoil a successful result. Prism glasses or frosted lenses may help to decrease symptoms as the disease ameliorates. Correction of coexistent eyelid retraction and eyelid fullness should also be deferred to the inactive phase. Occasional cases of retraction have been helped with guanethidine 10% (bethanidine or thymoxamine), but this is rarely used because of its predisposition to chemical keratoconjunctivitis.

MANAGEMENT OF THE INACTIVE PHASE OF GRAVES' DISEASE

Once the disease has been clinically inactive for 6 to 12 months, elective surgery may be considered to treat the various resultant ophthalmic disorders: exophthalmos, extraocular muscle dysfunction, eyelid retraction, and dermatochalasis. It is essential that surgery follow the above sequence because the correction of each preceding problem will alter the clinical state of each following problem (i.e., orbital decompression for exophthalmos will influence motility, motility surgery will influence eyelid retraction, and correction of retraction will influence a future blepharoplasty). Any procedure in this sequence may be omitted if it is not clinically indicated. Long-term results are often unpredictable if surgery is carried out in the active phase of Graves' disease.

SURGICAL DECOMPRESSION OF THE ORBIT
JAMES ORCUTT, M.D.

As noted earlier, in the active phase of thyroid ophthalmopathy, decompression may be an emergency proce-

dure in the treatment of optic neuropathy or corneal exposure that is not responsive to steroids. In the inactive phase, orbital decompression may be indicated for motility disturbances, pain, choroidal folds, recurrent luxation of the globe, and cosmesis.

Patients considering cosmetic decompression must be counseled thoroughly about the risks of decompression and alternative procedures, including levator recession and canthoplasty. Surgery should be undertaken only when the patient is willing to accept the risks of vision loss and diplopia to obtain symptomatic improvement.

Any wall or combination of walls of the orbit can be removed to decompress the orbit. The orbital roof is rarely removed because an extradural craniotomy is required and there is a risk of postoperative pulsatile exophthalmos. Removal of the lateral wall may be combined with removal of other walls to reduce exophthalmos, but does not adequately decompress the orbital apex in most cases of optic neuropathy. The approach to the lateral wall is described in the chapter on orbital tumors (Chapter 15). The membranous bone of the lateral wall may be removed with a burr, leaving the anterior portion of the lateral wall. The most easily decompressed walls are the orbital floor and medial wall. The floor and medial wall can be decompressed through either a transantral approach or an anterior orbital approach. The advantages of the anterior approach over the transantral approach include better exposure and a lower risk of developing diplopia. The incidence of diplopia is greater with the transantral approach, but this approach is more likely to result in adequate decompression in patients with optic neuropathy from a crowded orbital apex. The number of walls removed can be graded according to presence of optic neuropathy.

The orbital rim incision for decompression of the orbital floor and medial wall is described. The surgeon has the additional options of a subciliary, lower eyelid crease or lower swinging flap approach (see Figs. 15–13 and 15–15).

The incision is made along the lower orbital rim. Lymphedema will occur if the incision is extended beyond the lateral canthus or the lateral portion of the incision is turned upward. The incision is carried through orbicularis muscle to the orbital rim (Fig. 6–5). An incision is made through the periosteum to bone. The periorbita is elevated from the orbital floor using a periosteal elevator. A burr is used to open the orbital floor medial to the infraorbital nerve. The bone between the infraorbital nerve canal and the medial wall is then removed by cracking with a hemostat (Fig. 6–6). The bone is carefully removed from around the infraorbital nerve and temporally to the lateral wall of the maxillary sinus. Care is taken to remove bone to the posterior wall of the max-

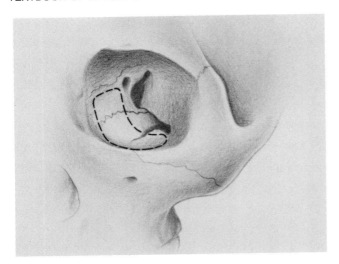

FIG. 6–5. Demonstration of the site of bone removal in decompression of the orbital floor and medial wall through either an anterior orbital or transantral approach.

illary sinus. Attention is then directed to the medial wall. Ethmoidal air cells and the lamina papyracea are removed with a hemostat to the level of the ethmoidal arteries (Fig. 6–6). The ethmoidal arteries are visualized by retracting the periorbita from the medial wall, and the arteries will be seen tenting the periobita as they penetrate the lamina papyracea. The ethmoidal air cells are removed until the orbital apex is reached. Several incisions are then made in an anterior-posterior direction in the periorbita along the medial and inferior walls to allow orbital fat to prolapse into the ethmoid and maxillary sinuses, respectively. The orbital rim periosteum

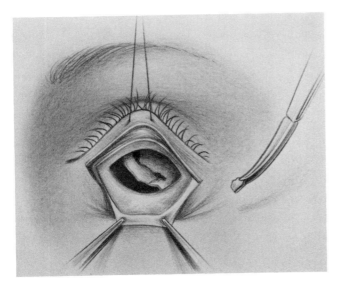

FIG. 6–6. Decompression of the orbital floor and medial wall through an anterior orbital approach.

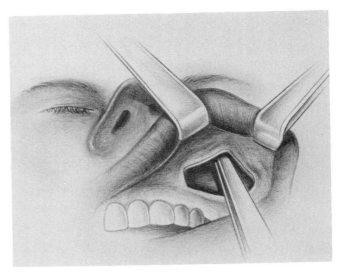

FIG. 6–7. Transantral decompression. An incision in the upper buccogingival sulcus is carried to the anterior maxillary wall. After elevation of the periosteum, a maxillary antrostomy is performed. The maxillary roof is removed and the bony excision is extended to the ethmoid air cells. This should stop short of the ethmoidal arteries.

is closed with interrupted 4-0 chromic catgut sutures. The skin is closed with a continuous 6-0 monofilament suture. If indicated, generally both orbits are decompressed at the same time to provide symmetry.

Transantral decompression requires an incision in the upper buccogingival sulcus to expose the anterior maxillary wall. The incision is placed under the upper lip above the roots of the maxillary teeth (Fig. 6–7). The incision is carried to the periosteum, which is then elevated from the maxillary wall, and a maxillary antrostomy is performed and opened with a rongeur. The maxillary sinus roof is opened with a punch after removal of the mucosa. The maxillary roof is removed piecemeal, with a small rongeur preserving the infraorbital nerve (Fig. 6–8). The excision of bone is then carried medially to perform an ethmoidectomy using a bone punch. Ethmoid air cells are removed to the level of the ethmoidal arteries and posterior to the orbital apex (Fig. 6–8). Slits are then made in the periorbita to allow orbital fat to prolapse into the sinuses. A nasoantral window is created and the antrum is packed with antibiotic gauze. The tissue overlying the maxillary sinus is closed with 3-0 absorbable suture. The packing is removed the following day through the nose.

Complications of orbital decompression include diplopia, vision loss, hemorrhage, infection, numbness in the distribution of the infraorbital nerve, eyelid edema, inadequate decompression, and cerebrospinal fluid leak. Diplopia is commonly present in thyroid patients before surgery. However, if a cosmetic decompression is being

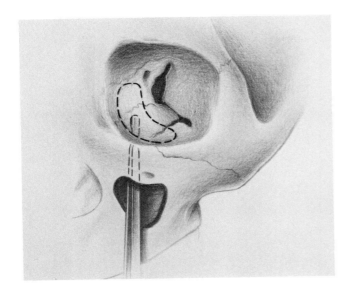

FIG. 6–8. Demonstration of the site of bone removal in decompression of the orbital floor and medial wall through a transantral approach.

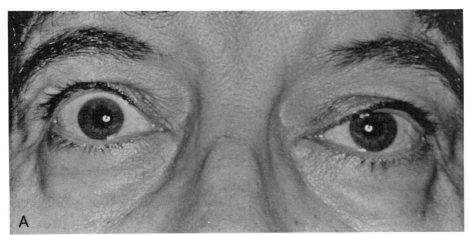

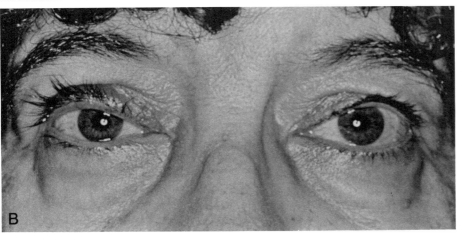

FIG. 6–9. A, Preoperative retraction of the right upper eyelid secondary to overcorrected blepharoptosis surgery. B, Appearance 5 years after recession of the right levator aponeurosis with two pedicle tarsal rotation flaps. (From Kohn, R.: Treatment of eyelid retraction with two pedicle tarsal rotation flaps. Published with permission from Am. J. Ophthalmol., 95:539–544, 1983. Copyright by the Ophthalmic Publishing Company.)

contemplated in a patient without diplopia in primary gaze or downgaze, the risk of development of diplopia may be as high as 33%. A transantral approach is more likely to produce diplopia than the anterior orbital approach.

Vision loss is a rare complication of orbital decompression. The risk of vision loss can be minimized by careful dissection, hemostasis, and close postoperative visual evaluation.

Decompression for optic neuropathy must include posterior ethmoid removal. The major cause of inadequate decompression is incomplete removal of the posterior ethmoid wall. Cerebrospinal fluid can leak when bone is removed above the level of the ethmoidal arteries. Should a cerebrospinal fluid leak occur, it can be covered with an orbicularis muscle patch. The patient should be placed on oral antibiotics to reduce the risk of brain abscess or meningitis.

EXTRAOCULAR MUSCLE SURGERY
ROGER KOHN, M.D.

The extraocular muscle most commonly infiltrated in Graves' disease is the inferior rectus. This is followed in frequency by the medial rectus, superior rectus, and lateral rectus. One or more muscles may be involved in each case. This leads to a variety of vertical, horizontal, and mixed motility disturbances in Graves' disease.

Surgical decisions generally follow conventional strabismus guidelines. One exception to this is the amount of recession applicable to these fibrotic muscles. In Graves' disease, the recession is not strictly limited by the equator of the globe. Some cases may require recession 1 to 2 mm beyond the equator, traction sutures fixating the globe in overcorrection, or adjustable sutures. The details of these techniques can be found in most strabismus texts.

EYELID RETRACTION SURGERY

The appearance of eyelid retraction in patients with Graves' disease may be a manifestation of true retraction or pseudoretraction from proptosis. Factors that contribute to true upper and/or lower eyelid retraction may include Müller's muscle contraction from adrenergic

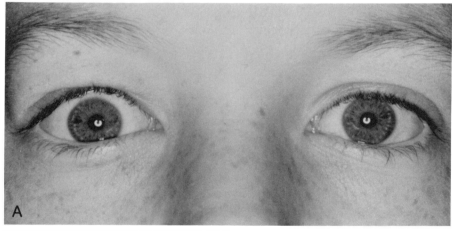

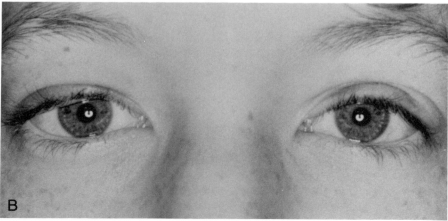

FIG. 6–10. A, Preoperative retraction of the right upper eyelid secondary to overcorrected blepharoptosis surgery. B, Appearance 4 years after recession of the right levator aponeurosis with two pedicle tarsal rotation flaps. (From Kohn, R.: Treatment of eyelid retraction with two pedicle tarsal rotation flaps. Published with permission from Am. J. Ophthalmol., 95:539–544, 1983. Copyright by the Ophthalmic Publishing Company.)

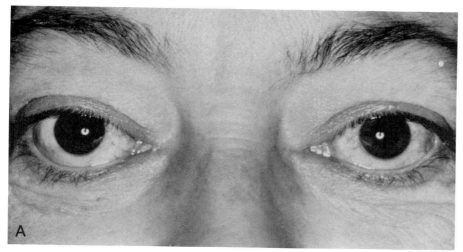

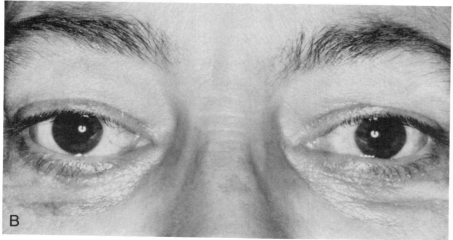

FIG. 6–11. A, Preoperative retraction of both lower eyelids secondary to previous vertical extraocular muscle surgery for Graves' disease. B, Appearance 4 years after bilateral recession of the inferior eyelid retractors with two pedicle tarsal rotation flaps. (From Kohn, R.: Treatment of eyelid retraction with two pedicle tarsal rotation flaps. Published with permission from Am. J. Ophthalmol., 95:539–544, 1983. Copyright by the Ophthalmic Publishing Company.)

stimulation, infiltration of the levator palpebrae superiorus muscle, and overaction of eyelid retractors as a compensation for restricted vertical extraocular muscles.

Surgery for eyelid retraction is directed at weakening the relationship between the tarsus and the eyelid retractor. Cases of mild retraction of the upper eyelid can be managed by recessing the levator aponeurosis to a more superior tarsal position. As this frequently proves insufficient, various levator aponeurosis tenotomy and recession procedures have been devised. When either a conjunctival or a cutaneous approach is used, these techniques allow the levator aponeurosis to retract freely or utilize soft tissue attachment or sutures tied loosely into the tarsus. This type of surgery has been somewhat unpredictable, and the effects may diminish with time. Similarly, lower eyelid retraction has been managed by recession of the inferior aponeurosis (capsulopalpebral head of the inferior rectus muscle) beyond the tarsus with no insertion, soft tissue insertion, or loose suture insertion.

To augment and quantify levator aponeurosis recession, materials such as lamellar auricular cartilage, sclera, Gelfilm, Gelfoam, collagen film, and orbicularis oculi muscle have been interposed between the levator aponeurosis and the tarsus. These substances contract to various degrees, adding scar tissue and an element of unpredictability.

Upper eyelid retraction has also been treated by lengthening the levator aponeurosis with partial myotomy and by decreasing sympathetic input with Müller's muscle excision. These techniques appear to be effective, although postoperative contracture again varies.

Lower eyelid retraction has also been managed with lateral canthal sling procedures, lower eyelid fascia lata slings, and recession of the retractors with or without an interposed spacer. Although effective, postoperative retraction varies with these techniques.

A procedure has been developed in which either the levator aponeurosis or the inferior aponeurosis may be

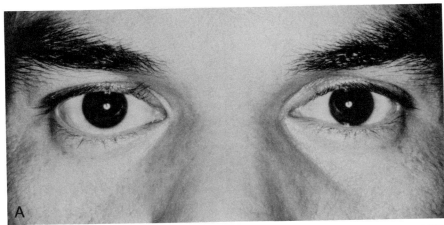

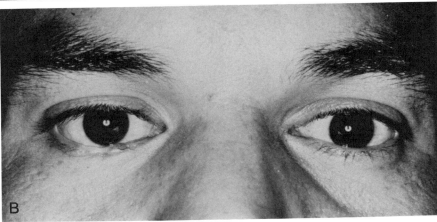

FIG. 6–12. A, Preoperative retraction of the right lower eyelid secondary to previous vertical extraocular muscle surgery. B, Appearance 5 years after recession of the right inferior eyelid retractor with two pedicle tarsal rotation flaps. A 4 mm gap in the eyelashes resulted from the close proximity of the surgical dissection to the eyelash follicles. (From Kohn, R.: Treatment of eyelid retraction with two pedicle tarsal rotation flaps. Published with permission from Am. J. Ophthalmol., 95:539–544, 1983. Copyright by the Ophthalmic Publishing Company.)

recessed beyond the tarsal border while remaining directly attached to the tarsus by means of an extended framework created by two pedicle tarsal rotation flaps. This establishes efficient transfer of muscle contracture into eyelid movement, thus aiding surgical quantification and predictability. This procedure has proven effective and predictable in treating eyelid retraction from Graves' disease and various other causes (Figs. 6–9 to 6–11). The only adverse effect occurred in one case of lower eyelid retraction in which the close proximity of the surgical dissection to the eyelash follicles resulted in a 4 mm gap in the eyelashes (Fig. 6–12).

Technique for Correction of Upper Eyelid Retraction.
Mark the area of intended incision with methylene blue at the position of the desired eyelid fold (Fig. 6–13A). Subjacent to this, a local anesthetic is administered so that there is analgesia without akinesia. Make an incision through the skin and orbicularis oculi muscle to the anterior tarsal surface (Fig. 6–13B). Separate the preseptal orbicularis oculi muscle from the orbital septum. If the septum has not been opened by previous surgery, open it in its entirety, exposing the levator aponeurosis below

with intervening orbital fat. The levator aponeurosis, along with subjacent Müller's muscle and conjunctiva, are disinserted as one complex.

Two pedicle flaps are fashioned from the upper border of the tarsus, with bases placed medially and laterally (Fig. 6–13C). These pedicles are 2 mm wide and curve somewhat centrally to provide easier rotation (Fig. 6–13D). The width of the interval between the flaps should be the same as the width of the levator aponeurosis to be recessed. Conjunctival tissue subjacent to these tarsal flaps may be removed by sharp dissection.

In patients with Graves' disease or previous vertical motility surgery, recess the entire levator aponeurosis along with subjacent Müller's muscle and conjunctiva as one complex. If the retraction has resulted from overcorrection due to blepharoptosis surgery, resuture the conjunctiva to the superior tarsal border; this is followed by recession of only the portion of levator aponeurosis involved in the previous resection.

Each end of the levator aponeurosis or the levator aponeurosis complex is sutured to its corresponding tarsal pedicle with a 6-0 Vicryl mattress suture (Fig. 6–13E). This can be adjusted by tying temporary knots and ob-

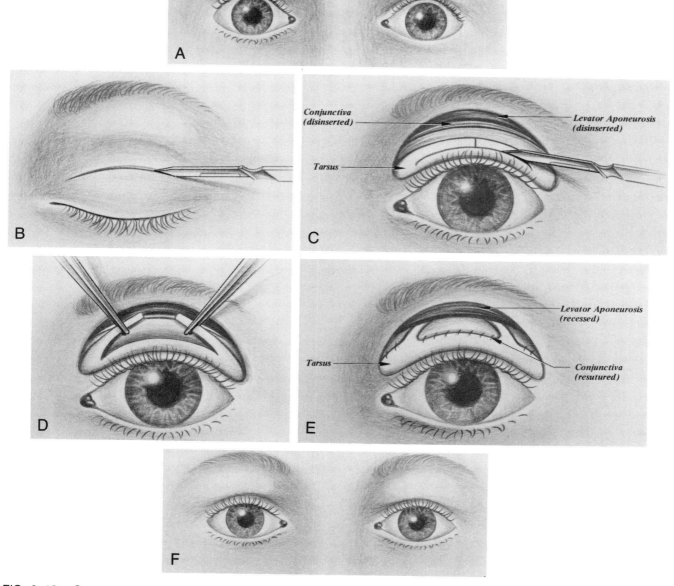

FIG. 6–13. Correction of eyelid retraction with two pedicle tarsal rotation flaps. A, Preoperative appearance demonstrating bilateral upper eyelid retraction with scleral show. B, An incision is made at the position of the desired postoperative eyelid crease. C, Levator aponeurosis is isolated and recessed. Two pedicle flaps are fashioned from the tarsus. D, The two pedicle tarsal flaps are rotated superiorly and, E, attached to the recessed levator aponeurosis. In overcorrected blepharoptosis surgery, the conjunctiva is resutured to the superior tarsal border. In Graves' disease, the conjunctiva is not resutured. F, Desired appearance after correction of eyelid retraction using this technique. (From Kohn, R.: Treatment of eyelid retraction with two pedicle tarsal rotation flaps. Published with permission from Am. J. Ophthalmol., 95:539–544, 1983. Copyright by the Ophthalmic Publishing Company.)

serving the position of the eyelid. At this stage, accuracy is further enhanced by turning off the surgical lights to minimize eyelid closure induced by light. Secure the eyelid 1 to 2 mm below the desired position to compensate for mild postoperative contracture. Once the correct position has been determined, tie the sutures permanently and cut (Fig. 6–13F). Close the incision with 7-0 silk running sutures, imbricating the distal levator aponeurosis if eyelid fold augmentation is desired. A modified Frost suture may be used to hold the upper eyelid in a position of mild overcorrection. At surgical closure, a resutured conjunctiva serves as a barrier, separating the pedicles from the globe. A recessed conjunctiva heals toward the tarsus, providing such a barrier later.

Technique for Correction of Lower Eyelid Retraction. Place the incision horizontally 3 mm below the lower eyelid margin. Extend the incision through the orbicularis oculi muscle to the anterior tarsal surface. The orbital septum, inferior aponeurosis (capsulopalpebral head of the inferior rectus muscle), and conjunctiva are disinserted and recessed as one complex.

The two tarsal flaps, each 2 mm wide, must be fashioned with care because the rudimentary lower eyelid tarsus measures only 4 or 5 mm vertically. Suture each end of the recessed complex to its correspondingly tarsal pedicle with a 6-0 Vicryl mattress suture. The lower eyelid should be secured 1 to 2 mm above the desired position to compensate for mild postoperative contracture. Close the incision with 7-0 silk running sutures. A modified Frost suture may be used to hold the lower eyelid in a position of mild overcorrection. The recessed conjunctiva heals toward the tarsus.

BLEPHAROPLASTY

The final surgical consideration for patients with Graves' disease is blepharoplasty. These patients often have dermatochalasis with prominent orbital fat as a result of orbital infiltration. Thus, upper and/or lower blepharoplasty will likely entail both skin excision and excision of appreciable herniated orbital fat. The details of this surgery are given in Chapter 9.

BIBLIOGRAPHY

Anderson, R. and Linberg, J.: Transorbital approach to decompression in Graves' disease. Arch. Ophthalmol. 99:120–124, 1981.

Baylis, H., Cies, W., and Kamin, D.: Correction of upper lid retraction. Am. J. Ophthalmol. 82:790–794, 1976.

Callahan, A.: Levator recession with reattachment to the tarsus with collagen film. Arch. Ophthalmol. 73:800–802, 1965.

Chalfin, J. and Putterman, A.: Müller's muscle excision and levator palpebrae recession in the treatment of thyroid upper eyelid retraction. Arch. Ophthalmol. 97:1487, 1979.

Collins, W.: Dural fistulae and their repair. In Neurological Surgery. Vol. 2. Ed. by J. Homans. Philadelphia, W.B. Saunders, 1973, 981–992.

Crawford, J. and Easterbrook, M.: The use of bank sclera to correct lid retraction. Can. J. Ophthalmol. 11:304–309, 1976.

DeSanto, L. and Gorman, C.: Orbital decompression in Graves' ophthalmopathy. Laryngoscope 83:945, 1973.

Dixon, R., Anderson, R., and Hatt, M.: The use of thymoxamine in eyelid retraction. Arch. Ophthalmol. 97:2147–2150, 1979.

Dryden, R. and Soll, D.: The use of scleral transplantation in cicatricial entropion and eyelid retraction. Trans. Am. Acad. Ophthalmol. Otolaryngol. 72:755–764, 1977.

Golding-Wood, P.: Transantral ethmoid decompression in malignant exophthalmos. J. Laryngol. Otol. 83:683–694, 1969.

Goldstein, I.: Recession of the levator muscle for lagophthalmos in exophthalmic goiter. Arch. Ophthalmol. 11:389–393, 1934.

Grove, A. et al.: Symposium on orbital diseases. Ophthalmology 86:854–873, 1979.

Grove, A.: Levator lengthening by marginal myotomy. Arch. Ophthalmol. 98:1433–1438, 1980.

Grove, A.: Upper eyelid retraction in Graves' disease. Ophthalmology 88:499, 1981.

Harvey, J. and Anderson, R.: The aponeurotic approach to eyelid retraction. Ophthalmology 88:513–524, 1981.

Henderson, J.: Relief of eyelid retraction: a surgical procedure. Arch. Ophthalmol. 74:205–216, 1965.

Kennerdell, J. and Maroon, J.: An orbital decompression for severe dysthyroid exophthalmos. Ophthalmology 89:467–472, 1982.

Kohn, R.: Treatment of eyelid retraction with two pedicle tarsal rotation flaps. Am. J. Ophthalmol. 95:539–544, 1983.

Kriss, J.: Graves' ophthalmopathy: etiology and treatment. Hosp. Pract. 10:125–134, 1975.

Leone, C. and Banjandas, F.: Inferior orbital decompression for dysthyroid optic neuropathy. Ophthalmology 88:525, 1981.

Linberg, J. and Anderson, R.: Transorbital decompression: indications and results. Arch. Ophthalmol. 99:113–119, 1981.

McCord, C.: Antral ethmoidal decompression through the eyelid approach. Ophthalmic Surg. 8:102, 1977.

McCord, C.: Orbital decompression for Graves' disease. Ophthalmology. 88:533, 1981.

McCord, C.: Current trends in orbital decompression. Ophthalmology 92:21–33, 1985.

McDougall, I. and Kriss, J.: New thoughts about the cause and treatment of the severe ocular manifestations of Graves' disease. Scott. Med. J. 19:165–169, 1974.

Moriarty, P.: The management of Graves' ophthalmopathy by surgical decompression of the orbit. Trans. Ophthalmol. Soc. U.K. 102:501, 1982.

Ogura, J. and Lucente, F.: Surgical results of orbital decompression for malignant exopthalmos. Laryngoscope 84:637, 1974.

Putterman, A. and Urist, M.: Surgical treatment of upper eyelid retraction. Arch. Ophthalmol. 87:401, 1972.

Putterman, A. and Urist, M.: A simplified levator palpebrae superiorus muscle recession to treat overcorrected blepharoptosis. Am. J. Ophthalmol. 77:368, 1974.

Putterman A.: Surgical treatment of thyroid-related upper eyelid retraction: graded Müller's muscle excision and levator recession. Ophthalmology 88:507–512, 1981.

Riddick, F., et al.: Update on thyroid diseases. Ophthalmology 88:467–564, 1981.

Rosenbaum, A.: Adjustable rectus muscle recession surgery. Arch. Ophthalmol. 95:817–820, 1977.

Scott, W. and Thalacker, J.: Diagnosis and management of thyroid myopathy. Ophthalmology 88:493–498, 1970.

Sergott, R., Felberg, N., and Savino, P.: The clinical immunology of Graves' ophthalmopathy. Ophthalmology 88:484–487, 1981.

Sergott, R. and Glaser, J.: Graves' ophthalmopathy. A clinical and immunologic review. Surv. Ophthalmol. 26:1–21, 1981.

Shammas, J., Minckler, D., and Ogden, D.: Ultrasound in early thyroid orbitopathy. Arch. Ophthalmol. 98:277–279, 1980.

Solomon, D.: The Eye in Endocrine Diseases, Especially Graves' Ophthalmopathy. In Mausolf, F.: The Eye and Systemic Disease, Second Edition. St. Louis, C.V. Mosby Co., 1980, 448–471.

Skinner, S. and Miller, J.: Permanent improvement of thyroid-related upper eyelid retraction from bethanidine. Am. J. Ophthalmol. 67:764–766, 1969.

Surks, M.: Assessment of thyroid function. Ophthalmology 88:476–478, 1981.

Trobe, J., Glaser, J., and Laflamme, P.: Dysthyroid optic neuropathy. Arch. Ophthalmol. 96:1199–1209, 1978.

Trokel, S. and Hilal, S.: Recognition and differential diagnosis of enlarged extraocular muscles in computed tomography. Am. J. Ophthalmol. 87:503–512, 1979.

Volpe, R.: The pathogenesis of Graves' disease: an overview. Clin. Endocrinol. Metab. 7:3–30, 1978.

Waldstein, S., West, G., and Lee, W.: Guanethidine in Hyperthyroidism. JAMA 189:609–612, 1964.

Werner, S., Coleman, D., and Franzen, L.: Ultrasonographic evidence of a consistent orbital involvement in Graves' disease. N. Engl. J. Med. 290:1447, 1974.

Zakarija, M., McKenzie, J., and Banovac, K.: Clinical significance of assay of thyroid-stimulating antibody in Graves' disease. Ann. Intern. Med. 93:28–32, 1980.

7

ECTROPION

Ectropion is a common eyelid malposition in which the eyelid is everted from its normal apposition to the globe (Fig. 7–1). The lower eyelid is involved much more frequently than the upper because of its more rudimentary tarsal support and gravitational factors.

Ocular changes resulting from ectropion may include cosmetic abnormalities, conjunctival inflammation, hypertrophy and keratinization, exposure keratopathy, and epiphora. Most cases are slowly progressive. Over time, this may result in a metaplasia of conjunctival goblet cells into stratified squamous epithelium with keratinization. Exposure-induced keratopathy may range from punctate staining and erosion to ulceration and perforation. Epiphora is a common and sometimes protective feature in ectropion. The lacrimal lacus is no longer in apposition to the punctum, and the punctum may additionally become stenotic from exposure-induced xerosis. When ectropion is present, punctal stenosis may increase tear retention on the globe and diminish corneal desiccation.

Subgroups in decreasing order of frequency include: involutional, cicatricial, mixed mechanism (involutional and cicatricial), punctal, paralytic, mechanical, and congenital.

Proper evaluation of ectropion should include a complete medical and ocular history, with particular reference to related trauma, previous ocular or adnexal surgery, burns, chronic skin diseases, epiphora, corneal irritation from exposure, and related loss of vision. A complete ophthalmic examination should be directed toward determining the etiologic subgroup; this dictates

proper management. The suspected etiology can be confirmed by simulating the surgically corrected eyelid position. Evaluation of the patient in an upright position discloses the full extent of eversion.

INVOLUTIONAL ECTROPION

The most frequent ectropion, involutional, characteristically occurs in older individuals and often presents with coexistent punctal ectropion and associated epiphora. This malposition arises from an orbital-tarsal disparity created by stretching and relaxing of the posterior (tarso-conjunctival) lamella. Weakness of the inferior eyelid retractors and the pretarsal portion of the orbicularis oculi muscle may coexist. These factors cause the eyelid to elongate and become unstable, sagging away from its normal position of intimate contact with the globe.

Various horizontal eyelid-shortening procedures have been used for this disorder. The classic Kuhnt-Szymanowski procedure was modified by Byron Smith to avoid such problems as unnecessary eyelid splitting, loss of lashes, and irregularities of the eyelid margin.

Smith Modification of the Kuhnt-Szymanowski Procedure. Following infiltration of local anesthetic, an infralash incision is placed extending from a position just lateral to the punctum to a position just lateral to the outer canthus (Fig. 7–2A). As the canthus is approached, the incision tapers in an inferotemporal direction. With this incision, a skin-muscle flap is undermined and mobilized temporally.

A pentagon-shaped segment is excised from the posterior lamella (containing the eyelid margin) (Fig. 7–2B). The extent of excision is dictated by the extent of horizontal laxity.

The posterior lamella is closed with three 5-0 silk sutures placed at the anterior, central, and posterior eyelid margin. The anterior lamella (skin-muscle flap) is pulled temporally, defining a redundant triangle by the extent of tissue overlap (Fig. 7–2C). This redundant tissue is excised and this layer is closed with running 7-0 silk

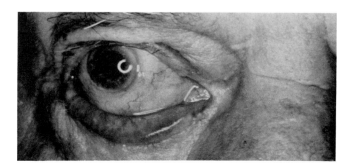

FIG. 7–1. Moderate ectropion of the right lower eyelid.

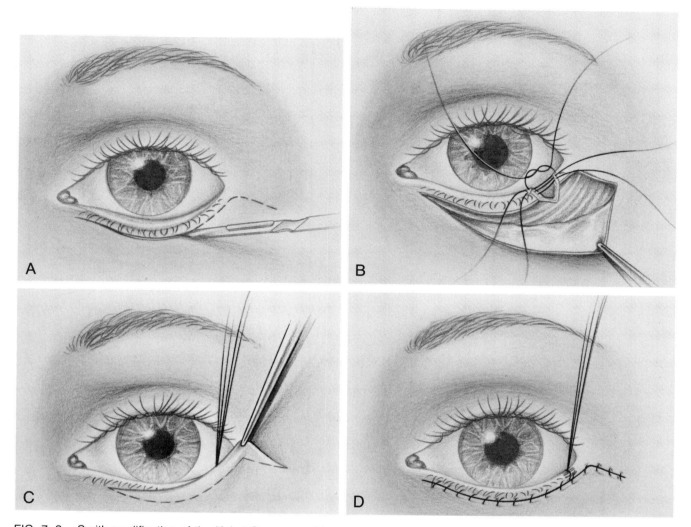

FIG. 7–2. Smith modification of the Kuhnt-Szymanowski procedure. A, Placement of infralash incision. B, Posterior lamella and eyelid margin excised in pentagonal manner. C, Anterior lamella pulled temporally, defining redundant tissue by the extent of overlap. D, Skin closure with running 7-0 silk sutures.

sutures (Fig. 7–2D). The skin sutures may be removed 6 days postoperatively, but the eyelid margin sutures should remain for 10 days.

Although a useful procedure, even the Smith modification has limitations because it involves unnecessary formation of skin flaps. For this reason, full-thickness horizontal eyelid shortening is recommended. This is best exemplified in the Bick procedure and the pentagonal full-thickness excision ("inverted house"). The choice of procedure depends on the extent of ectropion and the location of maximum eversion. The Bick procedure is most appropriate for the more common lateral ectropion, while the pentagonal excision is most appropriate for central or medial ectropion.

Bick Procedure. Using a marking pen, a line is drawn as an inferolateral extension of the upper eyelid on the lateral aspect of the lower eyelid (Fig. 7–3A). Local anesthetic is infiltrated subjacent to this, extending to the lateral orbital rim. According to this line, a full-thickness incision is made with Stevens scissors. The inferior crus of the lateral canthal tendon must be completely severed to maximally mobilize the eyelid and to ensure an optimal result. Once the crus has been severed, the lower eyelid is pulled laterally, overlapping the outer canthus. The degree of tissue overlap determines the extent of full-thickness eyelid excision (Fig. 7–3B). The redundant triangle is then excised.

The outer canthus is reconstructed with two 4-0 silk

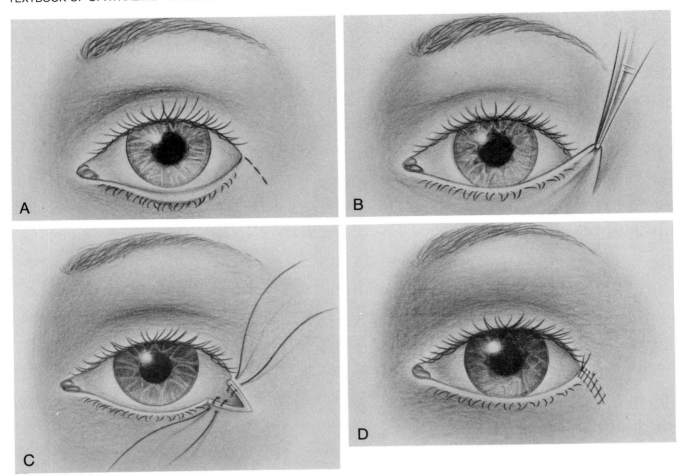

FIG. 7–3. Bick procedure. A, Skin incision line is an inferolateral extension of the upper eyelid upon the lateral aspect of the lower eyelid. B, Once the inferior crus of the lateral canthal tendon has been excised, the extent of full-thickness eyelid excision is defined by the degree of tissue overlap. C, Inferior crus of the lateral canthal tendon is reconstructed with two 4-0 silk sutures, engaging the lateral canthal tendon and periosteum at the lateral orbital rim, respectively. D, After closing tarsus with 6-0 Vicryl, the skin is closed with running 7-0 silk.

sutures designed to recreate the inferior crus of the lateral canthal tendon (Fig. 7–3C). The first suture joins the skin and tarsus at the superior lateral portion of the eyelid to the remainder of the lateral canthal tendon and its overlying skin. The second suture is placed inferior to the first, joining skin and tarsus to periosteum at the lateral orbital rim and its overlying skin. Tarsus is united to equivalent tissue laterally with 6-0 Vicryl followed by skin closure with running 7-0 silk (Fig. 7–3D). The skin sutures may be removed 6 days postoperatively but the two 4-0 silk sutures should remain for 10 days.

Pentagonal Excision. Two sides of a pentagon are marked with a marking pen in the position of maximum eversion (Fig. 7–4A). After infiltration of local anesthetic, sharp Stevens scissors are used to make an incision according to these lines. The amount of tissue to be excised is dictated by the extent of horizontal laxity (Fig. 7–4B). The remaining sides are next incised, and the result is a full-thickness pentagonal excision, which should not encroach upon the punctum or canaliculus.

The eyelid is reconstructed with three 4-0 or 5-0 silk sutures placed at the anterior, central, and posterior eyelid margins (Fig. 7–4C). Each suture should penetrate 2 mm deep into the tarsus and emerge 2 mm from each cut edge of the eyelid margin. Each suture should engage the anterior, central, and posterior aspects of the tarsal plate, respectively. The anterior suture should be placed carefully to avoid damage to the nearby eyelash follicles. As each of these sutures is placed, it should be tied

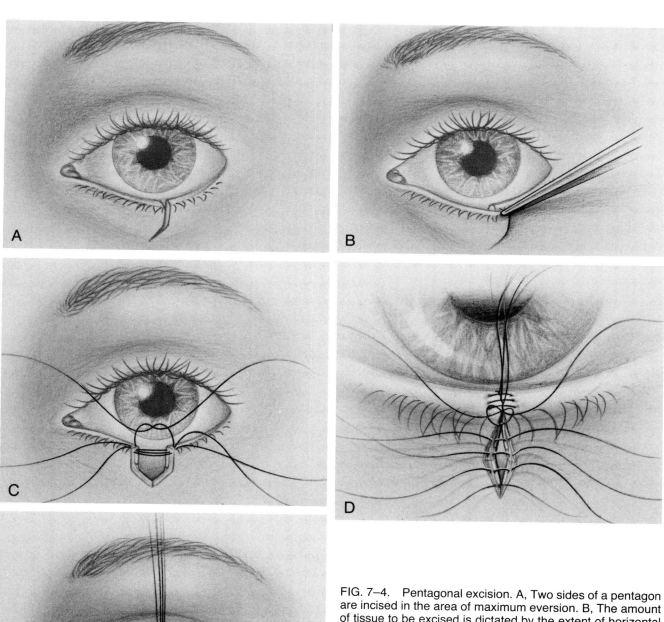

FIG. 7–4. Pentagonal excision. A, Two sides of a pentagon are incised in the area of maximum eversion. B, The amount of tissue to be excised is dictated by the extent of horizontal laxity. C, Eyelid margin is reconstructed with three 4-0 or 5-0 silk sutures. D, Magnified view of eyelid margin closure. Tarsus is approximated with 6-0 Vicryl sutures. E, Eyelid margin sutures may be placed under mild traction for 10 days, secured with tincture of benzoin and ¼-inch Steri-strips. This minimizes any tendency toward subsequent notching.

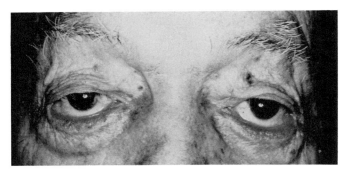

FIG. 7–5. Characteristic appearance of idiopathic cicatricial ectropion.

temporarily with a slip knot to determine the accuracy of apposition. Any suture that does not achieve optimal approximation should be replaced. To allow access to tissue, the sutures are permanently tied only after all three have been placed. The posterior sutures should be tied first and then tunneled underneath the anterior suture, which is tied last. This minimizes corneal epithelial disruption by the eyelid margin suture line. These sutures should be left long and secured to the opposing cheek or brow respectively to minimize postoperative notching tendency. Steri-strips and tincture of benzoin can be used to anchor these sutures. The tarsus is then approximated with 6-0 Vicryl mattress sutures (Fig. 7–4D) followed by skin closure with 7-0 silk. The skin sutures may be removed 6 days postoperatively but the eyelid margin sutures should remain under mild traction for 10 days (Fig. 7–4E).

CICATRICIAL ECTROPION

Idiopathic cicatricial ectropion characteristically occurs in fair-skinned individuals who often relate a history of frequent sun exposure (Fig. 7–5). It also may arise secondary to such underlying processes as trauma, previous eyelid surgery (Fig. 7–6), burns (thermal, radiation, or chemical), infections, chronic dermatitis (eczema, ichthyosis [Fig. 7–7], epidermolysis bullosa), or acute allergic dermatitis. The common denominator in these conditions is cicatrization, which causes vertical contracture in the anterior (skin-orbicularis) lamella. Cicatricial ectropion affects the lower eyelid more frequently because of its more rudimentary tarsal support.

While several cicatricial ectropions of dermatologic origin can be effectively managed with topical steroids, the remainder, like the other categories of cicatrical ectropion, must be surgically corrected. Unless emergent, surgical correction for such conditions should be deferred 6 to 12 months from the time the underlying process was stabilized to achieve optimal results. While the patient is awaiting surgery, the globe can be protected with lubricating ointment and drops, along with a moisture chamber and humidification.

The occasional circumscribed case (Fig. 7–8) can be managed with either Z-plasty, V- to Y-plasty, or pedicle transposition flaps (as covered in Chapter 2). Other cases require excision of scar tissue and placement of a free full-thickness skin graft.

Full-Thickness Skin Grafting—Recipient Bed. In the full-thickness skin graft procedure, two modified Frost sutures are placed at the eyelid margin to afford upward traction (Fig. 7–9A). An infralash incision is carried through the layer of scar tissue (usually superficial to the orbital septum) by sharp and blunt dissection. Fibrotic bands encountered should be lysed and all scar tissue excised until the eyelid margin assumes a normal position (Fig. 7–9B). The resultant elliptical cutaneous defect will then be covered by a full-thickness skin graft (Figs. 7–9C and D). Donor sites in descending order of preference include upper eyelid, retroauricular, supraclavicular, and upper-inner arm skin. Although the upper eyelid provides the best tissue match, it is not uniformly useful because it is often coexistently foreshortened and, if used, additionally requires a contralateral upper blepharoplasty to achieve postoperative upper eyelid symmetry. Retroauricular full-thickness skin grafts are therefore commonly used.

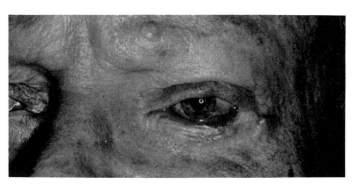

FIG. 7–6. Secondary cicatricial ectropion from prior removal of a basal cell carcinoma from the left lower eyelid.

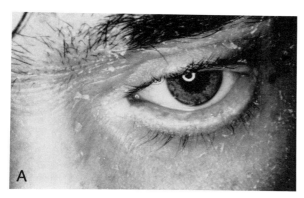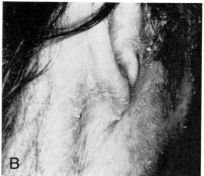

FIG. 7–7.   A, Secondary cicatricial ectropion from ichthyosis. B, Potential retroauricular donor site is composed entirely of ichthyotic skin.

Full-Thickness Skin Grafting—Donor Site. Once the donor site has been selected (Figs. 7–10A and B), it should be marked with methylene blue 25% larger than a template taken from the recipient bed (Fig. 7–10C). This allows for the expected contracture of the graft postoperatively. If a retroauricular site is chosen, exposure of the donor area is enhanced by placing a suture between the pinna and preauricular tissue, temporarily retracting the ear forward. The donor site should not involve any hair-bearing tissue. Lidocaine (Xylocaine) should be infiltrated subcutaneously to tense the donor site, thereby facilitating graft removal (Fig. 7–10D). An incision with a #64 Beaver blade according to the marked lines defines the extent of the donor tissue. The graft is removed by blunt and sharp dissection with Stevens scissors (Fig. 7–10E). The suture holding the pinna forward is released and the donor area is then closed with interrupted 4-0 silk. The graft should be defatted to the level of the rete pegs and horizontally fenestrated (Fig. 7–10F). It is then placed in the recipient bed, conservatively trimmed to proper size, and sutured with running 7-0 silk (Fig. 7–9C). Suturing is sometimes facilitated by

initially securing four corners with interrupted 6-0 silk. Careful hemostasis in the recipient bed is essential.

The postoperative dressing is important in maximizing apposition of this free skin graft to its recipient bed and blood supply (Fig. 7–9D). Several 4-0 silk-modified Frost sutures placed under stretch will avoid graft infolding and maximize apposition. These traction sutures can be taped to the brow when the lower eyelid is grafted or taped to the cheek when the upper eyelid is grafted. The graft is covered with antibiotic ointment and Telfa wicks soaked in an antibiotic solution. This is further covered by an eyepad and fluff dressing and secured with Elastoplast supported by tincture of benzoin. Left in place for 36 hours, this dressing enhances juxtaposition of the graft to its recipient bed and minimizes the likelihood of infection. An alternative approach using long 4-0 silk sutures tied over a "bolster" is less efficacious. This tends to elevate the edges of the graft, sometimes permanently.

The entire dressing is removed 36 to 48 hours postoperatively. Keeping the original dressing beyond this point does not appreciably align the graft to its recipient bed and may predispose to infection. The traction sutures may be removed anywhere from 2 to 10 days postoperatively depending upon the severity of the underlying cicatricial process. All other skin sutures are removed at 6 days. During the first 48 hours postoperatively, the skin graft appears white. By 72 hours, it takes on a pink hue, transiently more intense than the surrounding tissue. Within several weeks, the grafted area becomes relatively indistinguishable from the adjacent skin (Fig. 7–11).

Any appreciable blood accumulation beneath the graft should be rapidly evacuated, with cautery applied to discernible bleeding sites. Any intercurrent infection is heralded by a purulent discharge. This should be treated by topical and systemic antibiotics as dictated by culture

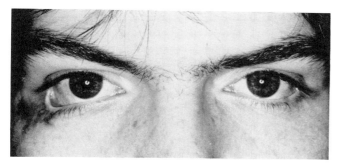

FIG. 7–8.   This focal case of cicatricial ectropion would be perfect for either Z-plasty or V- to Y-plasty correction.

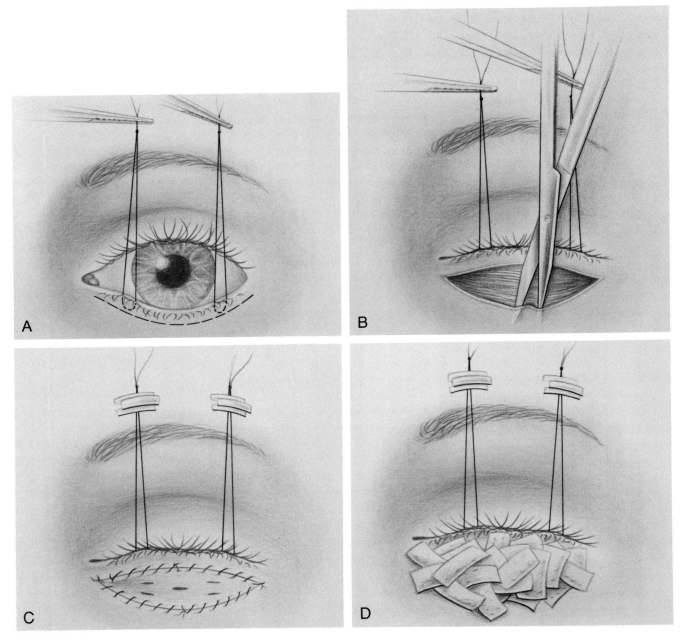

FIG. 7–9. Repair of cicatricial ectropion with full-thickness skin graft. A, Two modified Frost sutures are placed at the eyelid margin. An infralash incision is then made. B, The incision is carried through the layer of scar tissue and fibrotic bands by sharp and blunt dissection. C, Donor full-thickness skin graft is fenestrated and placed in the recipient bed. It is conservatively trimmed and then secured with running 7-0 silk. D, Postoperative dressing consists of Telfa wicks (shown here), eyepad, fluff dressing, Elastoplast, supported by tincture of benzoin, and Steri-strips.

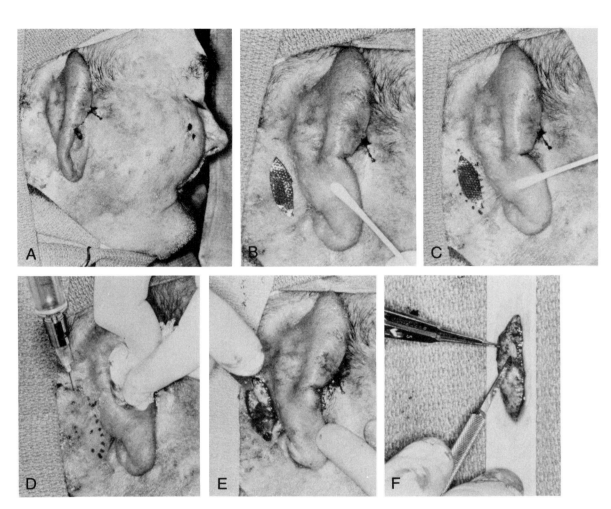

FIG. 7–10. A, Retroauricular area selected as donor site for retroauricular full-thickness free skin graft. B, Template from recipient bed placed over retroauricular donor site. C, Donor site marked 25% larger than template. D, Local anesthetic infiltrated subcutaneously to tense the donor site. E, Graft is removed by blunt and sharp dissection with Stevens scissors. F, The graft is defatted and horizontally fenestrated before placement in the recipient bed.

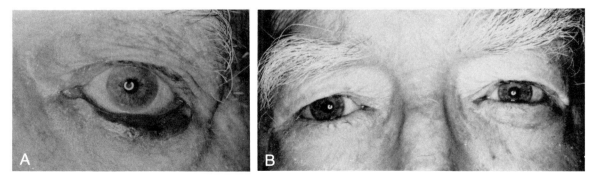

FIG. 7–11. A, Cicatricial ectropion before surgical repair. B, Cicatricial ectropion 6 weeks after placement of a full-thickness retroauricular skin graft.

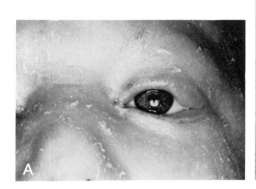
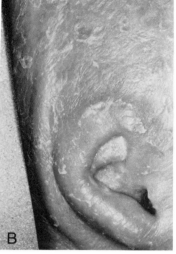
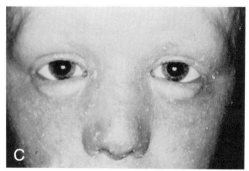

FIG. 7–12. A, Cicatricial ectropion from ichthyosis. B, Retroauricular donor site composed entirely of ichthyotic skin. C, Six weeks after placement of a full-thickness retroauricular skin graft. This graft was fashioned 50% larger than the recipient bed due to the ichthyosis.

and sensitivity studies. If ectropion recurs postoperatively, further scar excision and grafting are required, and the factors that led to the recurrence must be taken into consideration.

When the cicatricial process is severe (ichthyosis, burns), or recurrent, the graft should be 50% larger than its recipient bed (Fig. 7–12). Additionally, intermarginal adhesions can be placed for two months or longer to minimize postoperative shrinkage. Some grafts may form keloids that later require steroidal infiltration to minimize this process.

MIXED MECHANISM ECTROPION

In this category, long-standing cicatrization elongates the posterior lamella, resulting in an additional involu-

tional factor. If either the cicatricial or involutional element predominates, that cause alone can be surgically corrected (Fig. 7–13). Otherwise, these cases require a combined procedure. Horizontal eyelid shortening should precede full-thickness skin grafting to minimize the length of graft required.

PUNCTAL ECTROPION

Punctal ectropion (Fig. 7–14A) may be either isolated or secondary to any of the other ectropion subgroups. These patients demonstrate epiphora and often develop punctal stenosis. This is one of the most difficult categories of ectropion to repair satisfactorily.

Tarsoconjunctival Spindle Excision. Mild cases may be

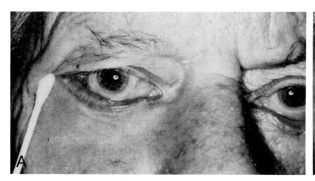
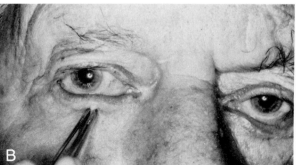

FIG. 7–13. Ectropion testing for, A, involutional component or, B, cicatricial component. In this case, the cicatricial component predominates.

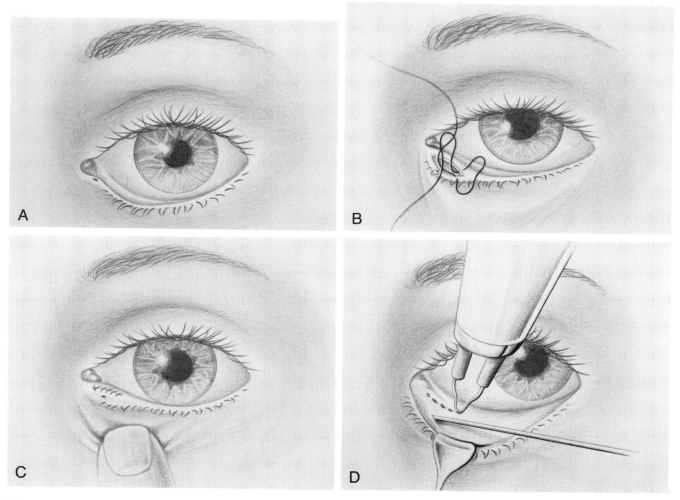

FIG. 7–14. A, Punctal ectropion. B, Tarsoconjunctival spindle excision and closure with 6-0 chromic catgut sutures. C, After spindle excision, the punctum should return to its normal position of apposition to the globe. D, Ziegler cautery may help cases more resistant to internal rotation.

managed by simply everting the eyelid, excising an infracanalicular spindle of tarsoconjunctival tissue parallel to the eyelid margin, and closing it with interrupted 6-0 chromic sutures (Fig. 7–14B). The spindle is placed 2 mm below the horizontal canaliculus with its center directly below the punctum. This should invert the malpositioned punctum and restore apposition to the globe (Fig. 7–14C).

In more severe cases, Ziegler cautery (Fig. 7–14D) and medial intermarginal adhesions may also be required. The most severe cases involve horizontal laxity and require Byron Smith's "lazy T" operation.

Lazy T Procedure. This procedure combines the infracanalicular tarsoconjunctival spindle excision with pentagonal horizontal eyelid shortening (Fig. 7–15A). The

latter must be performed just lateral to the punctum to achieve maximum effect (Fig. 7–15B). The merger of these two procedures appears as a T tilted on its side when viewed from the posterior aspect of the eyelid (Fig. 7–15C).

In all these procedures, canalicular protection is essential. If associated punctal stenosis is present, a one-snip procedure and placement of a Quickert-Dryden tube may restore lacrimal drainage (see Chapter 13).

PARALYTIC ECTROPION

This group characteristically presents as a flaccid ectropion accentuated laterally by the pull of atonic facial muscles (Fig. 7–16). The associated widened palpebral

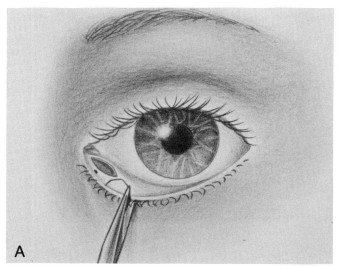

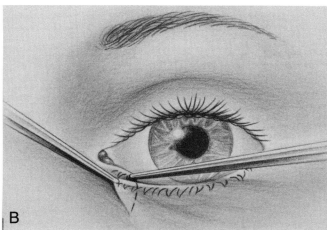

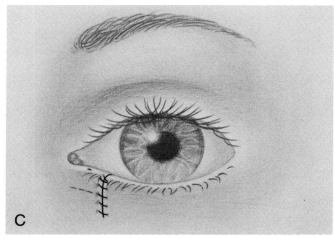

FIG. 7–15. Lazy T procedure. A, This procedure combines the infracanalicular tarsoconjunctival spindle excision with pentagonal horizontal eyelid shortening. B, Horizontal shortening is performed just lateral to the punctum. C, The juxtaposition of these two procedures produces a T configuration tilted on its side.

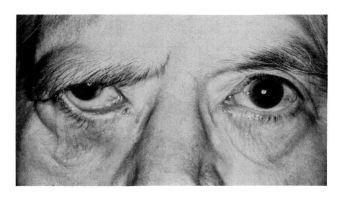

FIG. 7–16. Paralytic ectropion of the right lower eyelid resulting from right-sided peripheral VII nerve paralysis.

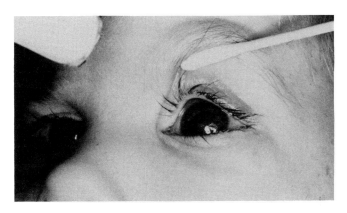

FIG. 7–17. Central corneal erosion from paralytic ectropion.

fissure, decreased lacrimal pump, and punctal malposition may cause epiphora and various degrees of exposure keratopathy (Fig. 7–17). Paralytic ectropion is caused by seventh-nerve dysfunction and can be self-limiting, as in most cases of idiopathic Bell's palsy, or permanent, as in trauma, parotid gland neoplasm, acoustic neuroma, stroke, or surgically related nerve damage.

In cases thought to be self-limiting, nonsurgical supportive measures such as artificial tears (lubricating drops and ointments), soft contact lenses, careful nocturnal patching, or a moisture chamber (Fig. 7–18) may prove useful. Sleeping close to a humidifier may be additionally helpful. The moisture chamber concept can be achieved in young children by placement of interlaced 4-0 silk modified Frost sutures to create temporary complete eyelid closure (Fig. 7–19). This suture technique can also be used intercurrently to inhibit the ulceration of a corneal erosion. When closure of longer duration is desired, lateral intermarginal adhesions should be considered. This involves denuding the opposing eyelid's posterior margins and joining them with 4-0 silk mattress sutures. These sutures are removed 2 weeks later. If nerve function returns, the adhesion can be severed, restoring the eyelid margins to their normal state.

Permanent cases of paralytic ectropion necessitate a more permanent surgical solution. Either Bick horizontal eyelid shortening or permanent lateral canthoplasty may fulfill this need. The former technique yields a more satisfactory cosmetic result. Patients should be examined intraoperatively in a sitting position to determine the extent of ectropion (Fig. 7–20); as the size of these procedures can be titrated to achieve the desired corneal coverage.

Lateral Canthoplasty. A lateral canthoplasty can be achieved by placing a "tongue" of lower eyelid tarsus into an upper eyelid tarsal groove. In this approach, local anesthesia infiltrates the lateral aspect of the upper and lower eyelid margins. With Stevens scissors, the lateral 5 mm portions of these eyelids are separated at the central gray line into anterior (skin-muscle) and posterior (tarsoconjunctival) lamellae. The marginal borders of these lamellae are excised. A 4 mm vertical incision is made through the posterior lamella at the medial aspect of the lower eyelid incision (Fig. 7–21A). This achieves upward mobilization of a "tongue" of tarsus. An analogous triangular segment of the posterior lamella of the upper eyelid incision is excised. The tarsal "tongue and groove" are then united with 5-0 Vicryl mattress sutures (Fig. 7–21B). If a permanent result is desired, the lateral lash margins may also be excised and united with 6-0 silk sutures. If a temporary result is desired, the lash margin should remain (Fig. 7–21C).

The Morel-Fatio spring and Arion prosthesis are not generally recommended due to frequent complications (infection, eyelid erosion (Fig. 7–22), blepharoptosis, ectropion), although the latter may be useful in selected cases because it imitates the action of a contracting orbicularis oculi muscle.

Arion Prosthesis. In this technique, after local anesthetic infiltration a somewhat curved vertical incision is made overlying the medial canthal tendon. The superficial head of this tendon is isolated, carefully protecting the subjacent lacrimal sac. A horizontal incision is made overlying the lateral orbital rim just lateral to the outer canthus (Fig. 7–23A). The insertion of the lateral canthal tendon into the lateral orbital tubercle is exposed.

The Silastic rod (Arion prosthesis) should be soaked in an antibiotic solution before placement. With a small needle, the rod is passed through the superficial head of the medial canthal tendon (Fig. 7–23B). A Wright needle is then passed in each eyelid horizontally from the lateral to the medial incision site (Fig. 7–23C). Each passage

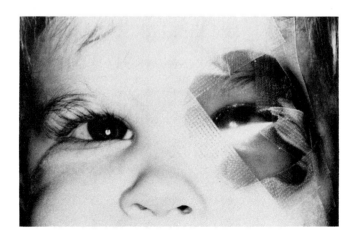

FIG. 7–18. A moisture chamber, composed of x-ray film cut into a circle and fashioned into a conical configuration, is set over this patient's left eye.

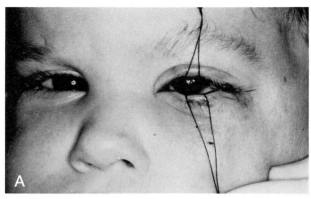

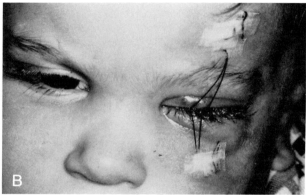

FIG. 7–19. Suture moisture chamber. A, Two 4-0 silk-modified Frost sutures are placed and tied long. B, The sutures are interlaced and secured to the cheek and brow respectively with ¼-inch Steri-strips and supported by tincture of benzoin.

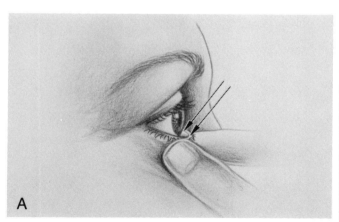

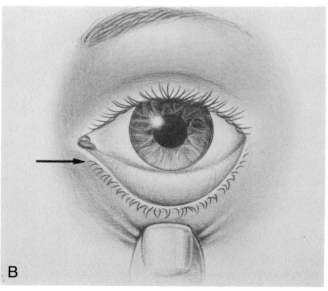

FIG. 7–20. A and B, The extent of ectropion and laxity should be evaluated in two planes.

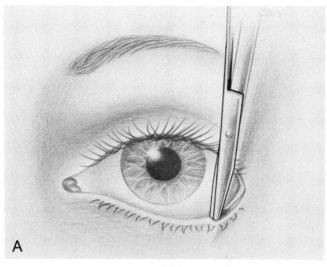

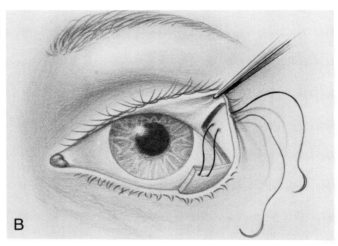

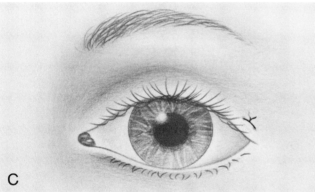

FIG. 7–21. Lateral canthoplasty. A, After separation of the lateral portion of the upper and lower eyelid margins, the marginal borders of the posterior lamella are excised. A 4-mm vertical incision is made through the posterior lamella of the lower eyelid incision. B, A tongue of tarsus is fashioned from the lower eyelid incision. An analogous groove is excised from the upper eyelid incision. The "tongue and groove" are united with 5-0 Vicryl mattress sutures. C, The resultant canthoplasty can be either temporary or permanent.

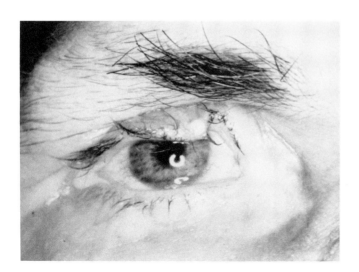

FIG. 7–22. Upper eyelid contour abnormality induced by partial erosion of eyelid tissue by a Morel-Fatio spring.

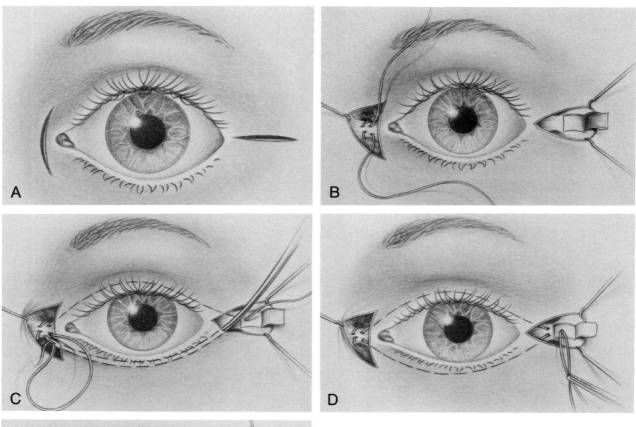

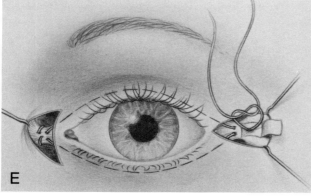

FIG. 7–23. Arion prosthesis. A, Vertical incision is made over-lying the medial canthal tendon, while a horizontal incision is made overlying the lateral orbital rim. B, Following deeper dis-section, a Silastic rod (Arion prosthesis) is passed through the superficial head of the medial canthal tendon. Periosteum is elevated anterior to the lateral orbital tubercle. C, A Wright needle may be used to extend the Silastic rod within the epitarsal space to the lateral orbital rim. D, The two ends of the rod are adjusted to proper tension at the junction of the lateral canthal tendon with the lateral orbital tubercle. E, The rod ends are tied in a slightly overcorrected position. 4-0 Mersilene sutures may give additional support.

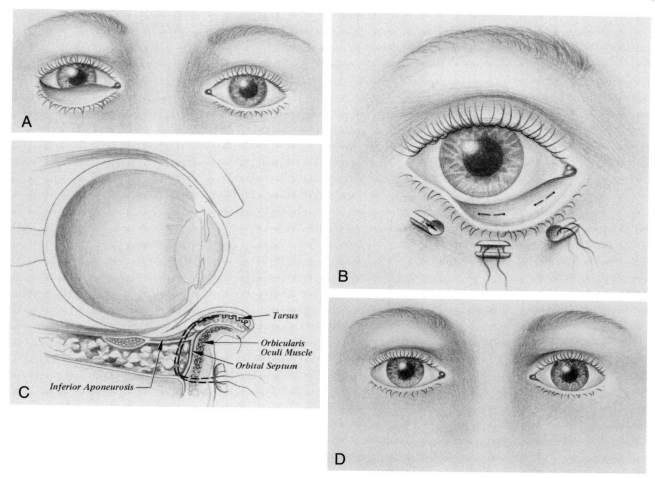

FIG. 7–24. Mechanical ectropion. A, Mechanical ectropion may arise from gravitational and other physical forces on the lower eyelid. B, Placement of three tarsal rotation sutures. C, Each suture passes through the conjunctiva into the base of tarsus. After replacing swaged-on needles with trochar 5 needles, each suture is passed vertically in a backhand manner, engaging inferior aponeurosis, septum, and periosteum at the infraorbital rim. The sutures emerge through lower eyelid skin and are tied over rubber bolsters titrating the tension on the knot. D, The sutures can be removed 6 to 8 weeks postoperatively.

should be in the epitarsal space 2 to 3 mm from the eyelid margin, emerging at the medial incision site. After each passage, the corresponding portion of the silastic rod is placed through the lumen of the Wright needle and becomes properly positioned as the needle is subsequently withdrawn. Both ends of the rod are secured under proper tension with 4-0 Mersilene sutures at the junction of the lateral canthal tendon with the lateral orbital tubercle (Fig. 7–23D). If this anchorage proves insufficient, securing the rod ends to a burr hole at the lateral orbital rim may provide additional support. The Silastic should be secured (Fig. 7–23E) in a slightly overcorrected position because it will stretch and migrate

somewhat toward the eyelid margins over time, thereby diminishing the result. Before closing, the rod should again be irrigated with an antibiotic solution. The skin incisions are closed with running 7-0 silk sutures.

The Arion prosthesis is predisposed to persistent infection or extrusion because it is an alloplastic foreign body implanted under some tension. Should either contingency arise, the rod should be surgically removed.

Cases with upper eyelid retraction from levator palpebrae superiorus action unopposed by a paralytic orbicularis oculi muscle may benefit additionally from levator recession surgery (see Chapter 6).

In paralytic ectropion, undercorrections are more

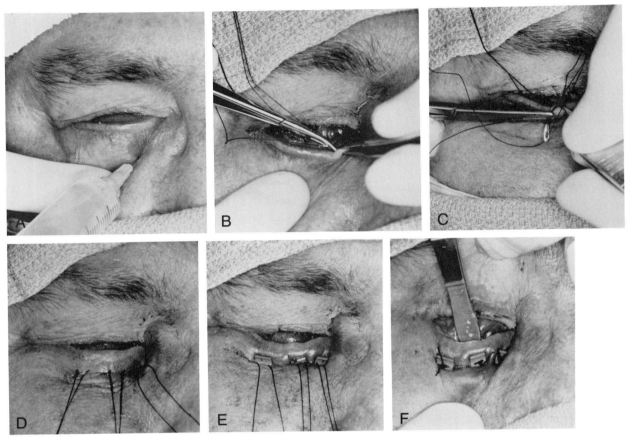

FIG. 7–25. Placement of tarsal rotation sutures. A, Local anesthesia by infraorbital nerve block. B, Swaged-on needle engaging the tarsal base. C, Trochar 5 needle used in a backhanded manner for deeper passage. D, Appearance after emergence of sutures through the skin. E, Placement of bolsters over the sutures. F, Once the sutures are tied, the ectropion resolves. Note the depth of the newly created lower fornix.

common than overcorrections; therefore optimum elevation should be the surgical goal. After surgery, these patients may still benefit from the supportive measures previously described.

MECHANICAL ECTROPION

Mechanical ectropion arises from gravitational and other physical forces exerted on the lower eyelid (Fig. 7–24A). Such forces may be intrinsic, such as eyelid tumors, inflammatory processes, or fluid accumulation (from sinus, thyroid, cardiac, or renal disorders), or extrinsic, such as proptosis or buphthalmos. If the ectropion is

chronic, it may persist despite elimination of its causal factors.

Residual mechanical ectropion can be managed effectively by placing tarsal rotation sutures. Three 4-0 sutures are passed symmetrically through conjunctiva into the base of the tarsus (Fig. 7–24B). After the swaged-on needles are replaced with Trochar 5 needles, each suture end is passed vertically, engaging inferior aponeurosis, septum, and periosteum at the infraorbital rim before emerging through lower eyelid skin. This passage should be in a backhanded manner to ensure that the needle passage does not come near the globe (Fig. 7–24C). The sutures are then tied over rubber bolsters, with tension dictated by the desired degree of eyelid rotation. After 6 to 8 weeks, a plane of cicatrization is established. The

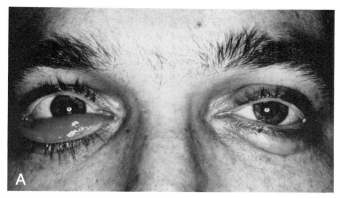

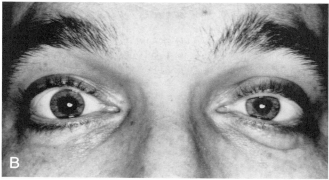

FIG. 7–26.   A, Mechanical ectropion of the right lower eyelid. B, Appearance 6 months after placement of temporary tarsal rotation sutures in the right lower eyelid.

sutures can then be removed without return of ectropion (Figs. 7–24D, 7–25, 7–26).

CONGENITAL ECTROPION

This exceedingly rare condition is reviewed in detail in Chapter 3.

BIBLIOGRAPHY

Arion, H.: Dynamic closure of the lids in paralysis of the orbicularis muscle. Int. Surg. 57:48–50, 1972.

Bick, M.: Surgical management of orbital tarsal disparity,. Arch. Ophthalmol. 75:386–389, 1966.

Callahan, A.: Reconstructive Surgery of the Eyelids and Ocular Adnexa. Birmingham, Aesculapius, 1966, 140–157.

Hamako, C, and Baylis, H.: Lower eyelid retraction after blepharoplasty. Am. J. Ophthalmol. 89:517, 1980.

Jones, L., and Wobig, J.: Surgery of the eyelids and Lacrimal System. Birmingham, Aesculapius, 1976.

Kohn, R.: Mechanical ectropion repair using tarsal rotation sutures. Ophthalmic Surg. 10:48, 1979.

Lee, O.: An operation for the correction of everted lacrimal puncta. Am. J. Ophthalmol. 34:575, 1951.

Leone, C.: Repair of ectropion using the Bick procedure. Am. J. Ophthalmol. 70:233, 1970.

Morel-Fatio, D, and Lalardrie, J.: Palliative surgical treatment of facial paralysis. The Palpebral Spring. Plast. Reconstr. Surg., 33:446, 1964.

Reeh, M., and Beyer, C., Shannon, G.: Practical Ophthalmic Plastic and Reconstructive Surgery. Philadelphia, Lea and Febiger, 1976, 123–132.

Smith, B., and Cherubini, T.: Oculoplastic Surgery. St. Louis, C.V. Mosby, 1970, 92–94.

Smith, B.: The "lazy T" correction of ectropion of the lower punctum. Arch. Ophthalmol., 94:1149, 1976.

Soll, D.: Management of Complications in Ophthalmic Plastic Surgery. Birmingham, Aesculapius, 1976, pp. 168–206.

Tenzel, R., Buffam, F., and Miller, G.: The use of the lateral canthal sling in ectropion repair. Can. J. Ophthalmol. 12:199–202, 1977.

Wood-Smith, D., and Guy, C.: Experience with the Arion Type Prosthesis of the Orbit. In Tessier, P., Callahan, A., Mustarde, J., Sayler, K. (eds.): Symposium on Plastic Surgery in the Orbital Region. St. Louis, Mosby, 1976.

8

ENTROPION

Entropion is another common eyelid malposition in which the eyelid is inverted, placing the cilia and eyelid margin in apposition to the globe (Fig. 8–1). The juxtaposition of stratified squamous cutaneous epithelium is the greatest hazard because it presents a recurring source of corneal epithelial disruption. The lower eyelid is involved much more frequently than the upper because of its more rudimentary tarsal support.

Subgroups in decreasing order of frequency include involutional, cicatricial, and congenital.

Proper evaluation of entropion should include a complete medical and ocular history with particular reference to related trauma, previous ocular or adnexal surgery, burns, corneal dysfunction, ocular pemphigoid (Fig. 8–2), Stevens-Johnson syndrome, chlamydial infection, and related loss of vision. A complete ophthalmic examination should be directed toward determining the etiologic subgroup to dictate proper management.

INVOLUTIONAL ENTROPION

Involutional entropion is the most common form and occurs only in the lower eyelid. Entropion is the product of eyelid margin instability resulting from several age-related factors, which may occur alone or in combination. These factors include: (1) horizontal laxity of the lower eyelid, (2) laxity of the inferior eyelid retractors, (3) overriding of the preseptal segment of the orbicularis oculi muscle upon the pretarsal segment, (4) laxity of the orbital septum, (5) atrophy and herniation of orbital fat resulting in a relative enophthalmos.

As the patient blinks, the lower eyelid elevates and the lower tarsal border moves away from the globe, causing intortion of the eyelid margin. The resultant foreign body sensation triggers further contraction of the orbicularis oculi muscle, which accentuates this process. Patients with involutional entropion also demonstrate lower eyelid retraction on downgaze.

The most effective operation for involutional entropion was devised by Jones, Reeh, and Wobig (Fig. 8–3). It anatomically corrects three of the causal factors by shortening (tucking) the inferior aponeurosis (lower eyelid retractor), tightening the orbital septum, and removing the overriding segment of preseptal orbicularis oculi muscle.

Shortening of the Lower Eyelid Retractors (Tuck of the Inferior Aponeurosis). The area of the intended incision

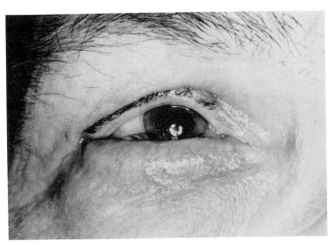

FIG. 8–1. Characteristic appearance of lower eyelid involutional entropion.

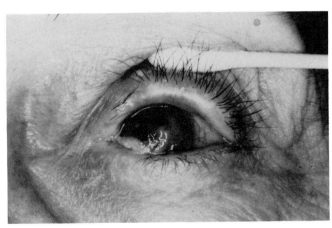

FIG. 8–2. Cicatricial entropion with symblepharon secondary to ocular pemphigoid.

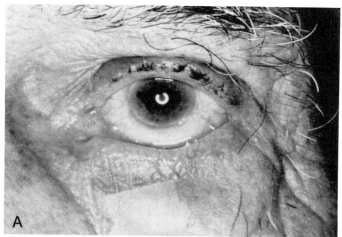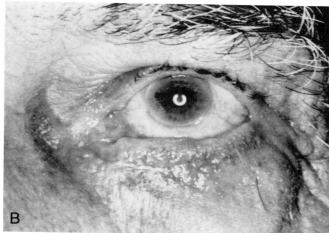

FIG. 8–3. A, Involutional entropion of the lower eyelid taped preoperatively to provide temporary symptomatic relief. B, The same patient 6 weeks after entropion repair using the tuck of the inferior aponeurosis (technique of Jones, Reeh, and Wobig).

is delineated with a marking pen. The mark is placed horizontally 4 to 5 mm below the eyelid margin, extending from a position just lateral to the vertical extension of the punctum to a position directly below the outer canthus. Subjacent to this, local anesthetic is infiltrated.

According to this line, an incision is made with a #64 Beaver blade (Fig. 8–4A). The medial third of the lower eyelid is not incised, preserving the "lacrimal pump" mechanism. This incision is extended to the lower tarsal border by blunt and sharp dissection with Stevens scissors. The uppermost 4 mm of preseptal orbicularis oculi muscle is excised in a horizontal fashion (Fig. 8–4B). This further exposes the tarsal border and the orbital septum below. With a conformer protecting the globe, hemostasis is obtained using electrocautery. A small strip of skin may be removed from the skin edges if dermatochalasis coexists.

Five 4-0 silk sutures are sequentially placed in the wound. Each suture joins the skin and lower tarsal border at the superior aspect of the incision, penetrates the orbital septum and engages the inferior aponeurosis, and finally emerges through the skin edge at the inferior aspect of the incision (Fig. 8–4C). The lower the suture engages inferior aponeurosis, the greater will be the resultant effect. Penetration of the inferior aponeurosis brings the needle into close proximity to the inferior rectus and adjacent sclera. To avoid the potential of scleral perforation, these sutures should be passed in a backhand fashion, with the concave side of the needle facing away from the globe. To ensure optimal position, all five sutures should be placed before tying (Fig. 8–4D).

Eyelid rotation is effected by tying the sutures with

imbrication (Fig. 8–4E). The degree of imbrication and suture tension is quantifiable based upon the amount of rotation desired. This can be checked by initially tying slip knots and observing the resultant rotation. Based on this, imbrication and suture tension can be adjusted. Once proper rotation is achieved, the slip knots are converted to permanent knots. At the close of surgery, the eyelid should be approximately 10% overcorrected. Lower eyelid retraction and diminution of the inferior cul-du-sac may be transiently present while sutures remain in place. The sutures are removed 10 days postoperatively, and earlier if overcorrection develops. Coordination of lower eyelid movement with downgaze should now be restored.

Other procedures devised for involutional entropion (Wheeler, Butler, Fox, Bick, etc.) have proven less uniformly successful and more prone to recurrence. Their descriptions have, therefore, been deleted from this text.

Involutional entropion can occasionally have a "spastic" component if it is the result of an apparent and self-limited focus of irritation. When causal factors such as recent ocular surgery or corneal epithelial disruption are found, the entropion can be managed conservatively. Mild cases may resolve by simply taping the involved eyelid in a somewhat everted position with vertically placed Steri-strips secured with tincture of benzoin. Should this prove insufficient, the Quickert three-suture operation should be considered.

Quickert Three-Suture Operation. In this technique, a barrier is established preventing the preseptal portion of orbicularis oculi muscle from overriding the pretarsal portion. Following direct infiltration of local anesthesia,

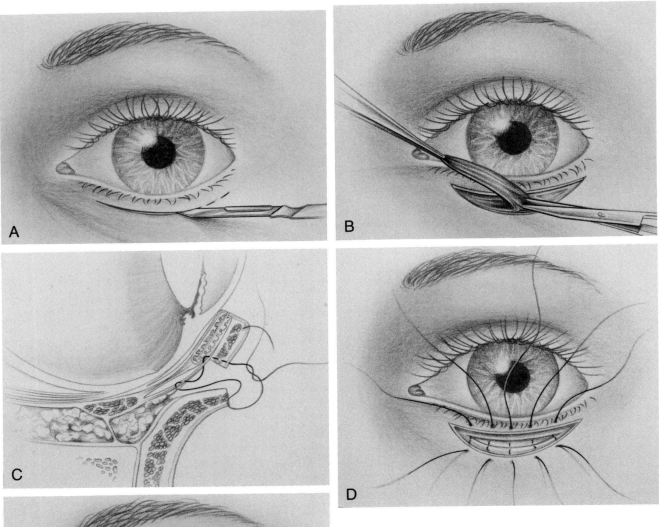

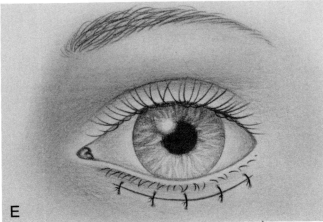

FIG. 8–4.   Technique of Jones, Reeh, and Wobig. Shortening of the lower eyelid retractors (tuck of the inferior aponeurosis). A, Incision line marked 4 to 5 mm below the eyelid margin and incised with #64 Beaver blade. B, The uppermost 4-mm section of preseptal orbicularis oculi muscle is horizontally excised. This also further exposes the lower tarsal border and orbital septum. C, Lateral view depicting suture placement. Each suture joins the skin and lower tarsal border at the superior portion of the incision. Sutures then penetrate septum and engage the inferior aponeurosis before emerging through the skin edge at the inferior portion of the incision. D, Appearance of the eyelid following suture placement, before tying. E, The sutures are tied with imbrication. The degree of imbrication and suture tension is quantifiable and determines the extent of rotation.

three 4-0 chromic catgut mattress sutures are placed at the medial, central, and lateral aspects of the lower eyelid (Fig. 8–5A). Each suture pass enters on the conjunctival surface immediately below the tarsal border, emerging on the skin surface 5 mm below the eyelid margin (Fig. 8–5B). Suture tension determines the degree of correction (Fig. 8–5C). A mild overcorrection is desired initially (Fig. 8–5D). These sutures dissolve at 6 weeks, or can be removed earlier if an overcorrection is developing. Any subsequent recurrence should be managed with a tuck of the inferior aponeurosis.

CICATRICIAL ENTROPION

Cicatricial entropion results from scar-induced vertical foreshortening of the posterior (tarsoconjunctival) lamella. It most commonly affects the lower eyelid, although either eyelid may be involved. Causal factors include infection (trachoma, severe herpes zoster), inflammatory processes (Stevens-Johnson syndrome, pemphigus, ocular pemphigoid), trauma, previous eyelid surgery, and burns (thermal, radiation, chemical). In some of these situations, the meibomian glands may undergo

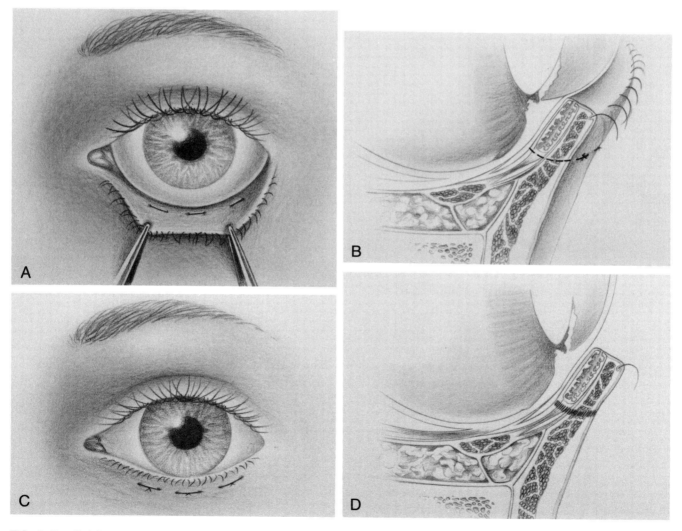

FIG. 8–5. Quickert three-suture operation. A, Three 4-0 chromic catgut mattress sutures are placed at the medial, central, and lateral aspects of the lower eyelid. B, Each suture enters the conjunctival surface immediately below the tarsal border, emerging on the skin surface 5 mm below the eyelid margin. C, Suture tension determines the extent of correction. D, A plane of cicatrization is established, maintaining the surgically corrected position.

metaplasia into a pilosebaceous unit. Aberrant distichiatic lashes may result, accentuating the patient's symptoms (Fig. 8–6A).

Wies Procedure. The principal reconstructive operation in cases of cicatricial entropion is the Wies procedure (Fig. 8–6B). This involves tarsal fracturing with sutures holding the newly malleable eyelid in an everted position. The result is achieved by transferring posterior lamellar cicatricial forces to the anterior lamella. A plane of cicatrization is established to ensure a lasting effect.

The closer to the eyelid margin that the incision is placed the more effective will be the rotation. This is limited to the extent that it must not compromise the marginal vascular arcade.

In either eyelid, the area of the intended incision is delineated with a marking pen. The mark should be placed horizontally 3 to 4 mm from the margin encompassing the central 80% of the eyelid (less if the entropion is anatomically limited) (Fig. 8–7A). It must be lateral to the canaliculus. Accordingly, local anesthetic is infiltrated. A Snellen clamp should be placed to fixate the eyelid and protect the subjacent globe. Following the marked lines, a full-thickness blepharotomy is performed within the confines of the clamp. Hemostasis is obtained as the clamp is gradually loosened and removed. The blepharotomy is extended to its full demarcation (Fig. 8–7B).

If the cicatrization is severe, additional segments of skin and tarsus can be excised before placement of sutures. Five 4-0 silk sutures are placed to achieve outward rotation. In the upper eyelid, these sutures join the skin edge at the lower limb of the incision to the posterior tarsal border and skin edge at the upper limb of the incision (Fig. 8–7C). In the lower eyelid these sutures join the skin edge at the upper limb of the incision to the posterior tarsal border and skin edge at the lower limb of the incision. The sutures are tied with imbrication, the degree of which dictates the extent of rotation (Fig. 8–7D). It is desirable to achieve a 10% overcorrection at surgical closure. After suture removal 10 days postoperatively, a plane of cicatrization holds the eyelid in normal position.

Most cases of cicatricial entropion distinctly benefit from the Wies procedure. This operation is so effective in rotating the eyelid that the incised tarsal edge may occasionally prolapse. Should this develop, it can be repositioned by placing through it several 6-0 chromic catgut sutures. These sutures enter from the conjunctival surface and exit on the skin surface in a mattress fashion.

It is important to recognize that some cases of ocular pemphigoid and Stevens-Johnson syndrome may actually exacerbate following surgery. There is no way to determine the susceptible cases preoperatively.

Mucous Membrane Grafts. The most severe cases of cicatricial entropion involving the upper eyelid have coexistent distichiasis and do not benefit completely from the Wies procedure. These cases require excision of the cicatrized tarsoconjunctival tissue with mucous membrane replacement.

After infiltration of local anesthetic, a 4-0 silk suture is placed in the upper central eyelid margin in a modified Frost fashion. This is used as a "handle" to evert the somewhat rigid eyelid. From this position, the abnormal tarsoconjunctival tissue is excised (Fig. 8–8A). This may

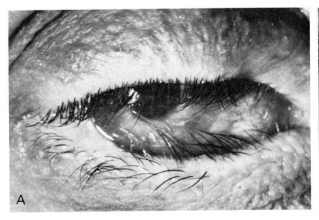
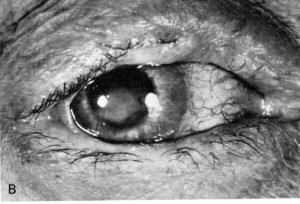

FIG. 8–6.   A, Preoperative appearance of a patient with ocular pemphigoid showing moderately severe trichiasis and distichiasis of both upper and lower eyelids. B, Same patient after marginal rotation of both upper and lower eyelids and elimination of aberrant lashes over the medial aspect of the upper eyelid. The patient is now asymptomatic.

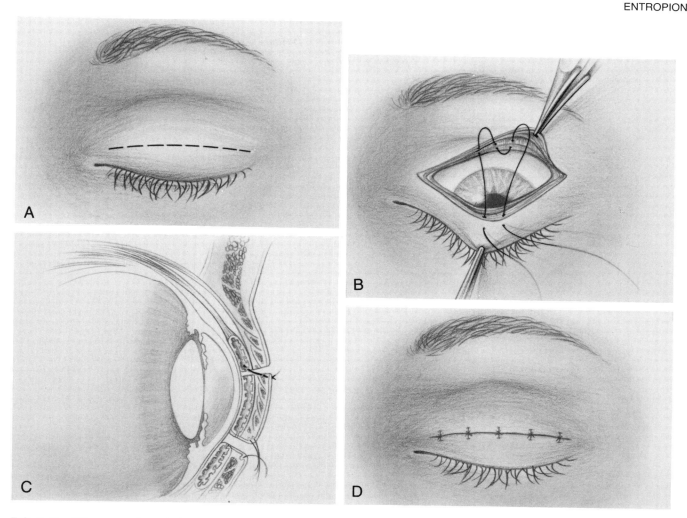

FIG. 8–7. Wies procedure. A, Incision line marked for upper eyelid cicatricial entropion is placed horizontally 3 to 4 mm from the eyelid margin. B, A full-thickness blepharotomy is performed, which will fracture the tarsal plate. This is facilitated by the use of a Snellen clamp, which also protects the subjacent globe. C, Five 4-0 silk sutures are placed. Each suture joins the skin edge of the marginal eyelid segment to the posterior tarsal border of the nonmarginal eyelid segment. The later suture bite can emerge through the overlying skin to facilitate tying. D, Sutures are tied with imbrication, the extent of which determines the degree of rotation achieved. A plane of cicatrization is established.

include the eyelid margin if it is involved. A 2 to 3 mm section of tarsus should always be left superiorly to support the graft (Fig. 8–8B).

In extreme cases such as Stevens-Johnson syndrome, it may be necessary to use a composite graft of nasal septal cartilage and subjacent mucous membrane. This tissue should be kept as thin as possible and should never be allowed to separate, thereby keeping the mucosa viable. Grafts should be 10 to 20% larger than the recipient bed to allow for expected shrinkage (Fig. 8–8C). Eye bank sclera and postauricular cartilage may be considered as alternative donor substances. These materials are less efficacious because they are devoid of mucous mem-

brane. If used, they should be contoured 50% larger than the recipient bed because of enhanced shrinkage.

Closure is facilitated by initially securing the corners of the graft with four interrupted 6-0 chromic catgut sutures. Two additional 6-0 chromic catgut sutures attach the graft to the distal levator aponeurosis. The graft edges are sutured to recipient tarsus with running 7-0 chromic catgut sutures (Fig. 8–8D). The 4-0 silk modified Frost suture should be secured to the cheek with tincture of benzoin and Steri-strips under mild tension for 10 days to augment the result.

Patients with Stevens-Johnson syndrome also require vigorous management with artificial tears (lubricating

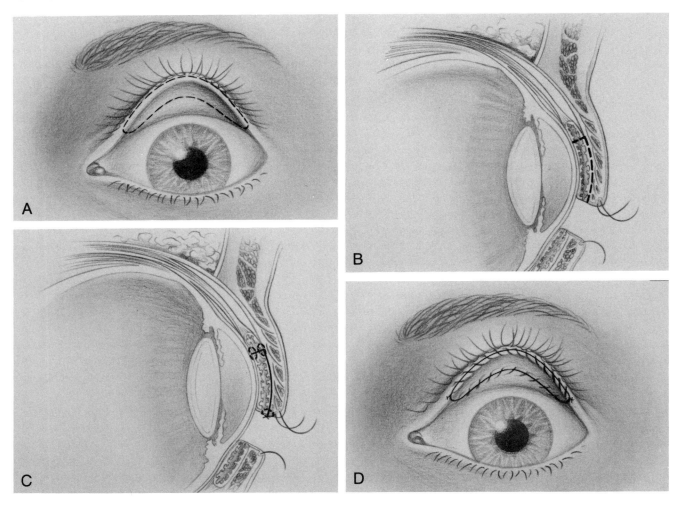

FIG. 8–8.   Placement of mucous membrane graft to treat severe cicatricial entropion. A, Anterior view demonstrating area of tarsus and conjunctiva to be excised. B, Lateral view demonstrating that the anterior eyelid lamella and normal lashes are left intact. A 2- to 3-mm strut of tarsus should remain for eyelid and graft support. C, In the upper eyelid, a composite graft of nasal septal cartilage and mucosa should be placed. Such grafts should be oversized by approximately 10 to 20% in anticipation of postoperative shrinkage. D, The graft is secured with interrupted 6-0 chromic catgut sutures at the corners. Additional 6-0 chromic sutures unite the graft to distal levator aponeurosis. The graft edges and eyelid margin are further secured with a running 7-0 chromic catgut suture.

drops and ointment) for an indefinite postoperative period.

Trichiasis and Distichiasis. Cases where trichiasis or distichiasis involve only a small portion of a properly positioned eyelid can be managed with cryosurgery. This technique is contraindicated when larger areas are involved because it might induce cicatricial entropion from contracture of the posterior lamella. Cryosurgery is also contraindicated when trichiasis or distichiasis is associated with entropion. In this situation, successful eyelash ablation would not diminish the deleterious effect of stratified squamous cutaneous epithelium upon the cornea. Application of one of the previously described entropion techniques obviates the eyelash problem by outwardly rotating the eyelid.

Cryosurgical technique is described in Chapter 11.

BIBLIOGRAPHY

Beyer, C.: Special procedures in the treatment of Stevens-Johnson disease and ocular pemphigoid. Trans. Am. Acad. Ophthalmol. Otolaryngol. 83:701, 1976.

Beyer-Machule, C., and von Noorden, G.: Atlas of Ophthalmic Surgery. New York, Thieme-Stratton, 1985.

Callahan, A.: Reconstructive Surgery of the Eyelids and Ocular Adnexa. Birmingham, Aesculapius, 1966.

Callahan, M., and Callahan, A.: Ophthalmic Plastic and Orbital Surgery. Birmingham, Aesculapius, 1979.

Dryden, R., Leibsohn, J., and Wobig, J.: Senile entropion: pathogenesis and treatment. Arch. Ophthalmol. 96:1883–1885, 1972.

Dryden, R., and Soll, D.: The use of scleral transplantation in cicatricial entropion and eyelid retraction. Trans. Am. Acad. Ophthalmol. Otolaryngol. 83:669–678, 1977.

Jones, L., Reeh, M., and Wobig, J.: Senile entropion: a new concept for correction. Am. J. Ophthalmol. 74:327–329, 1972.

Leone, C.: Nasal septal cartilage for eyelid reconstruction. Ophthalmic Surg. 4:68–71, 1973.

Quickert, M., and Rathbun, E.: Suture repair of entropion. Arch. Ophthalmol. 85:304–305, 1971.

Reeh, M., Beyer, C., and Shannon, G.: Practical Ophthalmic Plastic and Reconstructive Surgery. Philadelphia, Lea and Febiger, 1976.

Soll, D.: Management of Complications in Ophthalmic Plastic Surgery. Birmingham, Aesculapius, 1976.

Sullivan, J., Beard, C., and Bullock, J.: Cryosurgery for treatment of trichiasis. Am. J. Ophthalmol. 82:117, 1976.

Tenzel, R.: Repair of entropion of the upper lid. Arch. Ophthalmol. 77:675, 1967.

Tenzel, R., Miller, G., and Rubenzik, R: Cicatricial upper lid entropion. Arch. Ophthalmol. 3:999, 1975.

Wies, F.: Spastic Entropion. Trans. Am. Acad. Ophthalmol. Otolaryngol. 59:503, 1955.

9

BLEPHAROPLASTY

In recent years, patient interest in aesthetic surgery has clearly been on the increase. In many cases, the motivation is cosmetic, to turn the clock back a finite number of years. In other cases, the motivation is functional due to ocular fatigue or a compromised visual field. In a third group of cases, the motivation is sociologic, with a desire to alter the ethnic appearance of the eyelids. Whatever the motivation, it is essential that blepharoplasty candidates be completely evaluated and urged to approach surgical decisions with realistic expectations. Although their self-esteem may be enhanced, the procedure is not a panacea leading to social or professional success.

At the outset, the patient should relate to the surgeon his or her concept of the eyelid abnormality and the changes anticipated from surgery. A mirror may allow the patient to better communicate this information. This is followed by a complete medical and ocular history. Specifically, the surgeon should explore potential contributions from Graves' disease, diabetes, myxedema, renal dysfunction, cardiovascular disorders, hepatic dysfunction, trauma, previous surgery, inflammation, keloid formation, and allergies. Any intercurrent bleeding diathesis should be reviewed, as well as the use of aspirin or anticoagulants.

The ophthalmic examination should be complete and thorough, bringing any preoperative disorder to the patient's attention. Assessment of the best corrected visual acuity provides insight into the patient's visual function and serves as a baseline before surgical intervention.

Gravity is an important influence on blepharoplasty surgery. Laxity of the structures located superiorly may artifactually influence the appearance of the inferiorly located structures. Therefore, evaluation and surgical correction should proceed in this order: eyebrows, upper eyelids, lower eyelids. If no abnormality is demonstrable in one of these areas, that portion of the surgical correction should be deleted.

The brow position is assessed in relation to the supraorbital rim. Brows in men are usually horizontally configured; those in women are higher and more arched. Brow ptosis is the result of relaxation of scalp and forehead structures, along with atrophy of the brow fat pad.

A ptotic brow is usually more marked laterally due to diminished muscular attachment in this region. Brow ptosis can artifactually augment the upper eyelid hooding found in most of these cases (Fig. 9–1). For examination purposes, the contribution from brow ptosis can be negated by superimposing the brow hairline over the supraorbital rim. The relationship of periorbital structures to the orbital rims should be observed.

The height of the upper eyelid margins is noted, along with the presence and height of the eyelid folds. Males normally have a lower crease than females. It is important to identify those cases with superimposed true blepharoptosis with or without levator aponeurosis dehiscence. A quantitative assessment of vertical skin redundancy and horizontal full thickness eyelid laxity is essential. Likewise, a qualitative assessment of cutanous consistency and elasticity should be performed. Tumor and other contributing eyelid lesions must be recorded.

Evaluation of the orbicularis oculi muscle discloses cases with either hypertrophy or diminished function, the latter resulting from VII nerve palsy. While the patient is in an upright position, the quantity and location of prominent orbital fat are recorded. This fat must be distinguished from a large or prolapsed lacrimal gland. Any contribution from hypertrophy of the orbicularis oculi muscles should be noted.

The lower eyelids should be examined for malpositions (either entropion or ectropion). Failure to recognize lower eyelid laxity or scleral show before surgery may

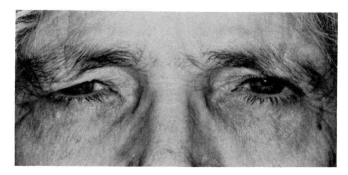

FIG. 9–1. Brow ptosis is superimposed on upper eyelid hooding from dermatochalasis in this patient.

predispose the patient to ectropion (and retraction) after lower-eyelid blepharoplasty. Laxity may be assessed by gently pulling the lower eyelid away from the globe and measuring the separation of bulbar from palpebral conjunctiva (Fig. 9–2A). It may also be estimated by pulling the lower eyelid toward the infraorbital rim, then releasing it (Fig. 9–2B). A lax eyelid will return slowly to its normal position. Coexistent lower eyelid laxity requires horizontal eyelid shortening in addition to blepharoplasty.

It is important to distinguish blepharochalasis from dermatochalasis. Blepharochalasis is a rare bilateral condition seen most commonly in young women. It is characterized by thin, atrophic, and wrinkled skin, only loosely attached to the orbicularis oculi muscle and levator aponeurosis below. It occurs most commonly in the upper eyelid, with orbital fat protruding forward through a weakened orbital septum. Blepharochalasis is occasionally familial and of unknown etiology, although some cases have followed recurrent episodes of angioneurotic edema.

Dermatochalasis is a common bilateral condition affecting both sexes equally. It is principally seen in the middle and older age groups and is characterized by vertical and horizontal redundancy of skin. This may be accentuated by brow ptosis and weakening of the orbital septum with herniation of orbital fat (Fig. 9–3). The upper and lower eyelids may be equally affected. Dermatochalsis is occasionally familial and may result from certain medical conditions (Graves' disease, myxedema,

renal dysfunction, cardiovascular disorders, hepatic dysfunction), periorbital cellulitis, and allergies. Patients in this group are the most likely to proceed with blepharoplasty.

Tear function analysis should be performed with the Schirmer$_1$ test. The quality of corneal wetting is assessed through the tear breakup time. Decreased tear production (less than 10 mm) or a short tear breakup time (less than 10 seconds) necessitates a more conservative procedure that will not predispose to exposure. Preoperative punctal ectropion should be noted.

The extraocular muscles are checked for the presence of full ductions, single vision, and Bell's phenomenon. Intraocular pressure recordings, slit lamp, and fundus examinations should follow. Visual fields are essential in assessing the degree of functional limitation. Preoperative photographs should be brought to surgery to help the surgeon tailor the procedure to individual circumstances.

Relative indications for correction of brow ptosis or blepharoplasty include cosmesis and functional impairment. The latter is documented by upper visual field changes from brow ptosis and/or upper eyelid pseudoptosis. Contact lens malpositions and significant eyelid asymmetry may also be indications.

Relative contraindications for blepharoplasty include tendency toward lower eyelid ectropion, eyelid retraction, lagophthalmos, keratitis sicca, recurrent erosion, and keloid formation. Contributing dermatologic conditions such as dermatitis, ichthyosis, or epidermolysis

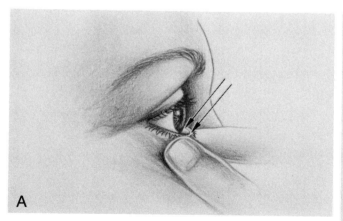

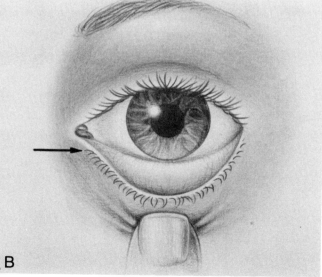

FIG. 9–2. Horizontal laxity can be evaluated by A, grasping the lower eyelid and gently pulling it away from the globe or B, retracting the lower eyelid toward the infraorbital rim, then releasing it.

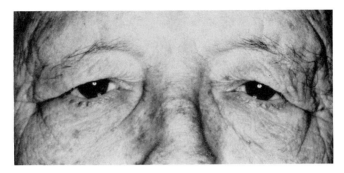

FIG. 9–3. Brow ptosis accentuating dermatochalasis. Correction of the brow ptosis must be the initial procedure in such cases to avoid an untoward result.

bullosa, affecting the periorbital area, should be treated primarily. Likewise, any medical etiology such as angioneurotic edema, congestive heart failure, or renal failure should be treated primarily.

Surgery should be avoided when the deformity is minimal, particularly in patients with a "surgiholic" tendency. Patients with a notable psychiatric overlay are not likely to benefit from this operation. It is imperative that candidates for blepharoplasty approach this operation informed and with realistic expectations.

SURGICAL APPROACHES

Local anesthesia is generally used for all forms of blepharoplasty to avoid the heightened risk of general anesthesia. Unless medically contraindicated, 2% xylocaine with epinephrine is locally infiltrated. The xylocaine affords analgesia and separation of tissue planes, while the epinephrine affords hemostasis and longer duration of action.

Brow Lift. A brow lift can be accomplished directly through a supraciliary incision or indirectly through a midforehead or coronal incision. Although the latter leaves a less demonstrable scar, it is more complex and may yield more complications. The large distance between the brow and the excision site may yield a poorer long-term result.

Supraciliary Brow Lift. The elliptical incision site is marked at that position where the brow is ptotic (Fig. 9–4A). This may involve anything from a segment to the entire brow. The lower limb of the intended incision site is marked at the upper border of the brow hairline. This is essential to camouflage the scar postoperatively. With the patient sitting up to demonstrate the full extent of brow ptosis, the distance of this line to its desired posi-

tion overlying the supraorbital rim is measured. The patient returns to his reclining position. The upper limb of the intended incision is marked 5 mm higher than the measured distance to allow for postoperative tissue stretching. Marks on both brows are compared to ensure symmetry. Subjacent to this, local anesthesia should be infiltrated.

According to the marked lines, a skin incision should be made with a #64 Beaver blade. This incision is carried through the subcutaneous tissue down to the level of the frontalis muscle. Redundant skin and subcutaneous tissue outlined by the incision are excised (Fig. 9–4B). Hemostasis is obtained with pressure and light cautery. The deeper layer is closed with interrupted 5-0 Vicryl vertical mattress sutures, engaging subcutaneous tissue and frontalis muscle with each bite (Fig. 9–4C). These sutures must not incorporate periosteum because this would immobilize the brow. The skin is closed with a running 7-0 silk suture (Fig. 9–4D). At closure, the wound edges should be slightly everted. This causes this somewhat thick skin to heal with a flat scar, partially concealed at the brow-forehead interface. The overcorrected brow stretches and assumes a normal position in the early postoperative period. Skin sutures should be removed by the sixth postoperative day (Figs. 9–5 and 9–6).

Upper Eyelid Blepharoplasty. The patient is asked to look up and down sequentially to demonstrate the eyelid crease. Men normally have a somewhat lower crease than do women. If this crease is properly positioned, the lower limb of the intended incision is marked there. This line may be placed 1 mm lower in anticipation of postoperative upward scar migration. If the patient's eyelid crease is too high, the lower limb of the intended incision is marked centrally 6 mm above the eyelid margin. This line should be curvilinear, tapering somewhat medially and laterally. The marks should not be placed too close to the canthi, to avoid postoperative webbing. With forceps, the central skin above should be pulled inferiorly to join this line. On a trial-and-error basis, a point should be identified above where the tissues just meet. This point should be marked, defining the central apex of the upper limb of the intended incision line. A curvilinear expansion of this point defines an upper line, joining the lower line medially and laterally (Fig. 9–7A). There is usually more redundant skin temporally; therefore it is often necessary to widen this junction, resulting in a "tail-like" configuration. The upper and lower lines are joined with forceps at various positions to test whether this positioning is correct. Titrations can be made to adjust for more or less excision. The upper eyelid marks are

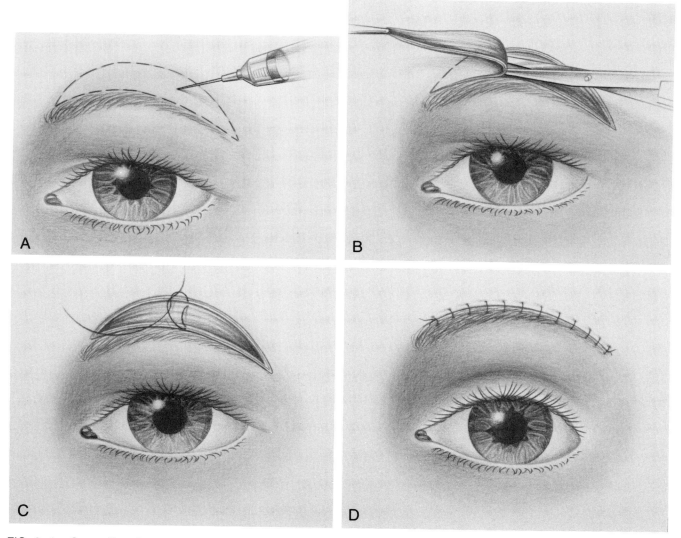

FIG. 9–4. Supraciliary brow lift. A, Elliptical incision site is marked with its lower limb at the upper brow hairline. B, Accordingly, skin and subcutaneous tissue are excised to the muscular layer. C, The Vicryl subcutaneous sutures engage the frontalis muscle in each pass. D, Skin closure with the wound edges slightly everted.

checked to ensure symmetry. Subjacent to this, local anesthetic is infiltrated.

According to the marked lines, a skin incision should be made with a #64 Beaver blade. Using blunt and sharp dissection with Stevens scissors, this tissue is excised (Fig. 9–7B). As a precaution against overcorrection, the skin may be saved for 24 hours by placing it within a saline solution in a refrigerator. With a conformer protecting the cornea, hemostasis is obtained with pressure and light cautery.

The skin edges are united with forceps at various positions to ensure that the redundancy has been optimally corrected. Any excess skin can be further trimmed.

Hypertropic orbicularis oculi muscle is sometimes encountered, diminishing access to the supratarsal area. A 2 to 3 mm wide strip may be excised horizontally from this site. If excessive or herniated orbital fat was detected preoperatively, the orbital septum should be opened completely (Fig. (9–7C). This opening should be at least 5 mm superior to the upper tarsal border to be above the area where levator aponeurosis and orbital septum are fused. The septum is usually weakest medially, at the position of maximum innervation and vascularity. In the upper eyelid, the principal fat pads are located medially and centrally (Fig. 9–7D). More fat is usually found within the medial pad. Lateral dissection should be

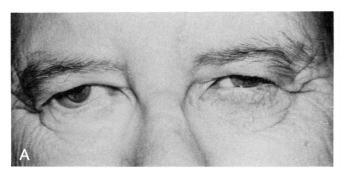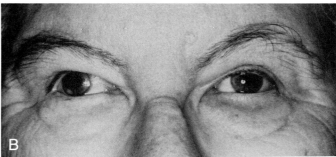

FIG. 9–5. A, Preoperative appearance of a patient with Möbius' syndrome (facial diplegia). B, Postoperative appearance of this patient after bilateral direct brow lift, upper eyelid blepharoplasty, and lower eyelid Bick procedure.

avoided to spare the lacrimal gland. Once orbital fat has been identified, it is freed by lysing its capsule and the various septae holding it in check. Gentle pressure on the globe prolapses a portion of this fat. Only the fat prolapsed in this manner should be excised. Any additional removal may result in enophthalmos. Hemostats are sequentially placed at the base of each herniated fat segment (Fig. 9–7E). The fat above the hemostat is excised and the hemostat tip is cauterized (Fig. 9–7F). After the hemostat is released, each fat pad is inspected for hemostasis before it is repositioned behind the orbital septum. The septum does not require closure.

Excision of herniated orbital fat provides better exposure of the levator aponeurosis. In the occasional case with coexistent blepharoptosis, the latter can be corrected at this point using either levator resection or levator dehiscence repair techniques (see Chapter 5).

The skin is closed with running 7-0 silk sutures. Supratarsal fixation can be used to ensure an ideal postoperative eyelid crease and to take up any residual der-

matochalasis. This is done by joining the skin edges with an intervening pass through the superficial fibers of the levator aponeurosis just above the tarsal border (Fig. 9–7G). After completion of an upper blepharoplasty (Fig. 9–7H), the eyelids should be parted 2 mm to allow for postoperative tissue stretching.

A dressing does not contribute to the surgical correction and may impede detection of postoperative hemorrhage, which is uncommon but significant. Ice in a sterile surgical glove may be applied intermittently for the next 4 hours to augment hemostasis. The sutures may be removed on the sixth postoperative day (Figs. 9–8 and 9–9).

The Oriental Eyelid. Clinical characteristics of the Oriental eyelid include a Mongolian eyelid fold (giving the appearance of an absent eyelid crease), an epicanthal fold, and a somewhat almond-shaped palpebral aperture. These changes are anatomically related to the position of the orbital septum and preaponeurotic fat pad (Fig. 9–10). In the Oriental eyelid, the abundant preaponeu-

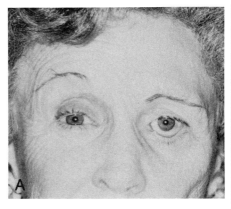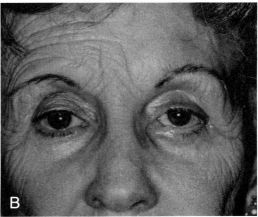

FIG. 9–6. A, Preoperative appearance of a patient with persistent left-sided Bell's palsy. B, Postoperative appearance of this patient after left direct brow lift, left upper eyelid blepharoplasty, and left lower eyelid Bick procedure.

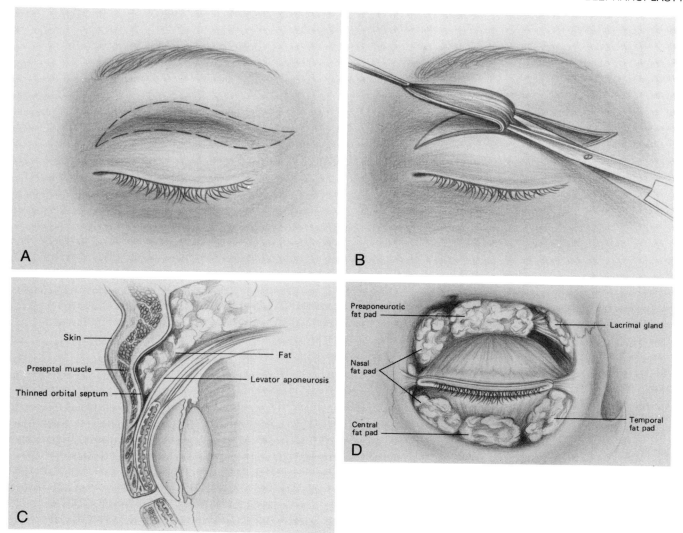

FIG. 9–7. Upper eyelid blepharoplasty. A, Elliptical incision line is marked at the area of desired eyelid fold. B, Skin or skin-muscle flap is excised accordingly. C, Lateral view of upper eyelid demonstrating the forward position of orbital fat behind a weakened orbital septum. D, Nasal and central fat pads are present in the upper eyelid, while nasal, central, and temporal fat pads are present in the lower eyelid.

rotic fat pushes the septum forward and downward anterior to a portion of the tarsal plate. This imparts a full appearance to these eyelids. These characteristics must be taken into account when Oriental patients seek to attain a more Occidental appearance through an upper blepharoplasty.

The surgical technique for Oriental upper blepharoplasty differs from conventional technique only in the amount of tissue that must be removed from the pretarsal space. It is necessary to thin this space considerably by removing all orbital fat found anterior to the tarsus. Ex-

cising a portion of the pretarsal orbicularis will help achieve this goal. Careful attention to skin closure with supratarsal fixation results in an eyelid crease that ensures a "western" appearance (Fig. 9–11) if this is desired.

Lower Eyelid Blepharoplasty. The area of the intended incision is marked in an infralash fashion. This horizontal line is placed 2 mm below the lower eyelid margin, extending from a position just lateral to the punctum to a position directly below the outer canthus (Fig. 9–12A).

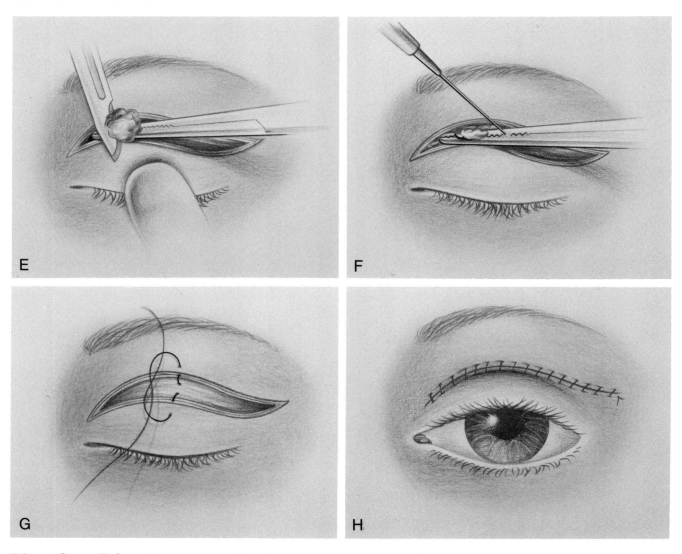

FIG. 9–7 Cont.   E, Curved hemostats are placed at the base of each herniated fat segment. F, After fat excision, the hemostat tip (base of fat pad) is cauterized. G, Skin closure involves fixation of superficial fibers of the levator aponeurosis just above the tarsal border. H, Skin closure completed with running 7-0 silk.

Laterally, this is then allowed to curve at a 25-degree angle in an inferolateral direction. The lower eyelid marks are checked to ensure symmetry. Subjacent to this, local anesthetic is infiltrated.

According to these lines, an incision is made with a #64 Beaver blade. Within the triangle demarcated by the incision, a skin flap (or a skin-muscle flap if the orbicularis oculi muscle is also redundant) is undermined by blunt and sharp dissection with Stevens scissors (Fig. 9–12B). A conformer is placed on the globe to protect the cornea and hemostasis is obtained with pressure and light cautery.

If excessive or herniated orbital fat was detected preoperatively, the orbital septum is opened in its entirety to expose the medial, central, and lateral fat pockets. Once the fat is identified, it is freed and mobilized by lysing its capsule and the septae holding it in check. Gentle pressure on the globe will prolapse a portion of this fat. Only the fat prolapsed in this manner should be excised. The medial pad contains the most fat; the lateral pad contains the least fat. Any excessive fat removal may result in enophthalmos. Curved hemostats are sequentially placed at the base of each herniated fat segment. The fat above the hemostat is excised and the hemostat

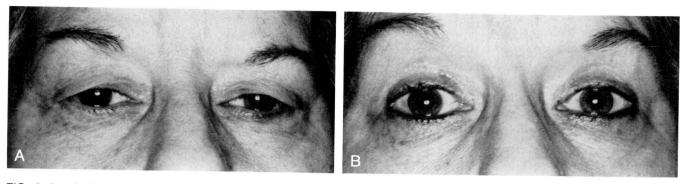

FIG. 9–8. A, Preoperative appearance of a woman with pseudoptosis from dermato-chalasis. B, Postoperative appearance following bilateral upper eyelid blepharoplasty.

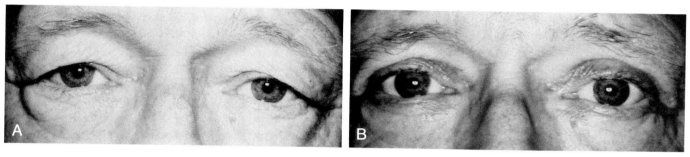

FIG. 9–9 A, Preoperative appearance of a man with pseudoptosis from dermatochalasis. B, Postoperative appearance following bilateral upper eyelid blepharoplasty.

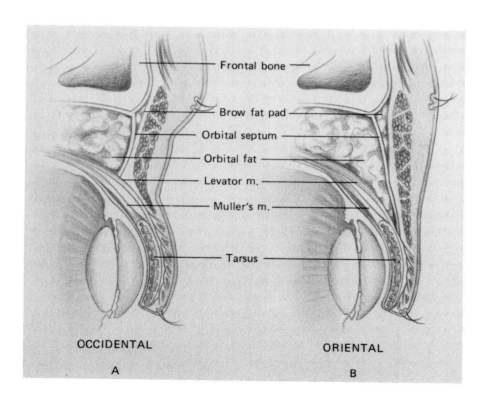

Frontal bone
Brow fat pad
Orbital septum
Orbital fat
Levator m.
Muller's m.
Tarsus

OCCIDENTAL

ORIENTAL

A

B

FIG. 9–10. Comparative anatomy of the (A), Occidental and (B), Oriental upper eyelid. Note that the orbital septum and subjacent orbital fat are positioned more anteriorly and inferiorly in the Oriental lid.

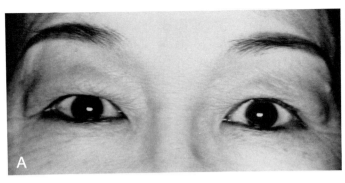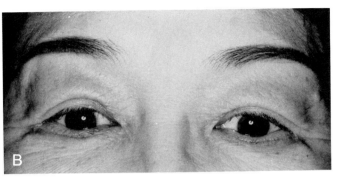

FIG. 9–11. A, Preoperative appearance of an Oriental woman who wished to have a more Western appearance in her upper eyelids. B, Postoperative appearance after bilateral upper eyelid blepharoplasty with supratarsal fixation.

is cauterized. After release of the hemostat, each fat pad is inspected for hemostasis before repositioning behind the orbital septum. The septum does not require closure.

The skin flap is mobilized laterally and draped over the incision (Fig. 9–12C). While the patient looks upward (stretching the inferior eyelid retractors), the amount of overlap defines the extent of redundant horizontal and vertical tissue to be excised. Because the lower eyelid has rudimentary tarsal support, vertical skin excision (under the cilia) should be conservative to avoid overcorrection. In case of coexistent horizontal laxity, the posterior lamella should be tightened with a triangular excision as in the Byron Smith modification of the Kuhnt-Szymanowski procedure (see Chapter 7). The skin is closed with running 7-0 silk sutures (Fig. 9–12D). Should a "dog ear" develop laterally, this may be corrected by taking wider suture bites on the side with more tissue.

A postoperative dressing does not contribute to the surgical correction and may impede detection of postoperative hemorrhage, which is uncommon but significant. Ice in a sterile surgical glove may be applied intermittently for the next 4 hours to augment hemostasis. The sutures may be removed on the sixth postoperative day (Fig. 9–13, 9–14 and 9–15).

Conjunctival Approach. As a general rule, the younger the lower blepharoplasty candidate, the greater is the contribution of prominent orbital fat and the lesser the contribution of dermatochalasis to the underlying defect. These patients may benefit from a conjunctival approach, which removes the causal orbital fat while leaving the skin intact. This avoids a cutaneous scar, leaves the orbital septum intact, and minimizes the chance of developing postoperative lower eyelid retraction.

Local anesthetic is infiltrated into the conjunctiva of the lower eyelid. With the lower eyelid fixated in an everted position, Stevens scissors are used to vertically incise the conjunctiva approximately 5 mm inferior to the lower tarsal border (Fig. 9–16A). The incision should run the full length of the tarsus, stopping just lateral to the punctum and canaliculus. Extending the dissection through the lower eyelid retractors exposes the three fat compartments (Fig. 9–16B). Once the fat is identified, it is freed and mobilized (Fig. 9–16C) by lysing its capsule and the septae holding it in check. Gentle pressure on the globe will prolapse a portion of this fat. Only the fat prolapsed in this manner should be excised. The medial pad contains the most fat; the lateral pad contains the least fat. Curved hemostats are sequentially placed at the base of each herniated fat segment (Fig. 9–16D). The fat above the hemostat is excised and the hemostat is cauterized. After the hemostat is released, each fat segment is inspected for hemostasis before repositing it. The lower eyelid retractors and conjunctiva are reapproximated with running 7-0 chromic catgut sutures (Fig. 9–16E).

A postoperative dressing does not contribute to the surgical correction and may impede detection of postoperative hemorrhage, which is uncommon but significant. Ice in a sterile surgical glove may be applied intermittently for the next 4 hours to augment hemostasis.

Blepharoplasty Complications. The most significant and potentially devastating complication from blepharoplasty is hemorrhage (Fig. 9–17). This is usually arterial, arising from inadequate cautery of a fat pad or its surrounding septae. A minor postoperative hemorrhage should be managed by observation and cold compresses. A major postoperative hemorrhage can compromise the blood supply to the optic nerve. This type of hemorrhage may be heralded by severe pain and ecchymosis, leading to proptosis, pupillary dilatation, and vision loss. Such a

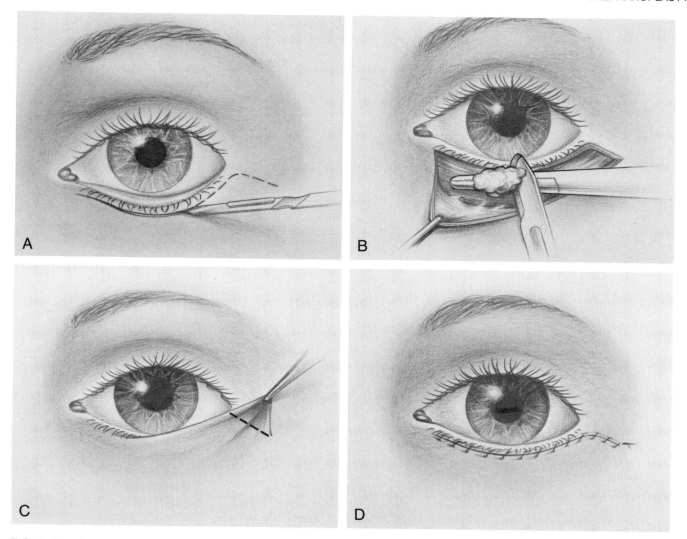

FIG. 9–12. Lower eyelid blepharoplasty. A, Infralash incision, which flattens somewhat at the outer canthus. B, Skin-muscle flap is undermined, orbital septum is opened, and herniated orbital fat is secured with hemostat and then excised. C, Skin flap is mobilized laterally and draped over the incision to define its excess. Overlapping tissue is excised, exercising particular caution as with any vertical excision. D, Skin closure.

development is a surgical emergency and should be managed by opening up the suture line in the involved eyelid, expressing out any blood clots, exposing the site of hemorrhage, and cauterizing until the surgical field is dry. If this proves inadequate, lateral canthotomy and cantholysis help to diminish intraorbital pressure. Placement of surgical drains or a hemovac is rarely required.

Infections after blepharoplasty are uncommon due to the extensive blood supply in the periorbital area. A bilateral infection is usually the result of surgical contamination because the same surgical instruments are serially brought from one side to the other. This usually becomes manifest within the first two days postoperatively. A unilateral infection is often the result of contamination after surgery. In either case, topical and systemic antibiotic therapy is dictated by culture and sensitivity findings. Moist heat may also hasten the resolution of these infections. Treatment must be adequate. Because the orbital septum has usually been surgically opened, the more severe cases can potentially lead to orbital cellulitis.

An undercorrected brow lift may later require a minor additional excision. This can be titrated to encompass a portion of the brow or the entire brow. An overcorrected

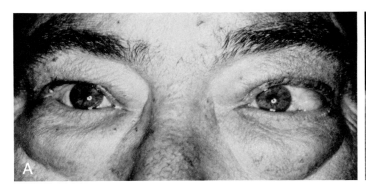 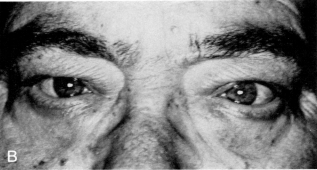

FIG. 9–13.   A, Preoperative appearance of a man with extensive herniation or orbital fat.
B, Postoperative appearance following bilateral lower eyelid blepharoplasty with extensive
removal of herniated orbital fat, including some contained under the left bulbar conjunctiva.

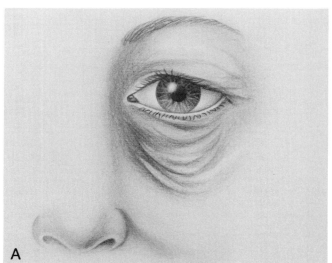 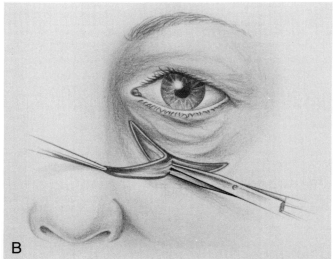

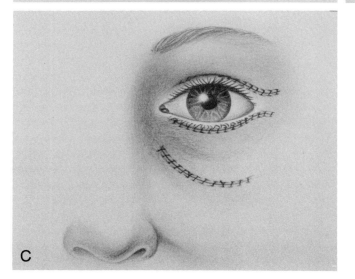

FIG. 9–14.   A, Extensive lower eyelid dermatochalasis with
"bag-on-bag" appearance, for which conventional lower
blepharoplasty is insufficient. B, Instead, a second (lower)
excision site is added in conformity with Langer's lines. C,
Skin closure after this extensive lower eyelid blepharoplasty
combined with upper eyelid blepharoplasty.

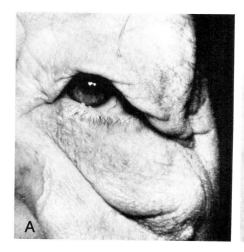
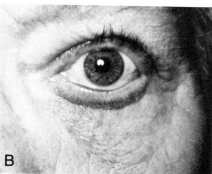

FIG. 9–15. A, Preoperative appearance of a patient with extensive dermatochalasis, including "bag-on-bag" appearance in the lower eyelid. B, Postoperative appearance following upper and lower blepharoplasty.

brow lift usually stretches adequately in the early postoperative period, obviating the need for additional surgery.

Undercorrected upper blepharoplasty may likewise require a minor additional skin or orbital fat excision. Overcorrected upper blepharoplasty may result in both cosmetic and functional problems. Cosmetically, the upper eyelid may appear excessively flat, with the eyelid margin too close to the brow. Functionally, lagophthalmos may occur, predisposing the patient to corneal erosion and ulceration. In minor overcorrections, lubricating drops and ointments can be used in the first few weeks after surgery until the tissues stretch sufficiently. Surgery is required for larger overcorrections.

If overcorrection is the result of overzealous skin excision, it is corrected by placing a full thickness skin graft. An obvious overcorrection recognized in the first 24 hours after blepharoplasty can be rectified by immediately replacing some of the skin that was excised and refrigerated. Most cases are recognized later and require a retroauricular full-thickness skin graft (as in cases of cicatricial ectropion). Overcorrections that are the result of an improper septal attachment are corrected by surgically freeing this attachment.

Undercorrections and overcorrections after lower blepharoplasty are treated in the same manner as for upper blepharoplasty (Fig. 9–18).

Excessive orbital fat removal may result in enophthalmos. This is difficult to treat effectively and should be avoided by judicious removal of fat during the original operation.

The upper eyelid may appear slightly ptotic while the supratarsal fixation sutures are in place. Upper eyelid height quickly normalizes after suture removal. Persistent blepharoptosis may represent a surgically induced aponeurotic injury. If this persists for 4 to 6 months, it should be assessed and treated along the guidelines for acquired blepharoptosis.

Lower blepharoplasty may result in ectropion, retraction, and/or scleral show. This occurs most commonly when the surgeon fails to recognize a lax lower eyelid preoperatively. Horizontal eyelid shortening should have been combined with lower blepharoplasty. If necessary, horizontal shortening can be performed as a secondary procedure. If ectropion is the result of excessive vertical skin excision, a skin graft is required. Gradually increasing ectropion may arise from inflammation of the septum or fat pad. This usually abates with time, although steroid injection may hasten this process. Retraction and scleral show may result from disruption of skin-muscle and/or septal planes. If these are persistent and significant, eyelid retraction repair may prove necessary (see Chapter 6).

Excessive scarring is associated particularly with brow lift. It can occur after blepharoplasty, especially in patients with a history of hypertrophic scar formation. Prominent scars should be treated with one or more steroid injections. Delivery of the steroid into a dense scar is facilitated by using an air-pressure delivery mechanism (Madajet, Panjet) rather than fine needles. Any persistent scar is excised with the wound carefully reapproximated. This may be followed by steroid injection to discourage further collagen deposition.

Webbing is usually avoided by keeping the suture lines properly distanced from the canthi. Any resultant web can be managed by a V- to Y-plasty. The apex of the V should be placed inferiorly, pointing toward the web. The base of the V extends to the superior portion of the web. To free the flap, the skin must be separated from the underlying orbicularis oculi muscle and repositioned in a Y configuration. This should eliminate the web.

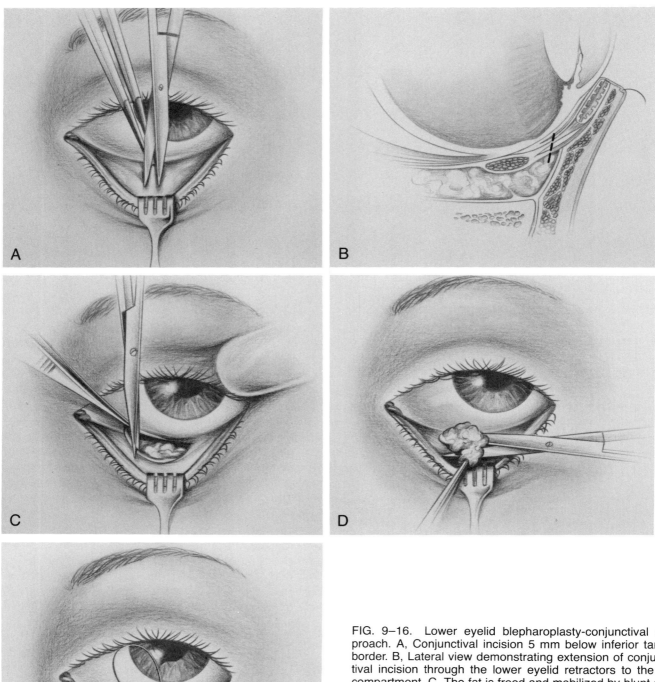

FIG. 9–16. Lower eyelid blepharoplasty-conjunctival approach. A, Conjunctival incision 5 mm below inferior tarsal border. B, Lateral view demonstrating extension of conjunctival incision through the lower eyelid retractors to the fat compartment. C, The fat is freed and mobilized by blunt dissection. D, Herniated orbital fat is clamped, excised, and cauterized at the base. E, The lower eyelid retractors and conjunctiva are reapproximated.

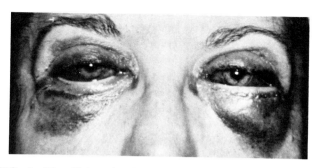

FIG. 9–17. Extensive hematoma after blepharoplasty, which cleared completely with supportive treatment.

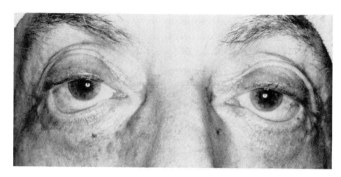

FIG. 9–18. Overcorrected lower eyelid blepharoplasty, which resulted in cicatricial ectropion and retraction.

BIBLIOGRAPHY

Beard, C.: Lower lid blepharoplasty. Ophthalmology 85:711, 1978.

Beyer, C.: Baggy lids. Int. Ophthalmol. Clin. 10:47, 1970.

Beyer, C.: Symposium: blepharoplasty procedures. Trans. Am. Acad. Ophthalmol. 85:702, 1978

Beyer, C., McCarthy, R., and Webster, R.: Baggy lids: a classification and newer aspects of treatment to avoid complications. Ophthalmic Surg. 11:169, 1980.

Beyer-Machule, C., and von Noorden, G.: Atlas of Ophthalmic Surgery. New York, Thieme-Stratton, 1985.

Bosniak, S., and Smith, B.: Advances in Ophthalmic Plastic and Reconstructive Surgery. New York, Pergamon Press, 1983.

Callahan, M., and Callahan, A.: Ophthalmic Plastic and Orbital Surgery. Birmingham, Aesculapius, 1979, pp. 124–133.

Castanares, S.: Forehead wrinkles, glabellar frown and ptosis of the eyebrows. Plast. Reconstr. Surg. 34:406–413, 1964.

Dryden, R., and Leibsohn, J.: The levator aponeurosis in blepharoplasty. Ophthalmology 85:718, 1978.

Edgerton, M.: Causes and prevention of lower lid ectropion following blepharoplasty. Plast. Reconstr. Surg. 49:367–373, 1972.

Johnson, C., Anderson, J., and Katz, R.: The brow lift 1978. Arch. Otolaryngol. 105:125–126, 1979.

Lemke, B., and Stasior, O.: The anatomy of eyebrow ptosis. Arch. Ophthalmol. 100:981–986, 1982.

Levine, M., and Boynton, J., Tenzel, R., and Miller, G.: Complications of blepharoplasty. Ophthalmic Surg. 6:53–57, 1975.

McCord, C.: Techniques in blepharoplasty. Ophthalmic Surg. 10:40–55, 1979.

Putterman, A.: Temporary blindness after cosmetic blepharoplasty. Am. J. Ophthalmol. 80:1081, 1975.

Reeh, M., Beyer, C., and Shannon, G.: Practical Ophthalmic Plastic and Reconstructive Surgery. Philadephia, Lea and Febiger, 1976.

Rees, T.: Technical aid in blepharoplasty. Plast. Reconstr. Surg. 41:497, 1968.

Rees, T.: Complications Following Blepharoplasty. In Tessier, P., Callahan, A., Mustarde, J.: Symposium on Plastic Surgery in the Orbital Region. St. Louis, C.V. Mosby, 1976, P. 455.

Rees, R.: Modern trends in blepharoplasty. Clin. Plast. Surg. 8: 1981.

Sheen, J.: Supratarsal fixation in upper blepharoplasty. Plast. Reconstr. Surg. 54:424, 1974.

Sheen, J.: A change in the technique of supratarsal fixation in upper blepharoplasty. Plast. Reconstr. Surg. 59:831, 1977.

Small, R.: Supratarsal fixation in ophthalmic plastic surgery. Ophthalmic Surg. 9:73, 1978

Small, R.: Extended lower eyelid blepharoplasty. Arch. Ophthalmol. 99:1402–1405, 1981.

Smith, B.: Post-surgical complications of cosmetic blepharoplasty. Trans. Am. Acad. Ophthalmol. Otolaryngol. 73:1162–1164, 1969.

Smith, B., and Nesi, F.: The complications of cosmetic blepharoplasty. Ophthalmology 85:726, 1978.

Soll, D.: Management of Complications in Ophthalmic Plastic Surgery. Birmingham, Aesculapius, 1976.

Stasior, O.: Cosmetic blepharoplasty: a search for perfection. Ophthalmology 85:705, 1978.

Steigler, L, and Crawford, J.: Blepharochalasis. Am. J. Ophthalmol. 77:100, 1974.

Tenzel, R.: Surgical techniques and problems in cosmetic blepharoplasty. Trans. Am. Acad. Ophthalmol. Otolaryngol. 73:1154–1161, 1969.

Tenzel, R.: Correction of brow ptosis. Ophthalmology 85:716, 1978.

Tenzel, R.: Cosmetic blepharoplasty. Int. Ophthalmol. Clin. 18:87, 1978.

Tenzel, R.: Surgical treatment of complications of cosmetic blepharoplasty. Clin. Plast. Surg. 5:517–523, 1978.

Waller, R.: Is blindness a realistic complication in blepharoplasty procedures? Trans. Am. Acad. Ophthalmol. Otolaryngol. 85:730, 1978.

Wiggs, E.: Blepharoplasty complications. Trans. Am. Acad. Ophthalmol. Otolaryngol. 81:603–606, 1976.

Wilkins, R.: Evaluation of the blepharoplasty patient. Ophthalmology 85:703, 1978.

10

EYELID TUMORS AND EYELID RECONSTRUCTION

In evaluating suspected eyelid and epibulbar tumors, one must consider the patient's age, sex, heredity, occupation, general health, previous therapy, and tumor growth characteristics.

The examination must be detailed. The lesion, or lesions, must be studied *in situ*, using magnification from loupes or a slit lamp when necessary. An assessment must be made of the appearance, size, shape, color, depth, firmness, mobility, location, and functional effect of the tumor. It is essential to note any juxtaposition of the tumor to vital structures (i.e., punctum and canaliculus). Destruction or alteration of eyelashes or meibomian gland orifices suggests the presence of a malignant neoplasm. Deeper orbital involvement with attachment or tissue fixation, altered extraocular muscle function, and bone or paranasal sinus invasion should also be evaluated.

Photographic documentation affords subsequent comparison for suspected clinical changes. It also provides a guide to facilitate placement of the definitive surgical site following biopsy.

Many eyelid malignancies, excluding basal cell carcinoma, have characteristic metastatic potential. Therefore, the preauricular, submandibular, and cervical lymph nodes must also be examined. Any suspected deep invasion mandates thorough radiologic study, including CT scanning. If the tumor is considered metastatic or part of a larger systemic disease, a complete oncologic and/or medical evaluation should be performed.

BENIGN EYELID TUMORS

Benign eyelid tumors are much more common than malignant tumors. Their treatment is directed at establishing a diagnosis (to rule out malignancy) and improving eyelid function and cosmesis.

Pseudoepitheliomatous hyperplasia is a rapid proliferation of epidermoid or squamous cells within the epidermis. It is often triggered by an irritative focus. An irregular hyperkeratotic nodule on the skin surface may result. These lesions grow rapidly, in contrast to the similar-appearing squamous cell carcinoma, which grows slowly over months or years.

Keratoacanthoma is a form of pseudoepitheliomatous hyperplasia. This relatively uncommon lesion grows rapidly with a characteristic central ulcerative crater containing keratin surrounded by hyperkeratotic margins. Some involute spontaneously; others may persist, damaging a portion of the eyelid and lashes in the process. Some of these lesions may resemble basal cell or squamous cell carcinoma; a biopsy is required for clear distinction.

Hyperkeratosis occurs in many nonspecific lesions in which excessive keratin is seen.

Papillomas are hyperkeratotic lesions in which a frond-like fibrovascular core is covered by epidermis. They may be single or multiple, sessile or pedunculated. Some papillomas may present as cutaneous horns. Papillomas are found particularly at the mucocutaneous junction, more commonly in the lower eyelid than the upper eyelid. When a papillomatous growth is of viral etiology it is called a *verruca* (Fig. 10–1).

Seborrheic keratosis (Fig. 10–2) denotes hyperkeratotic, crusty lesions that attach to the epidermis as a small plaque. They occur typically in elderly individuals and

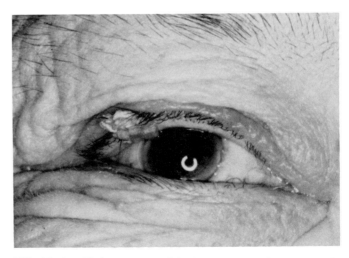

FIG. 10–1. Right upper eyelid with a verruca (papilloma of viral etiology). This one resembles a cutaneous horn.

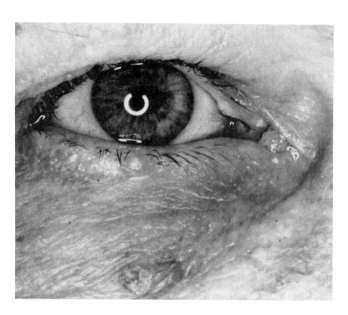

FIG. 10–2. Seborrheic keratosis of the right lower eyelid attached to the epidermis in plaque-like fashion.

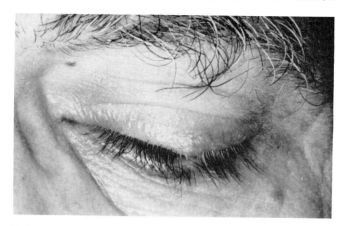

FIG. 10–3. Intradermal nevus just above the left upper eyelid lash line. This lesion appears nonpigmented.

may be pigmented. Histologically, seborrheic keratosis is composed of small, benign, epithelioid cells. Pseudocysts may form within their substance.

Molluscum contagiosum is a viral infection of eyelid epidermis, particularly involving the eyelid margin in children. These lesions appear waxy and nodular with central umbilication. A subjacent follicular conjunctivitis may result. They may be managed by surgical excision or limited cryotherapy application.

Actinic (senile) keratosis results from ultraviolet light exposure, which induces changes within the dermis and dysplasia in the overlying epidermis. It is particularly common in fair-skinned individuals (the same group that is predisposed to cicatricial ectropion and basal cell carcinoma). The clinical response may be multiple, discrete, somewhat pigmented lesions with a scaly texture. Actinic keratosis in its larger form may also present as a cutaneous horn. Few of these lesions undergo malignant degeneration into squamous cell carcinoma.

Eyelid *nevi* are common and may be intradermal, junctional, or compound. The occur commonly at the lash line and tend to grow slowly (Fig. 10–3). Nevi may present with varying degrees of pigmentation (Fig. 10–4), and at times may even be nonpigmented. The extent of pigmentation may be influenced by puberty and pregnancy. In these cases, the change is humorally mediated and not suggestive of malignancy. Changes in nevi pigmentation or size at other times may represent malignant degeneration and should be considered for diagnostic biopsy.

Intradermal nevi are confined to the dermis. They

have a smooth, somewhat elevated surface, and may occasionally be papillomatous. The presence of a hair within their substance strongly suggests benign histology. They rarely occur before puberty and have low malignant potential. Junctional nevi arise in the deeper layers of surface epithelium and subjacent dermis and have malignant potential. They appear as flat, smooth lesions with variable pigmentation. A compound nevus is composed of both dermal and junctional elements. This may occasionally undergo malignant change.

Less common varieties of nevi include the blue nevus and oculodermal melanocytosis (nevus of Ota). Blue nevi usually present at birth or within the neonatal period. They are characteristically somewhat elevated, with dark blue coloration. This nevus is located in the deeper layer of dermis and rarely enlarges. The nevus of Ota is a congenital pigmentation involving the periorbital skin,

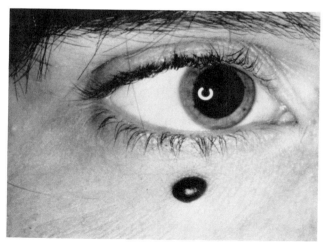

FIG. 10–4. Deeply pigmented nevus of the right lower eyelid.

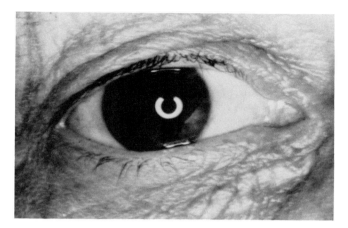

FIG. 10–5. Xanthelasma in characteristic location at the medial aspect of the eyelid.

conjunctiva, sclera, and/or uveal tract. An increased association has been found between oculodermal melanocytosis and later uveal melanoma.

Xanthelasmas are slow-growing, beige colored lesions found particularly at the nasal portion of the upper or lower eyelid (Fig. 10–5). They are commonly bilateral and occur in older individuals. Their presence in a younger patient may suggest hyperlipidemia and should be evaluated.

Hemangiomas are congenital hamartomatous lesions of variable location and presentation. They may present as a port wine stain representing telangiectatic intradermal capillaries. This stain appears at birth and remains unchanged. A port wine stain following the distribution of one or more branches of the fifth cranial nerve suggests Sturge-Weber syndrome. This condition may be associated with choroidal and/or cerebral hemangioma. In Sturge-Weber, if the upper eyelid is affected, glaucoma often occurs. These lesions are amenable to covering cosmetics. Surgery and irradiation are not recommended, but cosmetic tattooing has benefitted some patients.

Capillary hemangiomas are elevated red lesions composed of proliferative capillaries and endothelial cells. They often undergo a growth spurt from 6 to 12 months of age and variably involute thereafter. Most require no treatment. Larger capillary hemangiomas may resolve incompletely. Their size and location may predispose to deprivation amblyopia (from mechanical blepharoptosis) or anisometropic amblyopia (from induced astigmatism). Such hemangiomas should be treated. Surgical excision and radiation are not recommended because they incompletely resolve the problem and induce considerable scarring. Intralesional steroid injection has proven the most efficacious modality for capillary hemangiomas that

require treatment. Capillary hemangiomas are discussed in detail in Chapter 15.

Lymphangioma of the eyelid is often confused with capillary hemangioma. These two entities may sometimes coexist. Lymphangiomas are composed of lymph-filled spaces lined with endothelium and separated by thin septae. Germinal centers of lymphoid tissues are usually distributed throughout the tumor. An occasional hemorrhage into a lymphangioma may result in sudden enlargement of the lesion, causing marked proptosis. In severe hemorrhages, vision may be threatened and emergency anterior orbital decompression may be required.

Epithelial inclusion cysts are most prevalent at the canthi. They result from entrapment of epithelial cells below the skin surface. This ectopic tissue forms an epithelial lined cyst containing sloughed keratin. Its surgical excision should be complete within its epithelial capsule; otherwise extravasted keratin may incite a granulomatous inflammatory response.

MALIGNANT EYELID TUMORS

Malignant eyelid tumors in order of frequency include basal cell carcinoma, squamous cell carcinoma, sebaceous cell (gland) carcinoma, and malignant melanoma. Clinical changes suggesting malignancy may include loss of eyelashes; ulceration; changes in size, configuration, or color; or recurrence following prior excision. Malignant eyelid tumors may spread by local invasion or metastasis through blood vessels or lymphatic channels. Local spread may be horizontal (intralamellar) or vertical into the dermis or deeper layers. In general, the deeper the invasion, the greater is the metastatic potential. Some tumors may be multicentric, particularly sebaceous cell carcinoma.

BASAL CELL CARCINOMA

Basal cell carcinoma is distinctly the most common eyelid malignancy (90% of all primary eyelid malignancies). Its frequency of location, in descending order, is in the lower eyelid (50%), inner canthus (17–24%), upper eyelid, and outer canthus. These carcinomas are particularly prevalent in fair-skinned individuals, particularly those with a history of significant sun exposure. These tumors are usually slow-growing, invading bone or deeper orbital structures late in the disease. Deeper invasion is more characteristic of inner canthal neoplasms. Basal cell carcinomas rarely metastasize.

Basal cell carcinoma is composed of nests of small,

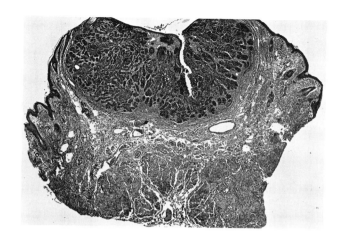

FIG. 10–6. Characteristic histologic appearance of basal cell carcinoma: small, ovoid, basaloid cells containing dark, uniform nuclei and scant cytoplasm. On fixation, it may retract into clefts, as in this complete surgical excision.

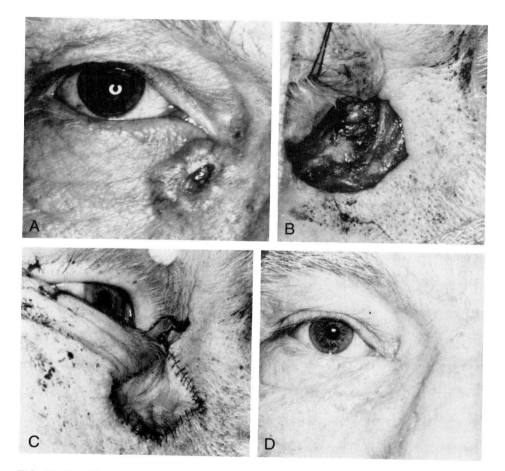

FIG. 10–7. Characteristic clinical appearance of basal cell carcinoma: elevated with overlying telangiectasia, extending to a necrotic, ulcerative core with an elevated, pearly margin. A, Preoperative appearance. B, Appearance following complete surgical excision. C, reconstruction with full-thickness retroauricular skin graft. D, Postoperative appearance.

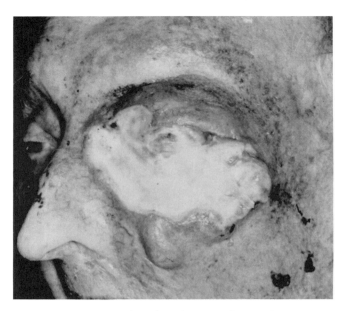

FIG. 10–8. Morpheaform basal cell carcinoma that was neglected by the patient.

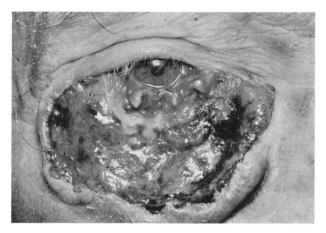

FIG. 10–9. Advanced basal cell carcinoma. Patient failed to appreciate the seriousness of this tumor.

ovoid, basiloid cells. These cells contain dark, uniform nuclei and scant cytoplasm (Fig. 10–6). During histologic fixation, basal cell carcinomas retract from the stroma, leaving clefts behind as a helpful diagnostic feature.

Three growth patterns are recognized: (1) nodular-ulcerative, (2) superficial, (3) morpheaform. Some basal cell carcinomas may be pigmented, suggestive of a nevus or melanoma. Other basal cell carcinomas may be cystic or papillomatous, or may resemble a chalazion. The basal cell nevus syndrome (Gorlin syndrome) is an uncommon variant. All suspicious lesions should undergo diagnostic incisional biopsy.

Nodular-ulcerative tumors are pale, elevated, and nodular with overlying telangiectasia. They often have a necrotic, ulcerative core with an elevated, pearly margin (Fig. 10–7). Clinically, these are the least aggressive and the slowest-growing basal cell carcinomas.

Superficial basal cell carcinomas rarely occur on the face. They are elevated, erythematous lesions that may have scaling patches.

Of the several types of basal cell carcinoma, the morpheaform (superficial sclerosing) is the most aggressive. These tumors are usually yellowish white, firm, nonulcerating lesions that may simulate scleroderma. The surface is often smooth and shiny; they grow as a plaque with overlying telangiectasia. They are relatively superficial, incite a significant fibrous response, and have poorly defined margins, spreading more widely than their clinical appearance suggests.

The morpheaform basal cell carcinoma is a particularly invasive, possibly lethal tumor (Fig. 10–8). It must be managed properly with complete removal to prevent residual tumor cells from growing at a deeper tissue plane (Fig. 10–9). Histologically, these tumors are composed of ribbons and cords of malignant epithelial cells that penetrate into deeper structures, becoming embedded in dense connective tissue (Fig. 10–10). They have the highest rate of recurrence among the basal cell group.

SQUAMOUS CELL CARCINOMA

Carcinoma *in situ* at the corneal-scleral limbus is usually superficial and grows in an exophytic manner. It can be directly excised in a lamellar manner.

Squamous cell carcinoma represents 5% of eyelid malignancies. It arises in the epidermis from actinic kera-

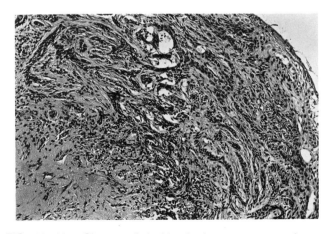

FIG. 10–10. Characteristic histologic appearance of morpheaform basal cell carcinoma: small spindle-shaped cells with scant cytoplasm separated by strands and sheets of connective tissue.

tosis and may be predisposed by excessive sun exposure. Such tumors may resemble keratoacanthoma, inverted follicular keratosis, seborrheic keratosis, pseudoepitheliomatous hyperplasia, and some basal cell carcinomas (Fig. 10–11A and B).

Squamous cell carcinoma is composed of large, pale cells with copious cytoplasm and focal areas of keratinization. It may spread by direct extension or metastasis to regional lymph nodes (preauricular, submandibular) and therefore is best managed by wide local excision. More radical excision or exenteration with lymph node dissection is reserved for extensive or deeply invasive squamous cell carcinoma.

SEBACEOUS CELL CARCINOMA

These are highly malignant tumors that arise from the meibomian glands within the tarsus, the glands of Zeis associated with the lash follicles, and the sebaceous glands within the caruncle. These tumors are composed of large atypical and pleomorphic sebaceous cells with foamy cytoplasm composed of lipid (Fig. 10–12). The nuclei may be large and irregular. The neoplasms may be multicentric (Fig. 10–13).

Sebaceous cell carcinomas arise most commonly in the upper eyelid and have a somewhat yellowish hue. Atypical, protracted, or recurrent chalazion-like lesions may harbor sebaceous cell carcinoma. A unilateral blepharoconjunctivitis with loss of lashes and/or alteration of meibomian gland orifices should also suggest the possibility of a meibomian carcinoma. A diagnostic incisional biopsy is warrented with consideration that these lesions may be multicentric. Fat stains should be specifically requested.

These tumors can spread by direct extension, vascular, dissemination, and lymphatic spread to the preauricular, parotid, or cervical nodes. Wide surgical excision is nec-

essary in most cases. Exenteration with lymph node dissection may be required for extensive or deeply invasive squamous cell carcinoma.

MALIGNANT MELANOMA

Malignant melanoma of the eyelid is rare. It may arise from pre-existing nevi or *de novo*. Some nevi may additionally arise from the conjunctiva and invade the skin secondarily (Fig. 10–14). Cutaneous melanomas are subdivided into (1) lentigo maligna (Hutchinson's freckle), (2) superficial spreading melanoma, (3) nodular melanoma. Hutchinson's freckle is an acquired pigmentation occurring on sun-exposed areas in older individuals. Nevi and Hutchinson's freckles may occasionally undergo malignant degeneration. Acquired melanosis of the conjunctiva is similar and may also give rise to malignant melanoma. Nodular melanomas tend to grow vertically and have a poor prognosis.

Clinically, pigmented basal cell carcinomas and seborrheic keratosis may resemble malignant melanoma.

Malignant melanomas are composed of atypical melanocytes of variable differentiation. When confined to the epithelium (conjunctiva or skin), they have a high cure rate. Deeper invasion has a poorer prognosis.

Because of their metastatic potential, the preoperative work-up for melanoma should include liver function studies and a liver scan, chest X-rays, and evaluation of regional lymph nodes.

Eyelid melanomas are managed by wide local excision (Fig. 10–15). Local conjunctival recurrence may respond to direct cryotherapy. Exenteration should be reserved for extensive or invasive melanoma.

BIOPSY

For lesions suspected as malignant, a biopsy is essential in establishing accurate diagnosis. Such tissue, ex-

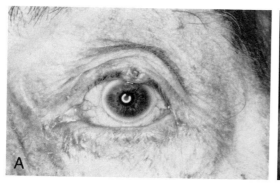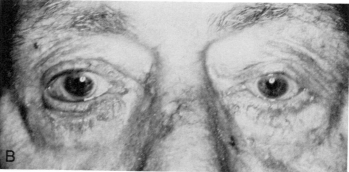

FIG. 10–11.   Squamous cell carcinoma of left upper eyelid. A, Preoperative appearance. B, Postoperative appearance following pentagonal excision and reconstruction.

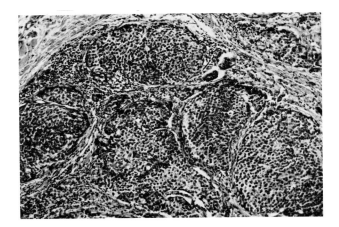

FIG. 10–12. A well-contained meibomian gland carcinoma.

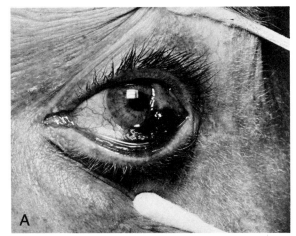

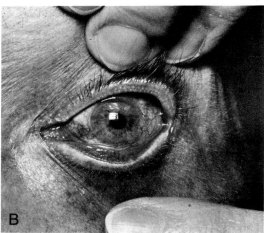

FIG. 10–14. Malignant melanoma of limbus with rapid growth and increasing pigmentation. A, Preoperative appearance. B, Postoperative appearance after tumor excision and placement of a conjunctival rotation flap.

amined histologically, provides diagnostic information on which to base subsequent therapeutic decisions. Fat stains assist the diagnosis of suspected sebaceous cell carcinoma.

An initial excisional biopsy is appropriate only for small circumscribed lesions that lend themselves to complete excision and simple reconstruction. Such specimens should have their corners labeled in case tumor is present at one or more margin.

An incisional biopsy is indicated in most other cases and should be directed at the most representative portion of the tumor. Specimens may be single or multiple, depending on the size and shape of the lesion and the condition of surrounding structures. It is important to remember that tumors developing from an epithelial surface may have an area of frank carcinoma surrounded by areas that show normal cellular architecture, or that represent various precancerous changes. The latter may ul-

timately develop into a true carcinoma. For this reason, multiple biopsy sites may sometimes be required.

When possible, the biopsy specimen should be large enough for study of the tumor and its interface with normal surrounding tissue. By furnishing an adequately sized specimen, the pathologist can accurately determine the nature of the lesion, along with its depth and breadth. Small specimens obtained by needle, punch, or aspiration biopsy may fail to accomplish this goal.

INCISIONAL BIOPSY TECHNIQUE

Before local anesthetic infiltration, the location and extent of the biopsy site is determined. Xylocaine 2% is infiltrated. A #64 Beaver blade or pair of sharp Stevens scissors is used to remove a representative specimen

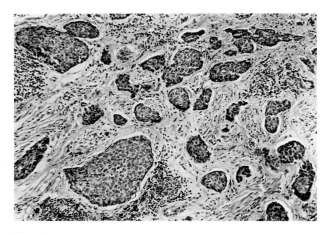

FIG. 10–13. Meibomian gland carcinoma with extensive, multicentric involvement of the eyelid.

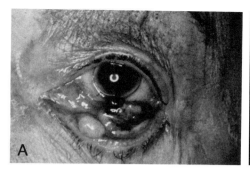
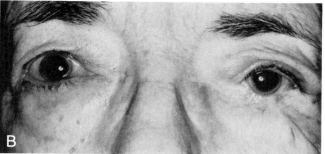

FIG. 10–15. Extensive malignant melanoma of the bulbar conjunctiva and entire lower eyelid. A, Preoperative appearance. B, Postoperative appearance after wide local excision, Mustarde cheek rotation, and buccal mucous membrane grafting. Vision and ocular motility were both preserved intact.

(Fig. 10–16). Hemostasis is obtained with pressure and light cautery. Small lesions are allowed to heal by granulation. Large lesions are closed with running 7-0 silk, ensuring that ectropion and notching do not result. The suture line should conform to Langer's lines if feasible.

MANAGEMENT OF EYELID MALIGNANCY

Once an accurate diagnosis has been established, the histology of the lesion, along with an assessment of the patient's overall medical status, dictates the proper mode of treatment. Although selected malignancies may benefit from cryosurgery, chemosurgery (Moh's technique), or radiation therapy, surgical excision is the treatment of choice whenever possible because it affords the lowest

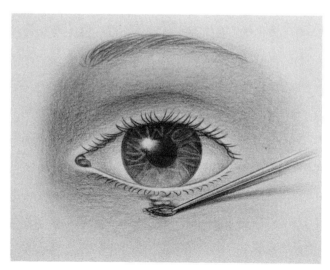

FIG. 10–16. Representative incisional biopsy in conformity with Langer's lines.

rate of recurrence and the most favorable functional and cosmetic result.

CRYOSURGERY

In this procedure, the lesion and adjacent tissue are frozen to $-30°$ C using a liquid nitrogen unit in a double freeze-thaw cycle. Cellular damage occurs during the thaw phase. It is essential to place a thermocouple to accurately monitor the temperature. Excessive cooling may damage surrounding normal tissue; insufficient cooling may leave viable tumor cells. Even when adequate freezing is achieved, the tumor recurrence rate is excessive (20%) with this technique, histologic control is absent, and it is not generally recommended. Cryotherapy is most useful for superficial basal cell carcinoma and the basal cell nevus syndrome. It is contraindicated for morpheaform basal cell tumors.

Following treatment, tissues become swollen and tender for several days. At times an eschar may result. Cryotherapy may cause skin depigmentation, loss of eyelashes, notching of the eyelid margin, and occasional canalicular stenosis.

MOH'S TECHNIQUE

Moh's fresh tissue technique (or chemosurgery technique if a zinc oxide fixative is used) is effective in removing extensive, recurrent, or deeply invasive tumors. In this process, tissue is surgically removed in small lamellar blocks of tissue. Histologic examination reveals the dimensional topography of the tumor in the process.

Any block with tumor present prompts additional specimens from adjacent or subjacent tissue blocks. This process continues until the malignancy has been entirely

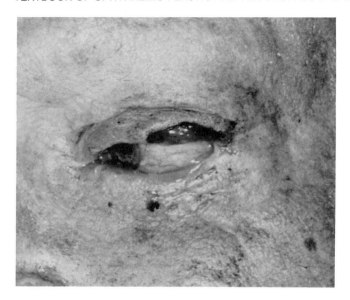

FIG. 10–17.   Upper eyelid appearance after a Moh's multi-stage excision.

removed. Although this method is histologically reliable, it is time-consuming and requires multiple separate surgical excisions, often on several different days.

In the past, reconstruction had been by way of spontaneous granulation, and often yielded a poor result (Fig. 10–17). Current reconstruction is now more thorough, achieving improved results. Yet neither of Moh's techniques achieves better histologic control than meticulous surgical excisional biopsy with frozen and paraffin section control. Therefore, surgical excisional biopsy followed by immediate reconstruction remains preferable.

IRRADIATION

Radiation therapy is limited by its lack of histologic confirmation and moderately high recurrence rate (5–10%), especially for sclerosing or morpheaform basal cell carcinoma. Deeply invasive tumors are even less responsive to radiation, obviating its use in most such situations.

Complications of radiation therapy may include epidermalization (keratinization) of the eyelid margin, loss of lashes, entropion, cicatricial ectropion, canalicular obstruction, cosmetic deformities, skin discoloration and atrophy, telangiectasia of the skin, and keratitis sicca. If the malignancy recurs after radiation therapy, it may then be deeply invasive and its margins may prove highly irregular, complicating subsequent surgical excision.

SURGICAL EXCISION

An accurate histologic diagnosis must precede definitive surgical excision. Surgery affords reliable, complete removal of the lesion with accurate histologic monitoring of the tumor margins. It has the lowest recurrence rate (2 to 3%), and in most circumstances yields the most favorable functional and cosmetic result.

The goal of surgical excision is to remove the tumor in a single piece, establishing adequate tumor-free margins. This is achievable in most cases. In those with bone or paranasal sinus invasion, it may not be possible to clear the tumor initially. In such cases, additional blocks of tissue may have to be submitted.

Complete removal of the tumor is the highest surgical priority, disregarding the juxtaposition of contiguous eyelid and periorbital structures (i.e., lacrimal drainage system). If adequate excision is compromised by more limited surgery, these structures will likely become invaded anyway by local tumor recurrence. Should essential structures be removed as part of the overall tumor excision, they are usually amenable to subsequent reconstruction (i.e., Jones tube).

The size of margin to be left depends on the type, size, and extent of the tumor, along with the condition of the surrounding skin. For small basal cell carcinomas, a 3 mm margin of normal-appearing skin may be adequate. For larger, more aggressive and/or multicentric tumors, wide local excision with an extensive margin may be required. According to these guidelines the excision site is defined with a marking pen. After xylocaine infiltration, an incision is made with either Stevens scissors or #64 Beaver blade. Lesions involving the eyelid margin are removed in the standard pentagonal manner. Taking additional marginal strips 1 to 2 mm in width may foster better histologic control.

If periosteum has been invaded by tumor, it must be removed along with the subjacent bony orbital wall. These tissues are examined in permanent section studies.

A close working relationship between surgeon and pathologist maximizes the diagnostic accuracy of tumor margins. To communicate effectively with the pathologist, the surgeon should provide a clear statement of the tumor site, differential diagnosis, and examination desired (paraffin sections only or frozen and paraffin sections). The tumor margins should be clearly labeled. This may be accomplished using sutures of different color or length, or a different number of sutures placed in each margin. An appropriate sketch showing the proper anatomic relationships further orients the pathologist. (If the tumor is sufficiently unusual or important, the pathologist should have the opportunity to examine the patient preoperatively.)

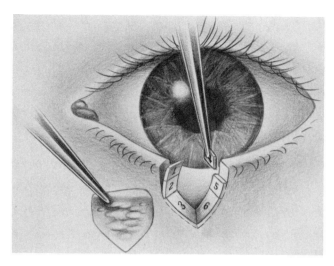

FIG. 10–18. Pentagonal excision of eyelid margin lesion. Additional frozen sections are 1 to 2 mm wide and should be consecutively numbered.

In tumors involving the eyelid margin, only the medial and lateral margins require study. The portion of tumor at the eyelid margin or conjunctival surface is of no significance because it does not contact other structures. In tumors involving the canthi, all margins, including the entire deep margin, must be examined.

Eyelid reconstruction should not proceed until the tumor has been *completely* excised as documented by frozen section results. This mandates frozen section studies performed by a pathologist concurrent with surgery. When frozen sections demonstrate residual tumor, the labeling sutures allow the pathologist to communicate its location to the surgeon. The surgeon must then take additional strips from the involved margin (including the deep margin, if involved). Subsequent specimens should be consecutively numbered and their location recorded (Fig. 10–18). Additional specimens must be removed from involved margins until all margins have been histologically cleared as documented by frozen sections. When all margins are reported as clear of tumor, the reconstruction can commence.

Out of necessity, surgical reconstruction must be based solely on frozen section information. In most cases this is confirmed by subsequent paraffin section studies. Occasionally the results of permanent sections and frozen sections may differ somewhat. If frozen sections indicate that the surgical margins are free of tumor, while the paraffin sections suggest the presence of residual tumor, a decision should be reached regarding further management.

In cases of basal cell carcinoma where "a few nests" of tumor cells remain, most will not lead to tumor recurrence. Such cases require observation, with further

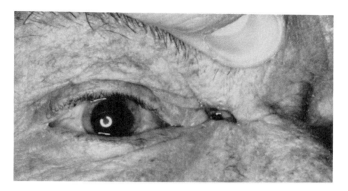

FIG. 10–19. Basal cell carcinoma of the inner canthus. This was previously incompletely excised, allowing recurrence to the level of the medial orbital wall.

surgery reserved for demonstrable clinical recurrence. An exception to this is the inner canthus. Should such a positive margin be discovered on permanent section, reoperation in the early postoperative period is recommended to completely clear the tumor (Fig. 10–19).

After the tumor has been excised, instruments should be resterilized and gowns and gloves changed to avoid transplanting tumor cells into the reconstruction site. This step is particularly important when dealing with malignant melanoma.

EYELID RECONSTRUCTION

In undertaking the reconstruction of any tissue, it is necessary to consider the anatomy and function of these tissues in their natural form (Fig. 10–20). Eyelid anatomy is considered in detail in Chapter 1. For reconstructive purposes, the eyelid may be divided into two planes: (1) the skin and orbicularis oculi muscle and (2) the tarsus and conjunctiva. These two segments meet at the mucocutaneous eyelid margin. The mucocutaneous junction at the eyelid margin is a precisely aligned area that prevents keratinized epithelium from coming into contact with the globe.

The tarsal plate forms the supportive framework for the eyelid and must be internally lined by mucous membrane to protect the subjacent cornea.

Retractor muscles in each eyelid insert into the respective tarsal plate, giving additional function and mobility, particularly in the upper eyelid. The retractors of the upper eyelid include the levator palpebrae superioris muscle and the less prominent Müller's muscle. The inferior aponeurosis is the lower eyelid retractor. It is a more rudimentary structure, but still must be considered to avoid lagophthalmos in lower eyelid reconstruction.

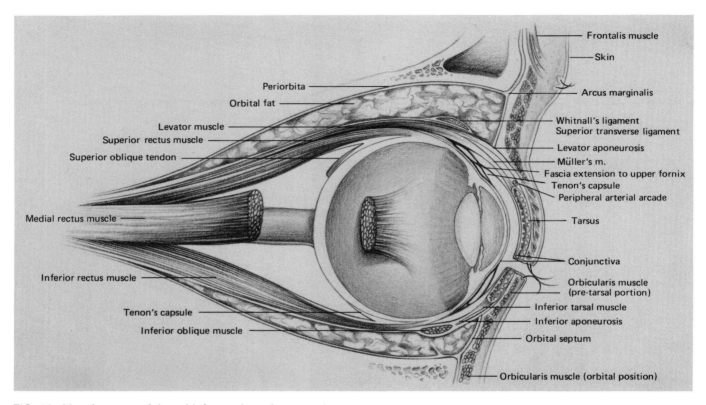

FIG. 10–20. Anatomy of the orbit from a lateral perspective.

The protractors of the eyelid are the palpebral (pretarsal and preseptal) portions of the orbicularis oculi muscle.

Eyelid defects requiring various reconstructive techniques may arise from eyelid colobomas, trauma, or tumor. Occasionally, extensive radiation, burns, or inflammation may result in large reconstructive defects as well. Eyelid colobomas were reviewed in Chapter 3. Principles of reconstruction after trauma were reviewed in Chapter 2. Surgical reconstructive techniques covered in this chapter apply to all categories, since the same surgical principles apply. The scope of reconstruction depends on the size and location of the defect, the structural integrity of the remainder of the periorbital structures, the elasticity of potential donor tissue (related to age), and the surgeon's experience.

Relevant lengths to be considered in adult eyelid reconstruction include upper eyelid, 34 mm; lower eyelid, 32 mm; palpebral fissure, 30 mm. The percentage of eyelid excision and reconstruction may be based on such figures, with slight variance in each case.

DEFECTS NOT INVOLVING THE EYELID MARGIN

Relatively small upper or lower eyelid defects not involving the eyelid margin can often be closed primarily.

If possible, the wound should be converted into an ellipse, orienting the suture line horizontally in conformity with Langer's lines. Such horizontal suture lines, however, should not be allowed to create vertical tissue insufficiency and ectropion. Undermining the wound edges may be required to close some defects. If the defect is too large to close horizontally without inducing ectropion, vertical closure may be considered.

Larger defects may result in relative or absolute tissue insufficiency. These situations may require sliding, transpositional, advancement, or rotational flaps, or free skin grafts to cover the defect and relieve tissue tension. The size and scope of a defect may, at times, require the combination of several reconstructive techniques (Fig. 10–21), described in Chapter 2.

DEFECTS INVOLVING THE EYELID MARGIN

When the eyelid margin is disrupted by trauma or tumor excision, the defect is artificially widened by the unopposed pull of the orbicularis oculi muscle away from the defect, toward the canthal tendons (Fig. 10–22). Marginal defects involving less than 30% (approximately 9 to 10 mm) of either eyelid afford reconstruction by

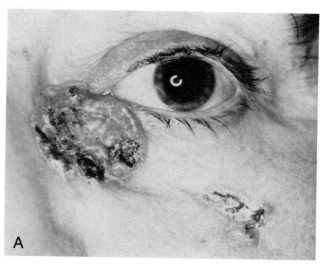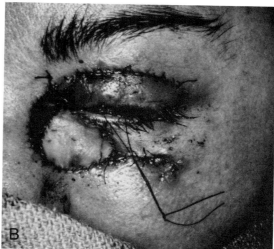

FIG. 10–21. A, Large morpheaform basal cell carcinoma of the left lower eyelid and inner canthus. B, Postoperative appearance after excision and reconstruction involving an upper eyelid pedicle flap combined with full-thickness retroauricular skin graft.

simply converting the defect into a pentagonal configuration and closing by direct approximation. All normal eyelid tissue should be preserved to minimize the scope of reconstruction.

Eyelid reformation is structured around reformation of the eyelid margin. Castroviejo forceps may be used to draw the edges of the eyelid margin defect gently toward one another to ascertain whether direct closure is feasible.

Eyelid Margin Closure. Three sutures are the corner-

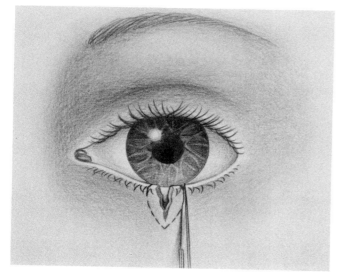

FIG. 10–22. Traumatic defect of the eyelid margin reconstructed into a pentagonal configuration.

stone of this reconstruction (Fig. 10–23A). The central eyelid margin suture of 4-0 silk is inserted at the gray line engaging the central portion of tarsus on each side of the defect. The anterior eyelid margin suture of 5-0 silk is inserted just anterior to the gray line engaging the anterior portion of the tarsus on each side of the defect. A similar posterior eyelid margin suture of 5-0 silk is inserted just posterior to the gray line engaging the posterior portion of tarsus. Each suture should penetrate 2 mm deep into the tarsus and emerge 2 mm from each cut edge of the eyelid margin (Fig. 10–23B). Placement of the anterior suture should carefully avoid damage to the nearby eyelash follicles.

As each of these sutures is placed, it should be temporarily tied with a slip knot to determine the accuracy of apposition. Any suture that does not achieve optimal approximation should be replaced. The central and posterior sutures should be tied first and then tunneled anteriorly underneath the anterior suture which is tied last. This minimizes corneal epithelial disruption by the eyelid margin suture line. These sutures should be left long and secured to the apposing cheek or brow respectively to minimize any postoperative notching tendency.

The tarsus (and subjacent conjunctiva) is then approximated with 6-0 Vicryl horizontal mattress sutures, followed by skin closure with running 7-0 silk (Fig. 10–23C). The skin sutures may be removed 6 days postoperatively, while the eyelid margin sutures may remain under mild traction for 10 days.

Application of proper reconstructive technique will obviate most postoperative problems (Figs. 10–24 and 10–25). Occasionally encountered complications include

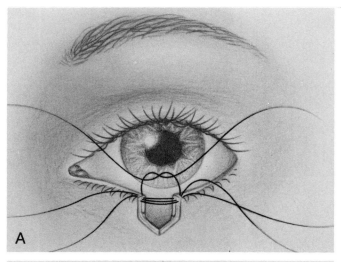

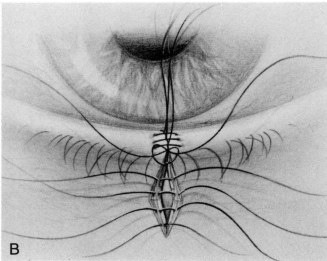

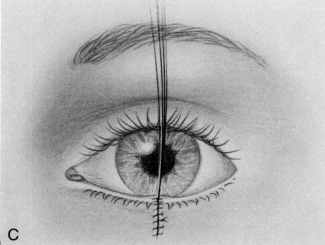

FIG. 10–23. Pentagonal closure of a full-thickness eyelid margin defect. A, Placement of three eyelid margin sutures. B, Central and posterior sutures should be tunnelled under the anterior suture, which is tied last. C, Following closure, the eyelid margin sutures may be placed under traction to avoid notching.

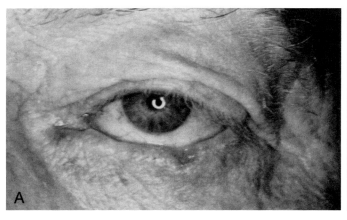

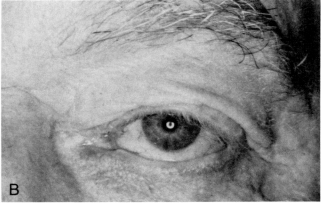

FIG. 10–24. Basal cell carcinoma of left lower eyelid. A, Preoperative appearance. B, Postoperative appearance after pentagonal excision and eyelid margin reconstruction.

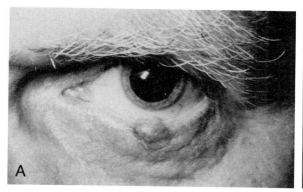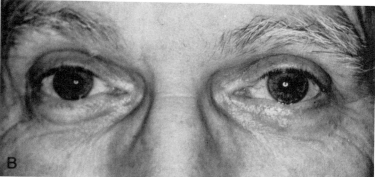

FIG. 10–25. Cystic basal cell carcinoma of left lower eyelid A, Preoperative appearance. B, Postoperative appearance after pentagonal excision and eyelid margin reconstruction.

eyelid notching, cicatricial ectropion, and trichiasis. A notch may be managed by simply excising the notch with revised closure of the eyelid margin. Cicatricial ectropion requires excision of the scar with reconstruction involving either a Z-plasty (see Chapter 2) or full-thickness retroauricular skin graft (see Chapter 7). Trichiasis, if limited, is responsive to cryotherapy. More extensive trichiasis requires eyelid rotation (Wies procedure).

Defects involving 30 to 50% (10 to 15 mm) of the eyelid margin additionally require a lateral canthotomy with lysis of the appropriate crus of the lateral canthal tendon. This should provide an additional 6 mm of eyelid mobility medially for reconstruction.

Canthotomy and Cantholysis. A straight hemostat is placed at the outer canthus, extending laterally toward the central portion of the lateral orbital rim. The hemostat is left in the closed position for approximately 10 seconds to enhance hemostasis. The hemostat is removed and replaced with Stevens scissors (Fig. 10–26A). A 5 mm cut is then made in the tract left by the hemostat blades. This divides the lateral canthal tendon into an upper and lower segment. Through this lateral canthotomy, the appropriate crus of the lateral canthal tendon is palpated with the tip of Stevens scissors. The scissors are then used to sever the desired crus from its attachment to periosteum at the lateral orbital tubercle (Fig. 10–26B). Once the crus has been divided, the eyelid demonstrates considerably more medial mobility.

Eyelid reconstruction may now begin with minimal tension on the suture line (Fig. 10–26C). The canthotomy may be closed with an interrupted 6-0 silk suture to reestablish the lateral canthal angle and running 7-0 silk (Fig. 10–26D).

Sliding tarsoconjunctival flaps and composite grafts may be used for 50% eyelid defects. Defects greater than

50% (16 mm or greater) can be preferentially reconstructed with Mustarde or Tenzel rotation flaps, or Hughes or Cutler-Beard eyelid sharing flaps. The larger defects (80 to 100%) are best closed using a Mustarde flap or a combination of several techniques. Eyelid sharing flaps for such large defects would otherwise adversely affect the function and appearance of the donor eyelid.

Sliding Tarsoconjunctival Flap. A sliding flap of tarsoconjunctiva may be used to reconstruct an eyelid defect approaching 50% (Fig. 10–27A). In this procedure, a lamellar tarsal flap is fashioned from adjacent normal eyelid. This flap is slid into the defect to reconstruct the posterior lamella. The anterior lamella is provided from a retroauricular full-thickness skin graft or a flap of skin adjacent to the defect.

Under local anesthesia, the involved eyelid is infiltrated with xylocaine, 2%. The eyelid is everted to afford exposure and a horizontal incision is made in the adjacent tarsus 2 to 3 mm above the eyelid margin (Fig. 10–27B). This incision should be intralamellar, not involving the full thickness of the tarsal plate. The length of this incision is dictated by the horizontal length of the adjacent defect. A vertical incision is then made at the distal end of the incision, extending to the upper border of tarsus. The attachment between this flap and conjunctiva should be meticulously preserved. All other attachments to levator aponeurosis and Müller's muscle should be severed.

This tarsoconjunctival flap is separated from overlying tarsus, mobilized into the adjacent defect, and secured with interrupted 5-0 Vicryl sutures joining tarsus to tarsus (Fig. 10–27C). The anterior lamella is provided by a full-thickness retroauricular skin graft (Fig. 10–27D). This tissue is harvested and sutured in place with interrupted 6-0 silk at the corners and running 7-0 silk for the remainder of the graft. A light-pressure dressing is

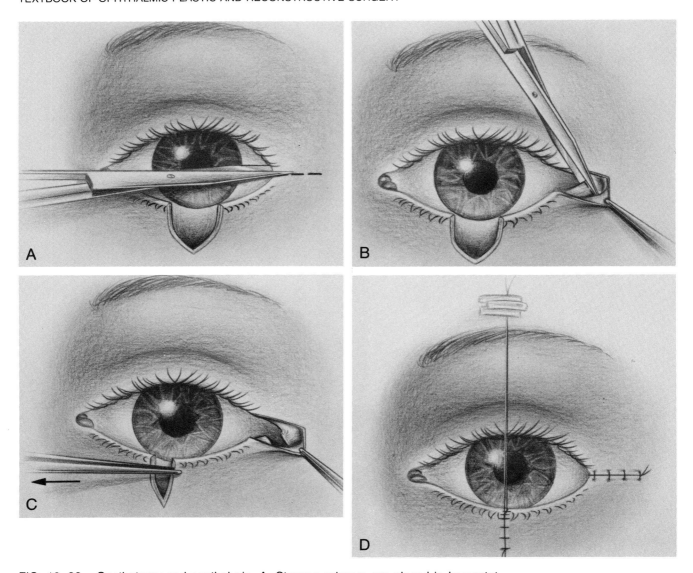

FIG. 10–26. Canthotomy and cantholysis. A, Stevens scissors are placed in hemostat tract at outer canthus. B, Following canthotomy, the appropriate crus of the lateral canthal tendon is severed, affording enhanced medial mobility of the eyelid, C. D, Reconstruction proceeds as in Figure 10–23.

provided and the skin sutures are removed 6 days after surgery.

Composite Grafts. Full-thickness defects involving up to 50% of an eyelid may be closed by free composite grafts from an uninvolved eyelid. This must follow a canthotomy or cantholysis to reduce the defect. If the recipient defect is 8 mm or less after canthotomy and cantholysis, a composite graft may be considered. Such a graft may be used only when sufficient tissue remains in the donor eyelid to allow its direct closure.

This technique is performed under local anesthesia. A composite full-thickness pentagonal graft is taken as a block from the donor eyelid and transplanted into the recipient bed. This graft should not be greater than 8 mm in vertical height (Fig. 10–28). Tissue manipulation must be delicate to avoid unnecessary vascular compromise to such a tenuous graft. The donor and recipient eyelids are both closed in two layers in a similar manner. Tarsus is joined at the eyelid margin with interrupted 5-0 Vicryl, and along its edge with interrupted or running 6-0 Vicryl. The skin is closed with running 7-0 silk.

A variation of this technique uses the eyelid margin and the posterior lamella (tarsus and conjunctiva) from the composite donor graft (Fig. 10–29). The remainder

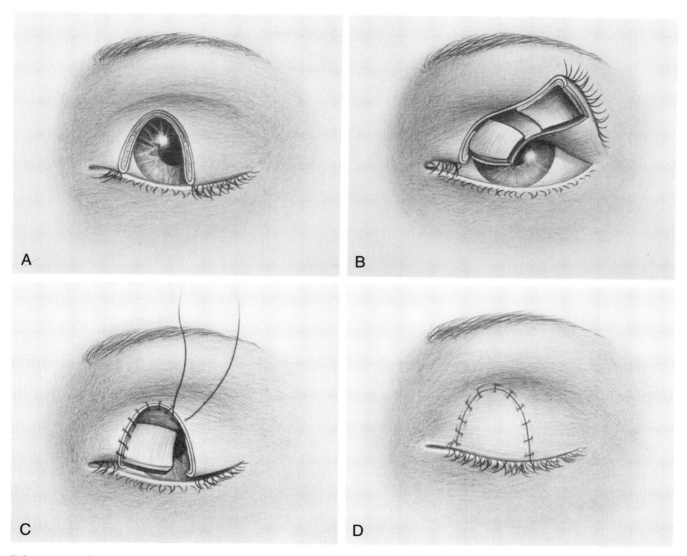

FIG. 10–27.   Sliding tarsoconjunctival flap. A, A 50% eyelid defect. B, Adjacent tarsus is incised in an intralamellar fashion. C, Tarsonconjunctival flap is mobilized and sutured into position. D, Anterior lamellar reconstruction is by full-thickness retroauricular skin graft.

of the anterior lamella is provided by a sliding or advancement flap of skin from an adjacent portion of the eyelid under reconstruction.

Mustarde Technique. The Mustarde technique is most effective when used for defects on the lateral half of either the upper or lower eyelid (reverse Mustarde procedure). It may be applied to larger defects, including reconstruction of the entire eyelid.

This is a one-stage procedure, usually performed under general anesthesia, that rotates the cheek and malar region toward the inner canthus. Care must be taken to free the skin flap completely and to carry the direction

of the flap into the curve of the eyelid to be reconstructed.

Before reconstruction, the remaining tarsal edges should be perpendicular to the eyelid margin. The area of cheek intended for rotation should be clearly designated with a marking pen. If the defect is in the lower eyelid, the scalpel incision (#64 Beaver blade) beyond the lateral canthus must be directed upward in a gentle, sweeping curve as a direct continuation of the direction of the lateral portion of the lower eyelid. The incision reaches its apex midway between the outer canthus and the sideburn area, at the height of the brow. It then extends in an inferolateral direction anterior to the hairline (Fig. 10–30A). Hair-bearing tissue must never be

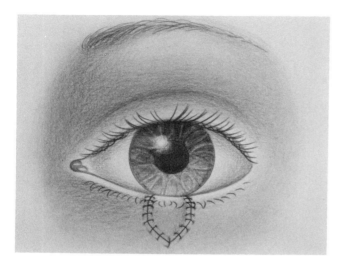

FIG. 10–28.   Full-thickness eyelid reconstruction with a composite graft.

incorporated into the flap; otherwise islands of hair will result.

Incision depth should be through the orbicularis oculi muscle medial to the lateral orbital rim and through the subcutaneous tissue lateral to that. The flap is then completely undermined by blunt and sharp dissection with Metzenbaum scissors. The flap should slip into a natural plane anterior to facial muscle fascia to achieve mobilization, rotation, and advancement. If the plane is too superficial, it may compromise blood supply; if too deep, it may injure branches of the facial nerve. In large reconstructions, it may occasionally be necessary to make a small horizontal back-cut at the lower end of the incision to facilitate rotation. The appropriate crus of the lateral canthal tendon must be severed as well as the lateral attachment of the orbital septum. Hemostasis is obtained with electrocautery. At this point, the anterior, skin-muscle layer of the new eyelid has been surgically defined.

In upper eyelid reconstruction, the flap configuration is the mirror image of that just described.

The posterior layer of the eyelid must be reconstructed with a mucous membrane lining. Reconstruction of the upper eyelid mandates an effective tarsal substitute. This is afforded by a composite graft of nasal septal cartilage and subjacent mucosa as described in Chapter 2. Such cartilage in the lower eyelid would provide excessive volume to this structure and inhibit its mobility. The posterior lamella of the lower eyelid should instead be reconstructed with a 0.3 mm buccal mucous membrane graft, also described in Chapter 2.

The skin muscle flap should be pulled medially to ensure that it is sufficiently mobile and to define the portion of the flap that will replace the eyelid. The mu-

cosal graft (with cartilage for upper eyelid reconstruction) should be sutured subjacent to the eyelid portion of the flap. It is essential that the mucosal surface be placed posteriorly to ensure its ultimate contact with the globe. The graft is initially secured with interrupted 5-0 chromic sutures at the corners. A running 6-0 chromic suture around its perimeter further secures the mucosa to the back of the skin-muscle flap. This suture must be meticulously placed at the eyelid margin to most effectively recreate the "gray line."

The cheek flap is rotated medially to reform the eyelid. To minimize tension at the anastomosis, the flap must be secured at its rotational apex in the region of the temple. This also minimizes subsequent eyelid retraction and sag. A 4-0 Supramid or Mersilene suture is used to join the dermis of the flap at its apex of rotation to the subjacent periosteum. A second suture of this type is placed, joining the deep surface of the flap to periosteum at the lateral orbital rim (Fig. 10–30B).

The eyelid margin is joined with two or three interrupted 4-0 silk sutures left long for postoperative traction (Fig. 10–30C). The tarsus may be united with interrupted 5-0 Vicryl mattress sutures, and the skin is closed with running 6-0 silk. An additional 4-0 silk suture taken with wide, deep bites may help reduce tension on the suture line. Any "dog-ear" that forms may be directly excised and closed with 6-0 silk.

The cheek rotation is closed in two layers. Multiple interrupted 5-0 Vicryl horizontal mattress sutures bring the cheek rotation into effective approximation. The skin is closed with running 6-0 silk sutures (Fig. 10–30D).

The relative tightness of the newly formed eyelid may temporarily preclude exposure of the fornix. If the fornix is accessible, the mucosal graft is sutured to the cut

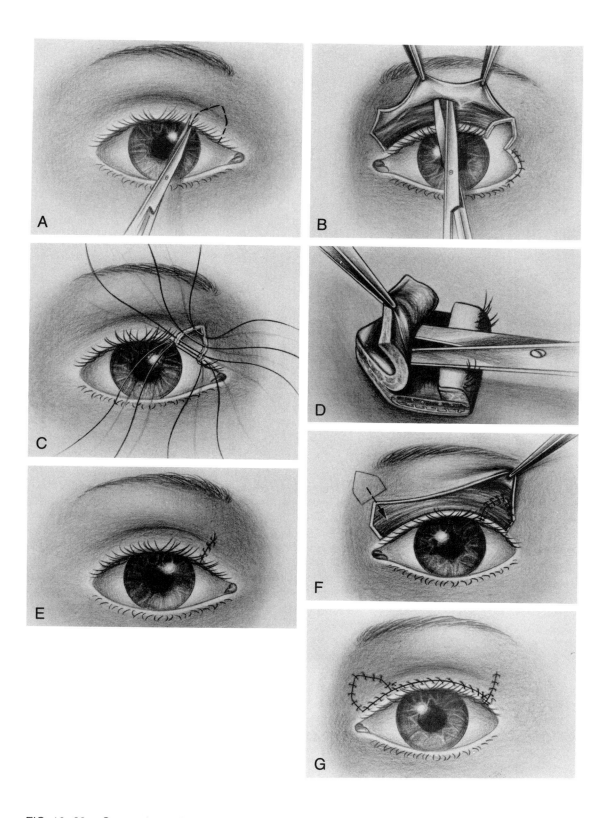

FIG. 10–29.   Composite graft variation. A, Composite pentagonal graft harvested from the donor right upper eyelid. B, Following tumor excision and lateral cantholysis, a skin flap is incised in the recipient left upper eyelid. C, Donor pentagonal defect is closed in the usual manner. D, The donor composite graft is split into anterior and posterior lamellae, leaving the eyelid margin intact. E, Donor eyelid reconstruction is completed. F, Posterior lamella of the graft is sutured into position and the skin flap is mobilized laterally to cover the defect. This leaves an anterior lamella defect at the medial aspect of the recipient eyelid. G, Pentagonal segment of skin from the donor graft is sutured into the medial aspect of the recipient eyelid.

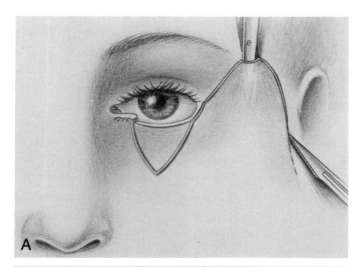

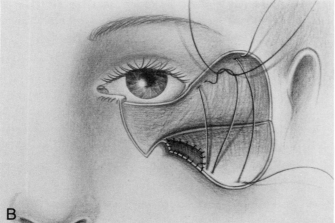

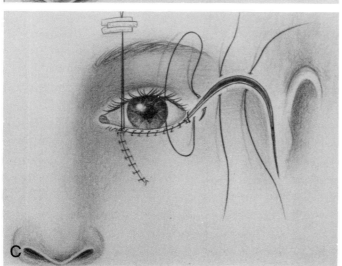

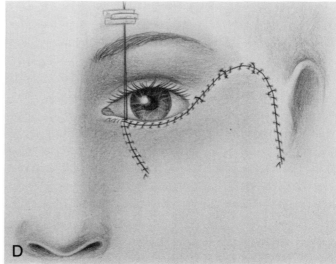

FIG. 10–30. Mustarde technique. A, Cheek rotation flap is marked, incised, and mobilized. B, Buccal mucous membrane graft is sutured to the portion of the flap that will become the new eyelid. 4-0 Supramid or Mersilene sutures are used to secure the flap to its apex of rotation and to periosteum at the lateral orbital rim. C, The eyelid margin is reformed and D, the skin is closed.

conjunctival edges with several interrupted 7-0 chromic catgut sutures.

The canthus may be closed with two interrupted 6-0 silk sutures to re-establish the lateral canthal angle. The more posterior suture is extended deeply to engage periosteum at the lateral orbital rim. This creates a collagenous tissue tract to re-establish the severed crus of the lateral canthal tendon. The 6-0 silk sutures are removed on the sixth postoperative day, while the 4-0 silk sutures remain under mild traction for 10 days (Fig. 10–31).

The Mustarde flap may be used in reverse for upper eyelid reconstruction.

Tenzel (Semicircular) Flap. This technique is effective in central eyelid defects involving as much as 75% of the eyelid margin. It is best performed with a segment of tarsus remaining on both sides of the defect. The Tenzel flap is similar to the Mustarde procedure, except for the shape of the flap (Fig. 10–32A). The Tenzel technique may be performed under local anesthesia because it uses

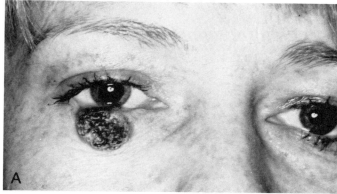

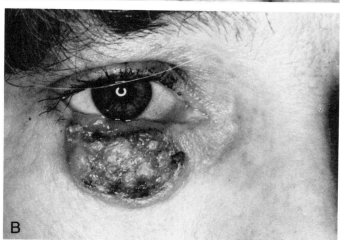

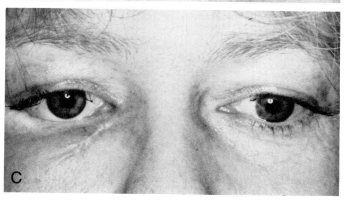

FIG. 10–31.   A, Basal cell carcinoma of the right lower eyelid. B, The same patient 2 years later when she decided to proceed with surgery. C, Postoperative appearance after tumor excision and Mustarde cheek rotation procedure.

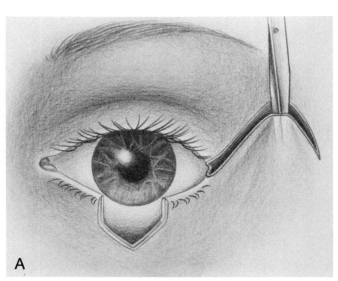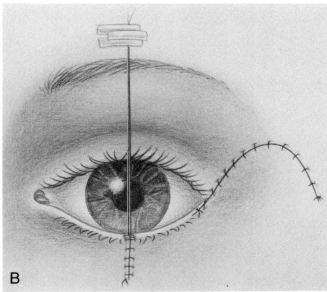

FIG. 10–32. Tenzel semicircular flap. A, Flap is marked, incised, and mobilized. B, The eyelid margin is reformed and the skin is closed.

a smaller flap with a higher arch to reconstruct a smaller defect. It does not extend as far laterally as the Mustarde. The incision, rotation, and suture placement, however, are identical (Fig. 10–32B). In the Tenzel procedure, if adequate conjunctiva remains, no mucosal graft is required.

The Mustarde and Tenzel procedures produce facial scars that can be moderately well camouflaged. Their most common feature is eyelid retraction. Diminution of the lacrimal pump, epiphora, entropion, ectropion, symblepharon, and necrosis of the flap may sometimes occur. These changes are more prevalent and pronounced in larger reconstructions.

Hughes Procedure. If an eyelid margin defect is in the medial or central portion, the vertical tarsoconjunctival advancement flap may be used. This two-stage procedure is appropriate for defects involving 40 to 80% of an eyelid. It should not be used when more than 5 to 7 mm of vertical height is required.

Although the Hughes procedure was devised to reconstruct a lower eyelid, using an upper eyelid posterior lamellar flap, it may be used in reverse to repair an upper eyelid if adequate tarsus is present in the donor lower eyelid.

It is important to realize that the eyelid defect considered for reconstruction may actually be somewhat smaller than is apparent because of the unopposed pull of the orbicularis oculi muscle. The actual size of the defect is accurately determined by firmly pulling the edges toward one another. A cantholysis may first be performed to reduce the defect size.

The Hughes procedure may be performed under local anesthesia. At the outset of reconstruction, the edges of the defect should be made perpendicular to the eyelid margin and the defect should assume a rectangular configuration. The upper eyelid is everted with either a 4-0 silk modified Frost suture or Desmarres retractor. With a #64 Beaver blade, a corresponding horizontal incision is made through the tarsoconjunctival surface of the everted upper eyelid to correspond in location to the lower eyelid defect (Fig. 10–33A). This should leave 3-4 mm of tarsus, along with the lashes undisturbed at the eyelid margin. Sufficient structural support should remain for the donor eyelid. Two vertical incisions are then extended from the ends of the horizontal tarsal cut toward the fornix. Tarsus must next be freed from its aponeurotic attachments (levator aponeurosis in an upper eyelid donor, inferior aponeurosis in a lower eyelid donor). The tarsal flap must be mobilized with only a thin attachment of conjunctiva.

The flap is then positioned in the recipient bed in a tongue and groove manner (Fig. 10–33B). Once placed into the defect, the tissues are joined with interrupted 5-0 chromic catgut. If tarsus is present in the recipient bed, the graft is united with tarsus-to-tarsus approximation. If tarsus is not present, the donor tarsus must be sutured to equivalent tissue. The eyelids may be further supported by anchoring to the adjacent canthal tendon.

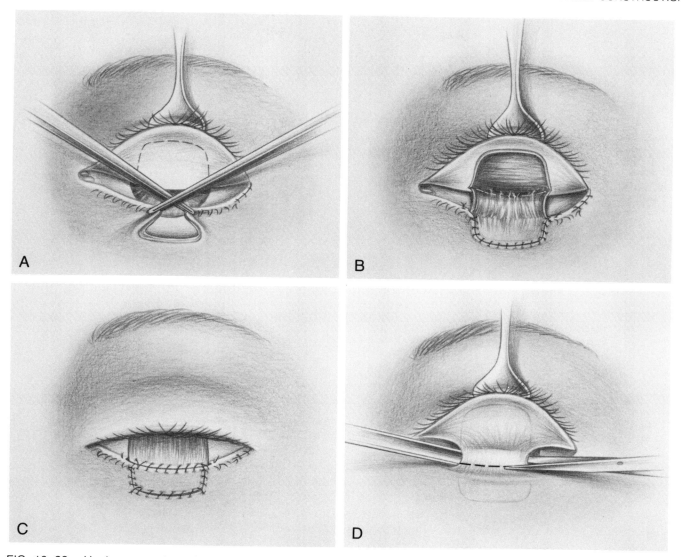

FIG. 10–33. Hughes procedure. A, Following a cantholysis, the upper eyelid donor tarsoconjunctival flap is marked to correspond with the lower eyelid defect. B, The flap is undermined, mobilized, and sutured into the recipient bed. C, Anterior lamella is provided by a free skin graft. D, After 2 to 3 months, the sharing graft is divided with the division set slightly in favor of the conjunctival surface to position more conjunctiva than skin at the reconstructed eyelid margin.

The anterior lamella is provided by a free skin graft (fenestrated), from either the contralateral upper eyelid or the retroauricular area (Fig. 10–33C). Details on graft harvesting were given in Chapter 2. The skin graft is sutured in place with interrupted 6-0 silk at the corners and running 7-0 silk for the remainder of the graft. The graft is covered with antibiotic and Telfa in the usual manner. A light-pressure dressing is placed.

Skin sutures are removed 6 days postoperatively. The sharing graft must be left in place 2 to 3 months. It is then carefully divided using direct infiltration with xy-locaine 2% (Fig. 10–33D). A blunt instrument (muscle hook or grooved director) is placed behind the donor flap. An incision is made with Stevens scissors 2 mm above the new lower eyelid margin. This incision should be slanted in favor of the conjunctival surface to position more conjunctiva at the eyelid margin than skin. The eyelid margin is then reformed with running 7-0 chromic catgut. The donor pedicle and donor bed are freshened and resutured in normal position with interruped 6-0 chromic catgut (Fig. 10–34).

Complications of the Hughes procedure may affect

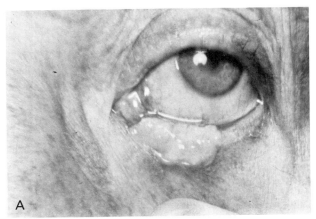

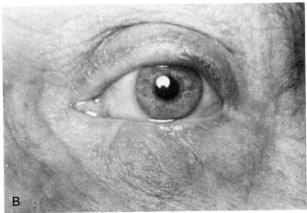

FIG. 10–34. Basal cell carcinoma. A, Preoperative appearance. B, Postoperative appearance after excision and reconstruction using Hughes procedure.

either the donor or recipient eyelid. Donor changes may include retraction, contour abnormalities, notching, ectropion, entropion, trichiasis, or loss of lashes. Retraction is caused by inadequate dissection and separation of the donor pedicle from the eyelid retractors. It may be corrected using the retraction techniques outlined in Chapter 6. The most common change in the recipient eyelid is entropion.

Cutler-Beard Procedure. The Cutler-Beard procedure is another two-stage procedure for the repair of large full-thickness rectangular defects. Although most commonly applied to reconstructing upper eyelid defects, it may also be used in reverse for lower eyelid defects. Tissues are advanced from the donor eyelid as one full-thickness flap to fill the recipient eyelid defect. The donor eyelid margin is left intact as a bridge overlying this advancement flap.

In an upper eyelid, the size of the defect may be reduced 6 mm through canthotomy and cantholysis. The residual horizontal defect (recipient bed) is accurately

determined by pulling the retracted edges toward one another.

The lower eyelid donor site is marked vertically 1 to 2 mm wider than the measured recipient bed. These marks are joined by a horizontal line 4 to 5 mm below the lower eyelid margin. This retains the vascular support to the remaining bridge at the lower eyelid margin. After local anesthetic infiltration, full-thickness incisions are made according to these lines with a #64 Beaver blade. A conformer may be used to protect the subjacent globe. It may be necessary to extend the vertical incisions somewhat farther inferiorly toward the fornix to afford adequate mobility to the donor flap (Fig. 10–35A). The conformer is now removed. The flap is carried under the marginal bridge to fill the upper eyelid defect. Donor and recipient tarsus are joined with interrupted 6-0 Vicryl (Fig. 10–35B). The distal end of levator aponeurosis is secured to donor tarsus with several interrupted 5-0 Vicryl sutures. Skin is closed with running 7-0 silk.

The skin sutures are removed 6 days postoperatively. The sharing graft must be left in place 2 to 3 months. It must then be carefully divided 1 to 2 mm below the desired position of the new upper eyelid margin. A blunt instrument such as a grooved director or muscle hook is placed beneath the bridge graft. After local anesthetic infiltration, an incision is made with Stevens scissors 2 mm below the desired upper eyelid margin to allow for postoperative contracture (Fig. 10–35C). This incision should be slanted in favor of the conjunctival surface to position more conjunctiva than skin at the eyelid margin. The new eyelid margin is reformed with running 7-0 chromic catgut. The donor pedicle and lower eyelid donor bed are freshened and resutured in position with interruped 7-0 chromic catgut sutures (Fig. 10–35D).

In this technique, if the donor eyelid margin bridge is too narrow, the blood supply may be compromised. Partial or complete necrosis may develop. This is the most devastating complication of the Cutler-Beard procedure, and requires later reconstructive techniques. Careful surgical planning and meticulous dissection are the best way to maximize perfusion of the bridge and obviate this problem. Additional problems may arise from instability of the upper eyelid, which may excessively pull the shared graft, resulting in entropion.

Cutler-Beard eyelid reconstruction may lead to cicatricial ectropion if vertical foreshortening occurs. This may require later correction by means of full-thickness skin graft. Eyelid laxity may result (involutional ectropion) if the donor segment was too wide or if canthal fixation is inadequate. These problems may be corrected by horizontal eyelid shortening (Bick procedure) or canthal tendon refixation respectively. Notching, which may occasionally occur, is managed by excision of the notched

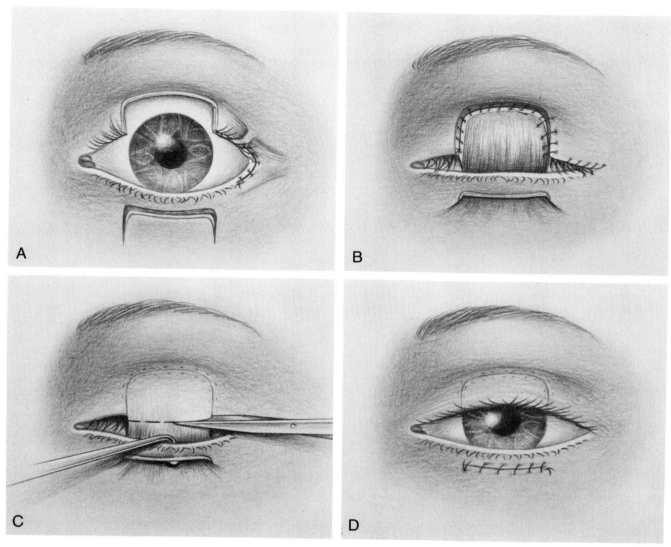

FIG. 10–35. Culter-Beard procedure. A, Following canthotomy and cantholysis, the donor full-thickness flap is incised in the lower eyelid to correspond to the colobomatous defect in the upper eyelid. B, The flap is carried under the marginal bridge to fill the upper eyelid defect. C, After 2 to 3 months, the sharing graft is divided with the division set slightly in favor of the conjunctival surface to position more conjunctiva than skin at the reconstructed eyelid margin. D, The donor pedicle and bed are freshened and resutured into position.

segment followed by direct closure of the eyelid margin. All these changes are more marked in the lower eyelid because of gravitational factors.

RECONSTRUCTION OF CANTHAL DEFECTS

Although the inner canthus forms an angle from the conjoined ends of the eyelids, it has a distinctly different appearance from the outer canthus and has unique reconstructive features. The inner canthus appears some-

what rounded due to the caruncle, which lies in the lacus lacrimalis. The puncta, canaliculi, and lacrimal sac must be considered when surgery is performed on the inner canthus. The position of the puncta as they relate to the tear lake is important. Symptomatic lacrimal obstruction resulting from reconstructive surgery may be corrected three months postoperatively. Consideration must also be given to possible cerebrospinal fluid leak resulting from midfacial trauma, as well as motility disturbance from entrapment of the medial rectus muscle in a medial wall fracture.

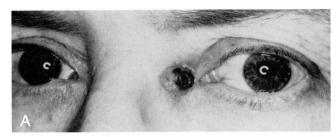

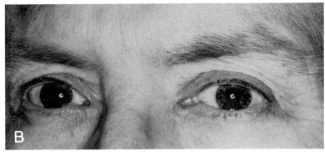

FIG. 10–36. Basal cell carcinoma at left inner canthus. A, Preoperative appearance. B, Postoperative appearance after tumor excision and primary canthal reconstruction.

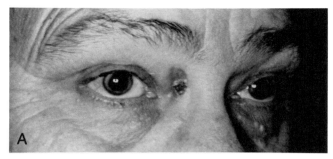

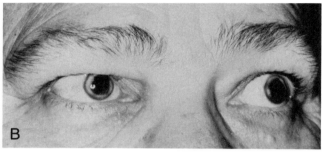

FIG. 10–37. Basal cell carcinoma at right inner canthus. A, Preoperative appearance. B, Postoperative appearance following tumor excision and primary canthal reconstruction.

The medial canthal tendon is complex. It embodies superficial and deep heads which attach to the pretarsal and preseptal orbicularis oculi muscle and activate the lacrimal pump mechanism.

The lateral canthus has a commissure that produces an acute angle. It has some mobility, unlike the medial canthus. The pretarsal muscles fuse into the lateral canthal tendon to insert at the lateral orbital tubercle. Fractures of the lateral orbit may induce vertical motility disturbances.

When reconstructive surgery is performed on the medial and lateral canthi, the goal is to restore both function and appearance to normal. The reconstructed canthi should have an appropriately positioned and angled commissure, containing relatively normal-appearing skin and inconspicuous scars.

Small canthal defects may be closed primarily in conformity with Langer's lines (Figs. 10–36 and 10–37). Larger canthal defects may result in relative or absolute tissue insufficiency. These situations may require sliding, transpositional, advancement, or rotational flaps, or free skin grafts to cover the defect and relieve tissue tension. The size and scope of a defect may sometimes require the combination of several reconstructive techniques. These procedures were covered in Chapter 2. Glabellar and midline forehead flaps may also be considered for large defects at the inner canthus.

Glabellar Flap. This is a modified V- to Y-advancement flap to cover inner canthal defects with glabellar tissue.

An inverted V is marked in the glabellar region with a longer arm extending to the lateral portion of the defect (Fig. 10–38A). Local anesthetic is infiltrated subjacent to this and a corresponding incision is made with a #64 Beaver blade. The flap is undermined, leaving a broad base of attachment. It is rotated into position and secured with interrupted 5-0 Vicryl mattress sutures and running 6-0 silk (Fig. 10–38B). The donor bed is closed with 6-0 silk, completing the inverted Y configuration. Skin sutures should be removed 7 to 10 days postoperatively. After surgery, the distance between the eyebrows may become slightly narrowed. These flaps afford only moderate cosmetic results.

Midline Forehead Flap. Large, deep defects 20 mm or more in diameter at the inner canthus require considerable tissue to cover them. In such cases, the midline forehead transposition flap offers a solution. Such flaps, however, require a second procedure to divide the flap and reinsert the donor pedicle.

This procedure requires careful calculation and measurement so that the flap, when brought down into position, fits properly and is not under undue tension. This flap may be as much as 2.5 cm in width. The length should not exceed 5 times its width. When the flap is transposed, its base will be located at the base of the nose.

Telfa may be used as a pattern, making certain that the length and width of the flap are correct before in-

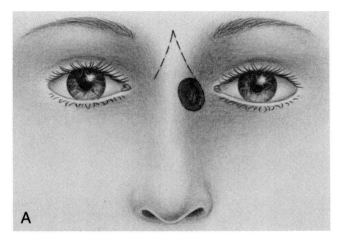

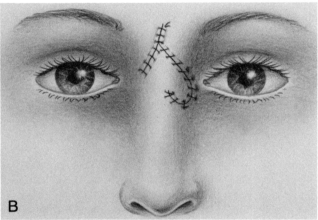

FIG. 10–38. Glabellar flap. A, Inverted V is marked at the glabella, with its longer arm extending to the lateral portion of the inner canthal defect. B, Advancement flap is rotated and sutured into position.

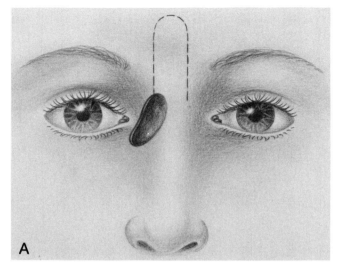

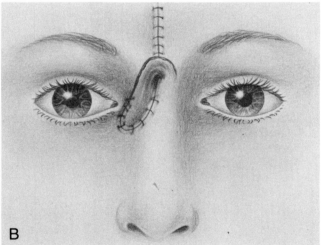

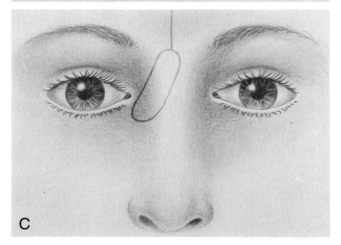

FIG. 10–39. Midline forehead flap. A, Donor pedicle is carefully positioned and marked at the central forehead. B, The flap is incised, undermined, and rotated into position to cover the defect. C, Eight weeks later, the pedicle is freed from its base and the base is returned to its original site.

cisions are made. The configuration of the flap is designated with a marking pen (Fig. 10–39A). The top of the flap may be tapered to facilitate later wound closure. Subjacent to the marked lines, local anesthetic is infiltrated. Once the incisions are made with a #64 Beaver blade, both sides are well undermined in the fatty layer with small Metzenbaum scissors. The flap is then rotated and sutured into the defect below with subcutaneous 5-0 Vicryl interrupted mattress sutures and skin 6-0 silk running sutures (Figs. 10–39B and 10–40). The forehead donor site is closed in a similar manner. Lateral undermining may be required.

After 8 weeks, the pedicle is freed and the epithelial edges are trimmed. The pedicle base is straightened and returned to its original site to prevent excessive narrowing of the eyebrows (Fig. 10–39C). The forehead wound may need to be modified somewhat to accommodate the return of a portion of the pedicle and to produce an

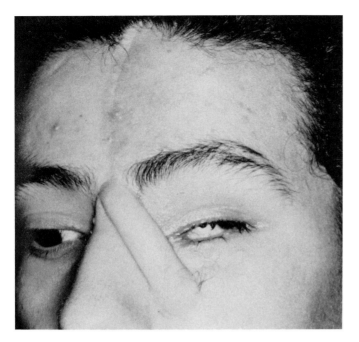

FIG. 10–40. Midline forehead flap positioned to cover defects at the inner canthus and medial aspect of the lower eyelid. Both the choice of reconstruction and its execution appear incorrect in this case, which was treated abroad.

acceptable scar. These incisions may be closed with running 6-0 silk.

This technique tends to produce a thickened medial canthus. Prominent scars are often left at both the canthus and forehead. Fair donor-recipient compatibility is usually seen in skin thickness, texture, and color.

RECONSTRUCTION IN CANTHAL DISPLACEMENT

HORIZONTAL CANTHAL DISPLACEMENT

When a canthal tendon has been disinserted from trauma or tumor excision, the adjacent canthus becomes flaccid and somewhat rounded. This is clinically less significant at the inner canthus, where the deep head of the medial canthal tendon may remain attached.

These conditions can usually be surgically corrected by repositioning the avulsed tendon with 2-0 Supramid sutures. The lateral canthal tendon is anchored to periosteum at the lateral orbital tubercle. The superficial head of the medial canthal tendon is anchored to periosteum at the anterior lacrimal crest. Bony fixation is sometimes required. If the canthal tendon is inadequate, the Supramid suture may instead be placed through the leading edge of tarsus. If the gap between tarsus and

periosteum is excessive, a periosteal flap may be advanced to join these structures. The subcutaneous tissue is closed with several horizontal mattress sutures of 5-0 Vicryl, and the skin is closed witn running 7-0 silk.

More severe cases may require bony wiring (see Chapter 3) or placement of a surgical piton (see Chapter 16).

In acute trauma, it is usually not necessary to move soft tissue as part of a canthoplasty. In old trauma, contracture is often more evident and may require C to U-plasty or Y to V-plasty, as well as canthal tendon shortening techniques.

Horizontal canthal displacement associated with periorbital fracture (LeForte II medially or trimalar laterally) may be managed by early open reduction of the fracture or later canthoplasty with canthal tendon shortening.

TRAUMATIC VERTICAL CANTHAL DISPLACEMENT

Vertical displacement of the inner canthus may result from sagittal maxillary fractures, whereas vertical displacement of the outer canthus may result from trimalar fractures. Acute displacements may be managed by open reduction and internal fixation. Later repair requires canthal Z-plasty with vertical repositioning of the canthal tendon.

In canthal Z-plasty (see Chapter 2), two of the three arms of the incision are marked adjacent to the canthus, approximately 2 to 3 mm away from the eyelid margin. The third arm is marked at the position where the canthus should be located. After infiltration of local anesthetic, corresponding incisions are made with a #64 Beaver blade. The two resultant flaps are undermined below the orbicularis oculi layer to afford later transposition.

The subjacent canthal tendon (lateral canthal tendon or superficial head of the medial canthal tendon) is isolated, disinserted, and secured with a 2-0 Supramid suture. To adjust for anticipated postoperative contracture, the Supramid suture is placed into periosteum 2 mm beyond (above or below) its normal point of attachment (lateral orbital tubercle or anterior lacrimal crest, respectively).

The two triangular flaps are transposed and sutured into their new position under minimal tension. Each flap is supported with a subcutaneous 5-0 Vicryl mattess suture at its leading edge, along with two additional mattress sutures along each side. The incisions are closed with one 6-0 silk suture at the leading skin edge, along with running 7-0 silk. Skin sutures should be removed on the sixth postoperative day.

BIBLIOGRAPHY

Abraham, J., Jabaley, M., and Hoopes, J.: Basal cell carcinoma of the medial canthal region. Am. J. Surg. 126:126, 1973.

Anderson, R., and Ceilley, R.: A multispecialty approach to the excision and reconstruction of eyelid tumors. Ophthalmology 85:1150–1162, 1978.

Aurora, A., and Blodi, F.: Reappraisal of basal cell carcinoma of the eyelids. Am. J. Ophthalmol. 70:329, 1970.

Beard, C.: Observation of the treatment of basal cell carcinoma of the eyelid. Trans. Am. Acad. Ophthalmol. Otolaryngol. 79:644, 1975.

Beard, C.: Management of malignancy of the eyelids. Am. J. Ophthalmol. 92:1–6, 1981.

Beyer-Machule, C., and von Noorden, G.: Atlas of Ophthalmic Surgery. New York, Thieme-Stratton, 1985.

Bullock, J., Beard, C., and Sullivan, J.: Cryotherapy of basal cell carcinoma in oculoplastic surgery. Am. J. Ophthalmol. 82:841, 1976.

Callahan, A.: Reconstruction of the eyelids with cartilage and mucosa from the nasal septum. Trans. Ophthalmol. Soc. U.K. 96:39, 1976.

Callahan, M., and Callahan, A.: Ophthalmic Plastic and Orbital Surgery. Birmingham, Aesculapius, 1979.

Cavanagh, H., Green, W., and Goldberg, H.: Multicentric adenocarcinoma of the meibomian gland. Am. J. Ophthalmol. 77:326, 1974.

Cole, J.: Histologically controlled excision of eyelid tumors. Am. J. Ophthalmol. 70:240, 1970

Cutler, N., and Beard, C.: A method for partial and total upper lid reconstruction. Am. J. Ophthalmol. 39:1–7, 1955.

Doxanos, M., Green, W., and Iliff, C.: Factors in the successful surgical management of basal cell carcinoma of the eyelids . Am. J. Ophthalmol. 91:726–736, 1981.

Doxanos, M., and Green, W.: Sebaceous gland carcinoma. Arch. Ophthalmol. 102:245–249, 1984.

Fraunfelder, F., Zacarian, S., Limmer, B., and Wingfield, D.: Cryosurgery for malignancies of the eyelid. Ophthalmology. 87:461–465, 1980.

Grove, A.: Staged excision and reconstruction of extensive facial orbital tumors. Ophthalmic Surg. 8:91–109, 1977.

Hecht, S.: An upside-down Cutler-Beard bridge flap. Arch. Ophthalmol. 84:760, 1970.

Hughes, W.: A new method of rebuilding a lower lid. Arch. Ophthalmol. 17:1008, 1937.

Iliff, C., Iliff, W., and Iliff, N.: Oculoplastic Surgery. Philadelphia W.B. Saunders, 1979.

Jacobiec, F., Braunstein, S., and Wilkinson R.: Combined surgery and cryotherapy for diffuse malignant melanoma of the conjunctiva. Arch. Ophthalmol. 98:1390–1396, 1980.

Jacobiec, F., Browstein, S., and Albert, W.: The role of cryotherapy in the management of conjunctival melanoma. Ophthalmology, 89:502–525, 1982.

Leone, C., and Hand, S.: Reconstruction of the medial eyelid. Am. J. Ophthalmol. 87:797, 1979.

McCord, C., and Cavanagh, H.: Microscopic features and biologic behavior of eyelid tumors. Ophthamolic Surg. 11:671–681, 1980.

McCord, C.: Oculoplastic Surgery. New York, Raven Press, 1981.

Mohs, F.: Chemosurgery for facial neoplasms. Arch. Otolaryngol. 95:62–67, 1972.

Mohs, F.: Chemosurgery for skin cancer: fixed-tissue and fresh-tissue techniques. Arch. Dermatol. 112:211–215, 1976.

Mohs, F.: Chemosurgery: microscopically controlled surgery for skin cancer—past, present, and future. J. Dermatol. Surg. 4:41, 1978.

Older, J., Quickert, M., and Beard, C.: Surgical removal of basal cell carcinoma of the eyelids utilizing frozen section control. Trans. Am. Acad. Ophthalmol. Otolaryngol. 79:658–663, 1975.

Putterman, A.: Viable composite grafting in eyelid reconstruction. Am. J. Ophthalmol. 85:237, 1978.

Reeh, M., Beyer, C., and Shannon, G.: Practical Ophthalmic Plastic and Reconstructive Surgery, Philadelphia, Lea and Febiger, 1976.

Robb, R.: Refractive errors associated with hemangiomas of the lids and orbit in infancy. Am. J. Ophthalmol. 83:52, 1977.

Soll, D.: Management of Complications in Ophthalmic Plastic Surgery. Birmingham, Aesculapius, 1976.

Stewart, W.: Ophthalmic Plastic and Reconstructive Surgery. San Francisco, American Academy of Ophthalmology, 1984.

Sullivan, J.: The use of cryotherapy for trichiasis. Trans. Am. Acad. Ophthalmol. Otolaryngol. 83:708, 1977.

Sullivan, J., Beard, C., and Bullock J.: Cryosurgery for treatment of trichiasis. Am. J. Ophthalmol. 82:117, 1976.

Tenzel, R.: Reconstruction of central one-half of an eyelid. Arch. Ophthalmol. 93:125, 1975.

Tenzel, R., Stewart, W., and Boynton, J.: Sebaceus Adenocarcinoma of the eyelid. Arch. Ophthalmol. 95:2203–2204, 1977.

Tenzel, R., Stewart, R.: Eyelid reconstruction by the semicircle flap technique. Ophthalmology 85:1164–1169, 1978.

11

CONJUNCTIVAL SURGERY

In dealing with the disorders that originate in the conjunctiva, I have subdivided the subject into problems associated with an intact globe and problems associated with an anophthalmic socket. The former is covered in this chapter and the latter in the following chapter.

PTERYGIUM

A pterygium is an elevated mass of conjunctival tissue, typically located at the nasal limbus. Various other locations may be occasionally encountered. When a pterygium is active, it is highly vascular, with the vascularity of its leading edge serving as a barometer of its aggressiveness.

Treatment is indicated when there is sufficient corneal overlap, cosmetic impairment, visual impairment, or induced astigmatism.

Bare Scleral Excision. This procedure is best accomplished with magnifying loops or operating microscope magnification. After adequate prepping of the periorbital area, a lid speculum is placed on the surface of the globe. Local anesthesia is administered in the form of topical tetracaine, followed by 2% lidocaine (Xylocaine) subjacent to the pterygium. The surgeon must note the vertical extent of the pterygium before infiltration because this demarcation may be obscured by the anesthetic (Fig. 11–1). With sweeping movements with a #64 Beaver blade in a medial direction, the portion of the pterygium overlapping the cornea is separated from the cornea. This separation should occur just at the level of Bowman's membrane.

Once the dissection has been carried to the limbus, the remainder of the growth can be excised in an elliptical manner with scissors, along with attached Tenon's capsule and conjunctiva. This excision should carefully avoid uninvolved conjunctiva, the plica semilunaris, and the subjacent medial rectus (Fig. 11–2) This leaves an elliptical area of bare sclera. The sclera and cornea are scraped free of connective tissue remnants, smoothing the cornea and limbus. Judicious cautery may be applied; sutures are not usually required. The conjunctiva should

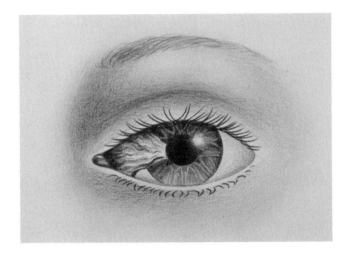

FIG. 11–1. Characteristic appearance and location of a pterygium.

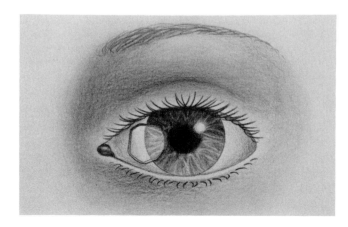

FIG. 11–2. In the surgical excision of a pterygium, be careful to avoid uninvolved conjunctiva, the plica semilunaris, and the medial rectus muscle. A bare scleral closure yields excellent results.

be left open, leaving an area of bare sclera. Normal conjunctiva will eventually grow to cover this defect.

Topical antibiotics are applied and the globe need not be patched. A course of postoperative β radiation (strontium 90, 3000 rads) delivered to the limbus may be useful in inhibiting recurrence. This technique is simple, minimally invasive, and results in few recurrences. Other techniques involving transposition of the pterygium or conjunctival grafting appear somewhat less efficacious.

RECURRENT PTERYGIUM

Recurrent pterygium is usually amenable to the bare sclera/β radiation technique described in the previous section. In situations of multiple or hypertrophic recurrences, grafting techniques may be required. An operating microscope is used, and the corneal extent of the pterygium is excised in a lamellar fashion to a depth of superficial or mid stroma. This superficial keratectomy is carried over the limbus into the superficial aspect of the sclera. Suitable donor material is harvested from eyebank tissue in a lamellar manner. This tissue is fashioned to conform in size, shape, and thickness to the configuration of the recipient bed, and sutured in place. Continuous 10-0 Ethilon sutures may be used for the cornea, while interrupted 8-0 Vicryl sutures may be used for the sclera. The graft is covered with a steroid and antibiotic ointment, which is continued in combination postoperatively. β radiation may inhibit further recurrence.

CARCINOMA IN SITU AND SQUAMOUS CELL CARCINOMA

Carcinoma in situ (Bowen's disease) and squamous cell carcinoma are occasionally found at the limbus and may resemble a pterygium. These lesions, though, may be somewhat more raised, vascular, irregular, or pigmented. Suspicious lesions should be biopsied.

Carcinoma in situ and squamous cell carcinoma are excised in the same manner as a pterygium, obtaining somewhat wider margins and histologic confirmation (both frozen and paraffin section) of cell type and tissue margins. Small defects may be left bare, while larger defects may require sliding, bipedicle ("bucket handle"), or full thickness conjunctival grafts.

CONJUNCTIVAL TRAUMA

Conjunctival lacerations are usually amenable to direct repositioning. Should significant tissue loss occur, ad-

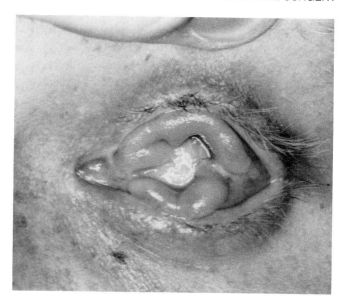

FIG. 11–3. Extensive corneal and conjunctival damage from an alkali burn.

jacent conjunctiva may be used to close the defect by means of advancement flap, transposition flap, or rotation flap techniques. Free conjunctival grafts may be useful for larger defects. These grafts may be obtained from the contralateral bulbar conjunctiva, if the other globe is uninjured. Still larger defects may require buccal mucous membrane grafts.

Chemical and thermal trauma to the conjunctiva are managed differently. Alkali burns have the worst prognosis (Fig. 11–3) because they rapidly penetrate tissue, particularly the cornea. In these cases, the highest ophthalmic management priority is caring for corneal injury and avoiding excessive exposure. Alkali burns must undergo immediate and copious irrigation. All necrotic conjunctival tissue should be debrided. The cul-de-sacs can be preserved with the use of a conformer, symblepharon ring, or stent. These may be made of Silastic, Telfon, or rigid acrylics. Once the suitable material has been selected, it must be carefully fitted and secured to avoid erosion of the surrounding friable tissues. Conjunctival, mucous membrane, or corneal grafting may later benefit selected patients.

SYMBLEPHARON

A symblepharon is an abnormal adhesion between the palpebral and bulbar conjunctiva (Fig. 11–4). It may follow surgery, trauma, thermal or chemical burns, inflammation (Stevens-Johnson syndrome, ocular pemphigoid [Fig. 11–5]), or infection (trachoma). Such cases

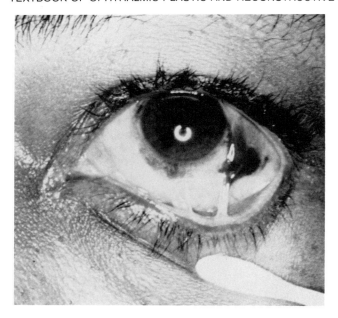

FIG. 11–4. A mild symblepharon attaching focal areas of palpebral and bulbar conjunctiva to one another.

may have coexistent xerophthalmia and kerato-conjunctivitis sicca from loss of goblet cells and accessory lacrimal glands, along with possible obliteration of the main lacrimal ducts.

This process may vary from small and isolated adhesions to severe scar tissue, encompassing the entire palpebral and bulbar conjunctiva, obliterating the cul-de-sacs. As with other scars, the condition should be stable for at least 6 months before surgical intervention.

When the symblepharon is small, correction can often be effected by simply excising the scar and transposing the remaining mucous membrane flaps (Fig. 11–6). Con-

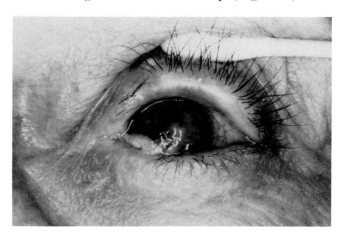

FIG. 11–5. Ocular pemphigoid with more severe symblepharon, cicatricial entropion, distichiasis, loss of conjunctival goblet cells, pannus, and corneal scarring.

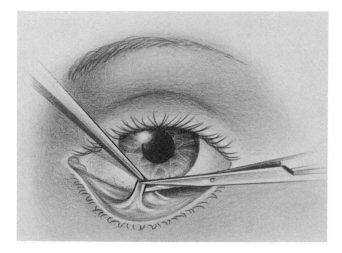

FIG. 11–6. Simple excision of a symblepharon. Often conjunctival transposition or Z-plasty adequately restores conjunctival integrity.

firmation of effective lysis of all adhesions is restoration of the fornices and return of full forced ductions. In many instances, the Z-plasty technique can be used, transposing conjunctiva across the line of contracture. The central axis should correspond to the symblepharon line of tension, usually perpendicular to the globe. The two sidearms are offset at 60-degree angles from both ends of the central axis line. The scar is excised along the central axis and the incised sidearms are transposed. The flaps may be secured with running 7-0 chromic catgut sutures. The postoperative use of a conformer, symblepharon ring, or stent is necessary to discourage recurrent symblepharon formation. These conformers, however, must be closely monitored for any effect or possible damage to the cornea.

If, after removal of the symblepharon, the defect is more extensive and the adjacent conjunctiva inadequate for repair, a full-thickness conjunctival graft should be used. This may be obtained from the upper cul-de-sac of the involved side or the contralateral side. Infiltrating 2% lidocaine (Xylocaine) subjacent to the donor site will provide analgesia and separate tissue planes, facilitating freehand removal. Once the graft is excised, it is soaked in an antibiotic solution and kept moist with saline solution. It is imperative that the epithelial surface remain on top for later identification. The donor graft is placed, epithelial side up, in the recipient bed and trimmed to fit the configuration, allowing for the expected 25% shrinkage. Suturing and conformer placement are as described in the previous paragraph (Fig. 11–7).

Other defects may require a full-thickness bipedicle conjunctival bridge flap. This is effected by removing a bridge of conjunctiva from the other cul-du-sac of the

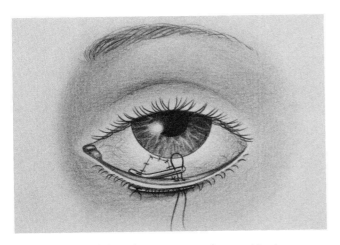

FIG. 11–7. Excision of a more extensive symblepharon may require placement of a conjunctival or buccal mucous membrane graft to fill the defect. This should be supported by a conformer, stent (pictured here), or symblepharon ring to minimize shrinkage and discourage recurrent adhesion.

same eye. It is incised down to the level of the limbus, leaving the medial and lateral attachments intact. This results in a "bucket handle" appearance. This flap is rotated toward the other fornix and sutured into the defect with 7-0 chromic catgut sutures. A "bucket handle" flap can also be used to cover corneal defects, when appropriate, as an alternative to the Gundersen flap.

Larger defects on the palpebral conjunctival surface require split-thickness buccal mucous membrane grafts, as described in Chapter 2 (Fig. 11–8). (Buccal mucosa should not be used on the bulbar conjunctiva because they tend to remain pink and become thickened.) These grafts should be 25% larger than the recipient bed to allow for expected shrinkage. They may need to be some-

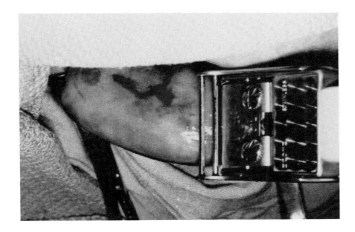

FIG. 11–8. Harvesting buccal mucous membrane graft with Castroviejo mucotome.

what larger in recurrent cases, or those following burns or inflammation.

Once the graft is sutured into position with 7-0 chromic catgut, it should be maintained in that position with a conformer, ring, or stent. This is of particular importance if the cul-de-sac is involved, in which case a conformer should be secured to the cul-de-sac and possibly to the periosteum of the overlying orbital rim. These sutures can be externalized over rubber bolsters to keep the fornix under mild stretch, while avoiding skin excoriation. Such fixation will help to discourage graft shrinkage and maintain the cul-de-sac.

In selected clinical situations, these techniques may be used in partial combination.

TRICHIASIS AND DISTICHIASIS

Distichiasis is a condition in which lashes arise from ectopic areas, away from the normal ciliary line. They often emerge from the meibomian orifices, posteriorly. These lashes are often small and lightly pigmented. Trichiasis occurs when aberrant lashes arising from the ciliary line come in contact with the globe. Both conditions may lead to corneal irritation, erosion, and ulceration in severe and untreated cases. Distichiasis and trichiasis may be idiopathic; secondary to trauma, previous surgery, or inflammatory conditions such as Stevens-Johnson syndrome or ocular pemphigoid; or associated with cicatricial entropion. In Stevens-Johnson syndrome and pemphigoid, the meibomian glands undergo metaplasia, producing irregular, distichiatic lashes.

In trichiasis and distichiasis, if a substantial number of lashes is involved, or there is associated cicatricial entropion, a Wies eyelid rotation procedure is required (see Chapter 8). Isolated distichiasis and trichiasis with a limited number of lashes involved, are effectively treated with cryotherapy. Epilation and diathermy are ineffective because the lashes will return in 2 to 3 months.

Lash follicles are more sensitive to the destructive effect of freezing than are the surrounding tissues. The cryodestructive effect is enhanced by a rapid freeze followed by a prolonged thaw. To achieve a therapeutic effect, this process should be repeated to achieve a double freeze-thaw cycle.

CRYOTHERAPY

After administration of direct infiltration anesthetic, a thermocouple is placed adjacent to the aberrant lashes and above the tarsus. A nitrous oxide delivery system

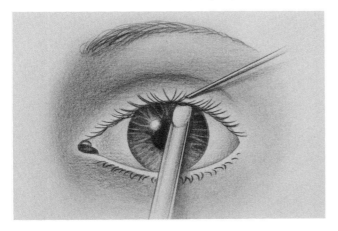

FIG. 11–9. Cryotherapy tip is placed on the conjunctival surface subjacent to the focal area of trichiasis or distichiasis slated for treatment. A thermocouple is placed to carefully monitor temperature.

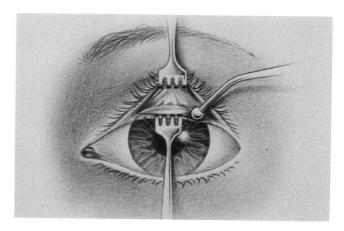

FIG. 11–10. In highly pigmented individuals, it is important to split the eyelid and treat only the posterior lamella to avoid skin depigmentation.

with a fine tip (Cryomedics) is used to freeze these lashes. The tip is placed on the conjunctival surface (Fig. 11–9), subjacent to the involved lashes, and the temperature is brought to −25° C as measured on the thermocouple. After this temperature is reached, the tissues are allowed to thaw slowly. This process is repeated to achieve a double freeze-thaw effect. During this procedure, the cornea should not be allowed to contact the cryotherapy area. Antibiotic ointment is applied and continued daily for 1 week. The treated lashes should slough spontaneously and permanently within the next 1 to 2 weeks.

Moderate inflammation with mild pain occurs for several days postoperatively. Transient blistering may sometimes occur. Minimal permanent scarring develops when treatment is properly applied and monitored. Distichiasis or trichiasis persist in approximately 10% of treated cases. Retreatment may be performed several months later.

Care must be taken in placing the cryo tip because treated normal lashes will be equally affected. The treatment should be more conservative in thin, atrophic eyelids to avoid necrosis from freezing. Temperatures lower than −25° C may cause areas of necrosis and notching of the eyelid margin.

This procedure is modified in highly pigmented individuals because focal areas of permanent depigmentation may result. In these circumstances, the eyelid should be split along the gray line. The cryo unit is applied to the posterior lamella only (Fig. 11–10). Because this approach reduces the treated area, less freezing is required to achieve the desired temperature. The eyelid margin is then reapproximated with 8-0 chromic catgut sutures in a running manner.

CHALAZION

A chalazion is the sequela of an unresolved internal hordeolum. It produces a lipogranuloma from obstruction and infection within the meibomian glands and can occur anywhere along the tarsal plate. Many chalazions abate after treatment with hot compresses and antibiotic ointment. After 6 weeks of these conservative measures, any appreciable residual chalazion may be amenable to minor surgical curettement. Early sebaceous cell carcinoma may sometimes appear similar to a chalazion. Suspicious lesions should be biopsied for histologic study.

Curettement of Chalazion. After adequate preparation, the area surrounding the chalazion is infiltrated with local anesthetic. Attention must be directed to the extent and location of the chalazion because the anesthetic may obsure its position. A small chalazion clamp is placed over the chalazion with the open side on the tarsoconjunctival surface (Fig. 11–11A). The eyelid is everted and a vertical incision (parallel to the meibomian glands) is made into the central aspect of the lesion with a #11 Bard-Parker blade (Fig. 11–11B). Care must be exercised to avoid incising the eyelid margin or extending more deeply beyond tarsus. If the chalazion is in the medial eyelid, the incision must avoid the canaliculi.

Stevens scissors may be used to spread the incised tarsus gently, adequately opening the chalazion. Applying pressure with applicator sticks gradually forces out the caseous material contained therein. A curette can be used to remove any residual inflammatory debris (Fig. 11–11C). The pseudocapsule surrounding the chalazion is excised with Stevens scissors and forceps to discourage recurrence. Hemostasis is obtained with cautery as the clamp is gradually loosened. No sutures are required,

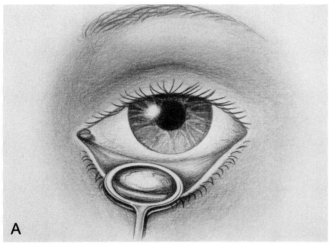

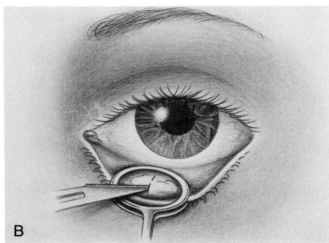

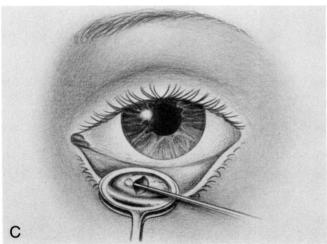

FIG. 11–11. Treatment of chalazion. A, A chalazion clamp is placed over the chalazion and the eyelid is everted. B, A vertical incision is made into the center of the lesion. C, Residual inflammatory debris is removed with a curette.

and an antibiotic ointment is applied to the tarsoconjunctival surface.

BIBLIOGRAPHY

Beyer-Machule, C., von Noorded, G.: Atlas of Ophthalmic Surgery. New York, Thieme-Stratton, 1985.

Leone, C.: Treatment of Conjunctival Diseases and Chalazion. In Stewart, W.: Ophthalmic Plastic and Reconstructive Surgery. San Francisco, American Academy of Ophthalmology, 1984.

Pearlman, G.: Recurrent pterygium and treatment with lamellar keratoplasty with presentation of a technique to limit recurrences. Ann. Ophthalmol. 2:703, 1970.

Reeh, M.: Corneal lamellar transplant for recurrent pterygium. Arch. Ophthalmol. 86:296–297, 1971.

Reeh, M., Beyer, C., and Shannon, G.: Practical Ophthalmic Plastic and Reconstructive Surgery. Philadelphia, Lea and Febiger, 1976.

Sullivan, J., Beard, C., and Bullock, J.: Cryosurgery for treatment of trichiasis. Am. J. Ophthalmol. 82:117, 1976.

Vastine, D., Stewart, W., and Schwab, I.: Reconstruction of periocular mucous membrane by autologous conjunctival transplantation. Ophthalmology 89:1072–1081, 1982.

12

ACQUIRED ANOPHTHALMOS AND RELATED DISORDERS

Before elective removal of a blind, painful eye, certain facts must be considered. With the eye left in place, motility is always better than that achieved with an evisceration or enucleation prosthesis. Pain in severely diseased or traumatized eyes is sometimes the result of uveitis and responds to topical atropine 1% treatment. Other cases may benefit from retrobulbar alcohol injection. If the problem is also cosmetic, a scleral shell may be tried. This is particulalrly useful in cases of phthysis bulbi (Fig. 12–1).

In children, the presence of a globe, even a severely damaged or microphthalmic globe, has a trophic effect on bony orbital growth. Except in cases of malignancy, enucleation in children should be avoided or delayed if possible. Should it become necessary at an early age, a large implant will best stimulate growth of the bony orbit.

In cases of acute trauma to the globe, every attempt should be made to perform an optimal primary repair. This not only affords the possibility of some visual and/or cosmetic restoration, but also affords the patient time to adjust psychologically to the traumatic event.

If an eye must be surgically removed, a decision should be made as to whether the patient would benefit most from evisceration or enucleation. The choice of procedure is based on the surgeon's preference, with due consideration of the individual circumstances of each case.

EVISCERATION VERSUS ENUCLEATION

Evisceration is a procedure in which all intraocular contents are removed, leaving intact the scleral shell and its external attachments to the extraocular muscles, optic nerve, blood vessels, nerves, and orbital connective tissue. Removal of the cornea is optional, although most patients requiring evisceration are more comfortable without it.

Enucleation is a procedure in which the entire globe and an adjacent portion of the optic nerve are removed as one unit. This procedure results in significant anatomic and metabolic changes within the orbit. These changes include partial atrophy of orbital fat, redirection of orbital connective tissue septae, decreased support and altered insertion for the extraocular muscles, diminished support for the levator muscle, laxity of the lateral canthal tendon, and lower eyelid retraction.

Evisceration has significant cosmetic advantage over enucleation because it minimally alters orbital anatomy. Specifically, evisceration retains the continuity between the scleral shell, extraocular muscles, and orbital connective tissue. It helps maintain socket motility and minimizes superior sulcus defects. In cases where evisceration is indicated, it affords comfort, excellent cosmesis, and motility.

Evisceration may be performed for a blind and painful eye that harbors no tumor. Ultrasonography and/or CT studies should be performed on eyes with cloudy media to rule out an occult neoplasm. If a malignancy is suspected on the basis of clinical, radiologic, or ultrasonographic evidence, enucleation should be considered because it facilitates more complete excision of the tumor and enhances histologic accuracy, including tissue margins. Enucleation is also the preferred procedure for phthysis bulbi or after severe intraocular trauma.

Sympathetic ophthalmia is rare. Enucleation of the traumatically blind eye within two weeks of injury is considered the most effective way of avoiding this potential sequela. Evisceration with complete removal of uveal tissue may also be effective in preventing sympathetic ophthalmia.

Either evisceration or enucleation may be performed for endophthalmitis that is incompletely responsive to antibiotic therapy. Although enucleation opens a communication between the orbit and the subarachnoid space, such posterior extension of an infection is uncommon.

Whether evisceration or enucleation is chosen, both procedures have similar goals: (1) secure, central placement of an orbital implant of adequate size to minimize sulcus deformity and allow for a mobile prosthesis, (2) conjunctival fornices adequate for secure support and maintenance of a prosthesis, (3) a lower eyelid that is properly positioned and of adequate tone to support the prosthesis, (4) an upper eyelid demonstrating optimal

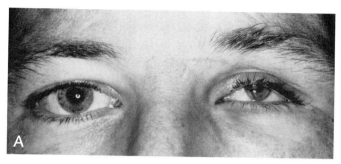
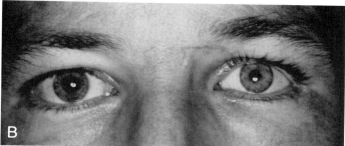

FIG. 12–1.   Phthysis bulbi of the left eye from previous trauma. B, Appearance with scleral shell in place.

height, fold, contour, and symmetry, without lag-ophthalmos, (5) a properly fitting prosthetic eye, matched to the contralateral intact eye. These parameters are all interrelated. Any dysfunction of one feature may alter the normal function of other features.

EVISCERATION SURGERY

To ensure surgery on the correct eye, the patient's chart and surgical consent are reviewed before surgery. An intraoperative ophthalmoscopic evaluation should be performed to confirm the correct eye, and the uninvolved eye is taped shut. Under general anesthesia, an eyelid speculum is placed on the involved side. A 360-degree peritomy is performed, undermining conjunctiva and Tenon's capsule 5 mm posteriorly (Fig. 12–2A). A limbal incision is made into the anterior chamber with a 75M Beaver blade (Fig. 12–2B). When corneal removal is desired, the cornea should be completely excised at the limbus with corneal-scleral scissors (Fig. 12–2C and D).

A cyclodialysis spatula is placed posterior to the iris, separating the ciliary body from the sclera. As the spatula extends posteriorly, the choroid is further separated from sclera (Fig. 12–2E). Resistance may be encountered at the scleral spur and optic nerve. The spatula is exchanged for an evisceration spoon, which is used to remove the entire uveal tract and its contents (lens, zonules, vitreous, retina). Any remaining uveal pigment can be removed by forceps, curette, or applicator stick. Hemostasis is obtained with pressure. Occasionally, persistent bleeding at the optic nerve head requires direct cautery. Once hemostasis is obtained, the orbital tissues should be irrigated with an antibiotic solution.

A sterile 18 to 20 mm spherical implant is rinsed in an antibiotic solution and placed within the scleral shell. The implant may be made of glass, silicone, or Teflon. Over the implant, the scleral pouch should be closed as a horizontal ellipse. To facilitate closure, small triangles of sclera may be excised at the 3 and 9 o'clock wound edges to help form the ellipse. The sclera is closed with interrupted 5-0 Vicryl sutures (Fig. 12–2F). The conjunctiva is later closed horizontally as a separate procedure with running 6-0 chromic catgut.

Sterile antibiotic ointment is placed on all suture lines and a conformer should be positioned postoperatively to help preserve the fornices and inhibit conjunctival shrinkage. This may be covered with a pressure dressing for 24 hours. After 4 to 6 weeks postoperatively, the patient may be fitted with a prosthesis. In most cases, the patient is comfortable with a prosthesis that is cosmetically pleasing and mobile. Safety glasses to protect the remaining eye are recommended after surgery.

In cases where corneal preservation is desired, the intraocular contents are removed through a 180 degree limbal incision. The cornea is later resutured with interrupted 8-0 Vicryl.

When evisceration is performed for endophthalmitis, the inner surface of the scleral shell should be irrigated with a broad-spectrum antibiotic solution. In such cases, a spherical implant is not placed, and a drain may be temporarily substituted until inflammation has resolved. If orbital volume later proves insufficient, a dermis fat graft may then be placed as a secondary implant.

Should an intraocular tumor be encountered during evisceration, the procedure must be converted to an enucleation to afford more complete removal.

After evisceration, sympathetic ophthalmia in the unaffected eye is rare. It can usually be obviated by complete removal of uveal tissue during evisceration surgery. The management of sympathetic ophthalmia is covered in uveitis textbooks.

ENUCLEATION SURGERY

As outlined in the section on evisceration, steps must be taken to ensure that surgery is performed on the

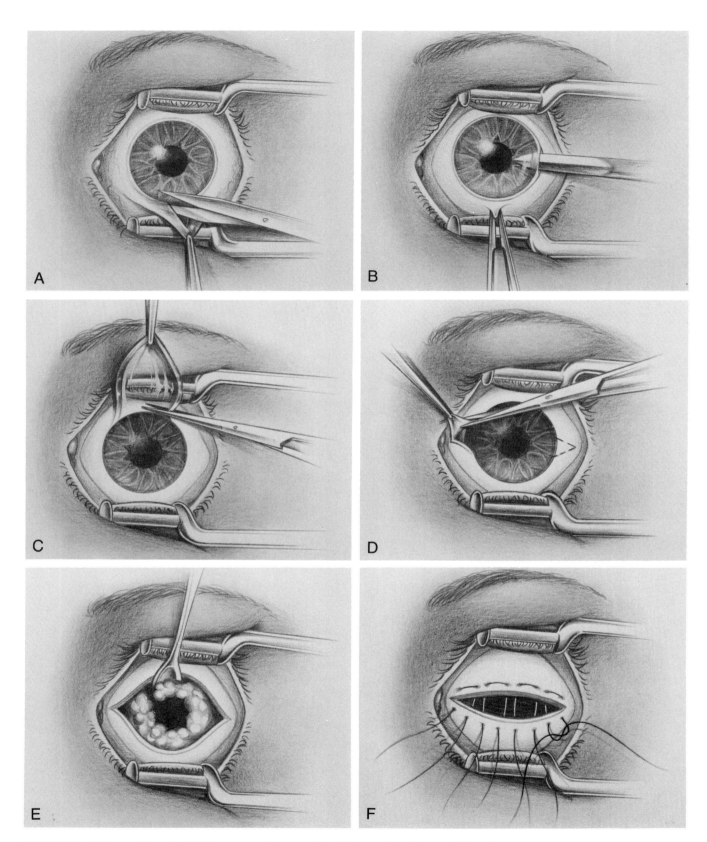

FIG. 12–2.   Evisceration. A, 360-degree peritomy undermining conjunctiva and Tenon's capsule. B, Limbal entrance into the anterior chamber with 75M Beaver blade. C, Complete excision of the cornea at the limbus. D, Scleral wound extensions at the 3 and 9 o'clock positions to facilitate later closure. E, Cyclodialysis spatula separates uvea from sclera. F, After placement of spherical implant, sclera is closed with Vicryl mattress sutures.

correct eye. This procedure is performed under general anesthesia with the uninvolved eye taped shut to prevent error in the surgical site. On the involved side, an eyelid speculum is placed and a 360-degree conjunctival peritomy is performed, undermining conjunctiva and Tenon's capsule posteriorly (Fig. 12–3A). The four rectus muscles are sequentially isolated with muscle hooks (Fig. 12–3B) and secured at their distal ends with double-armed 5-0 Vicryl sutures (Fig. 12–3C). These muscles are disinserted at the point of their scleral attachment, leaving a small stump of medial and lateral rectus muscle for traction. Then 5-0 Mersilene sutures on spatula needles are carefully and securely passed through these muscle stumps and tied long for traction (Fig. 12–3D).

Enucleation scissors are passed down the medial orbital wall. While the traction sutures gently draw the globe forward, the position and size of the optic nerve are carefully assessed by palpation with the scissors tip. The scissors are then opened, with the nerve placed between the blades. The scissors tip is then moved posteriorly toward the orbital apex to obtain a longer segment of optic nerve. This step may be critical in retinoblastoma, where a long portion of optic nerve (10 to 15 mm) must be obtained. In small children, the orbital apex may be too narrow to admit enucleation scissors. Long Metzenbaum scissors may be a useful alternative instrument in such cases. In enucleations not involving a tumor, severing the nerve at the apex is unnecessary and may injure the extraocular muscles, levator muscle, or their nerve supply.

After the nerve is severed, the globe is brought forward with the Mersilene traction sutures as the remaining attachments of the oblique muscles, short ciliary arteries, and soft tissue are removed (Fig. 12–3E). Hemostasis is obtained with 5 to 10 minutes of firm pressure applied to the orbital apex. Persistent bleeding may also require direct cauterization of the optic nerve stump. Once hemostasis is obtained, the orbital tissues should be irrigated with an antibiotic solution.

A sterile enucleation sphere should be rinsed in an antibiotic solution and placed in the posterior orbit within the muscle cone through a rent in the posterior layer of Tenon's capsule (Fig. 12–3F). These spheres may range from 14 to 16 mm in children to 18 to 22 mm in adults, depending on the size of the patient's orbit. In adults, a 22 mm sphere is preferable to avoid volume deficit and help obviate a later superior sulcus deformity. Glass, silicone, and Teflon are equally effective materials. They may be placed uncovered, or covered with eyebank sclera, sutured on their posterior side. Alternative implant configurations are the Iowa implant with four prominences and the Allen implant with an attached ring affording slots for extraocular muscle

insertion. Although the Iowa and Allen implants may enhance motility somewhat, they are much more prone to later migration and extrusion. Therefore, in most cases, enucleation spheres are recommended.

The four 5-0 Vicryl sutures secured to the distal ends of the rectus muscles are placed through Tenon's capsule and conjunctiva overlying the respective muscle and tied (Fig 12–3G). This enhances postoperative motility because they afford an extra "kick" to movement of the fornices.

A 5-0 Vicryl suture is positioned within posterior Tenon's capsule in a purse-string manner. The sphere should be maintained deep within the muscle cone as this suture is placed. This suture is pulled taut, tied, and cut. The more superficial layer of Tenon's capsule is next closed vertically with interrupted 6-0 Vicryl sutures (Fig. 12–3H). The conjunctiva is closed horizontally as a separate layer with running 7-0 chromic catgut (Fig. 12–3I). This three-layer closure affords wound strength in three different directions, minimizing the chance of postoperative extrusion.

Sterile antibiotic ointment is placed on the conjunctival suture line and a conformer should be placed postoperatively to help preserve the fornices and inhibit conjunctival shrinkage (Figs. 12–3J and 12–4). This may be covered with a pressure dressing for 24 hours. After 4 to 6 weeks postoperatively, the patient may be fitted with a prosthesis. In most cases, the patient is comfortable with a prosthesis that is cosmetically pleasing and somewhat mobile. Safety glasses to protect the remaining eye are recommended after surgery.

When enucleation is performed for an intraocular tumor, it should be performed with sharp dissection in an extremely gentle manner, avoiding excessive elevation of intraocular pressure ("no touch"). A cryo-ring is applied to the sclera to protect the surrounding tissues and to allow the tumor (usually a melanoma) to be frozen, thereby interrupting blood flow from the tumor. The enucleation proceeds while the tumor is maintained in a frozen state. This process helps to minimize potential surgically induced hematogenous spread of tumor cells.

In cases or tumor, the optic nerve and sclera should be inspected carefully for gross evidence of tumor extension. This examination should be correlated with later histologic information to determine whether radiation, chemotherapy, or more radical surgery is required in a particular case.

COMPLICATIONS AFTER EVISCERATION AND ENUCLEATION

Problems that may be encountered after either evisceration or enucleation include implant extrusion, infec-

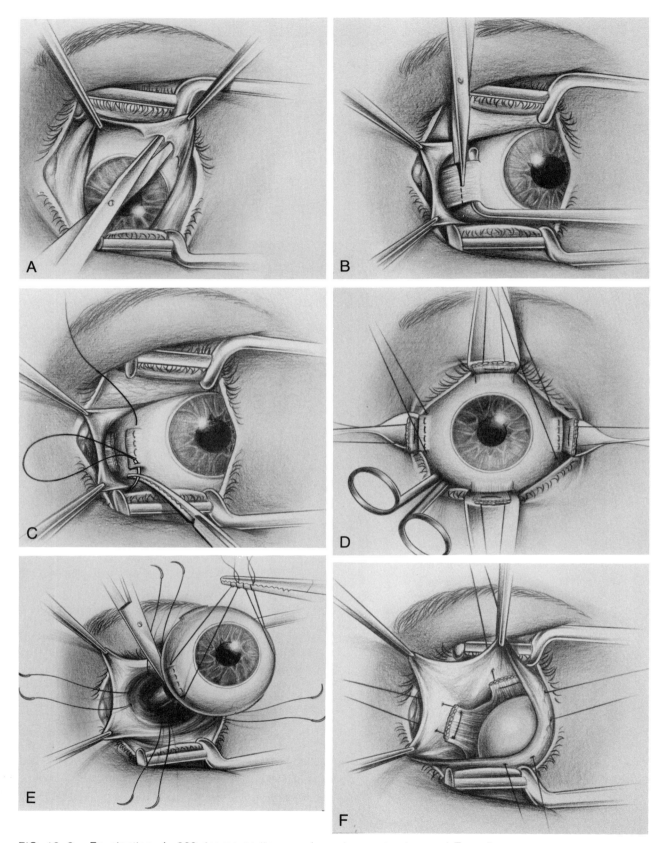

FIG. 12–3. Enucleation. A, 360-degree peritomy undermining conjunctiva and Tenon's capsule. B, The four rectus muscles are sequentially isolated and, C, secured with 5-0 Vicryl sutures. D, Following muscle disinsertion, the medial and lateral rectus muscle stumps are fixated with 5-0 Mersilene traction sutures. E, The optic nerve is severed and the globe is brought forward with the traction sutures. Any remaining globe attachments are severed. F, An enucleation sphere is placed in the posterior orbit, within the muscle cone through a rent in posterior Tenon's capsule.

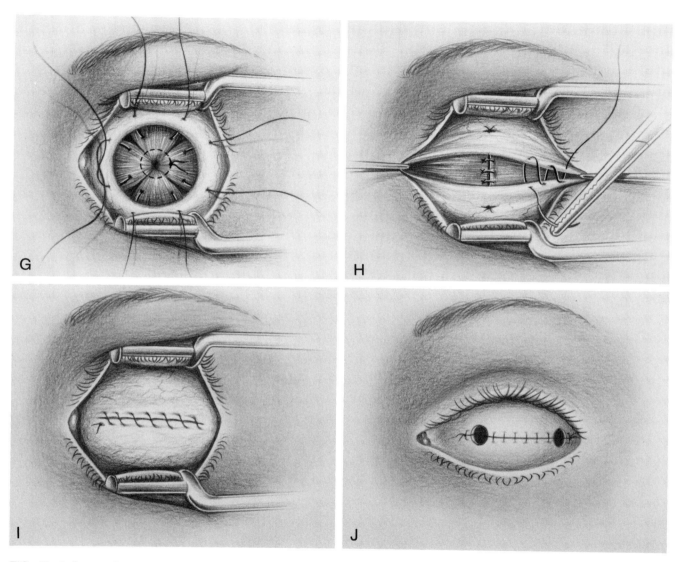

FIG. 12–3 Cont.   G, Previously placed Vicryl sutures are externalized through Tenon's capsule and conjunctiva. H, Three-layer closure: posterior Tenon's capsule purse string closure, superficial Tenon's capsule vertical closure, conjunctival horizontal closure. I, Conjunctival closure completed. J, A conformer is placed to preserve the fornices.

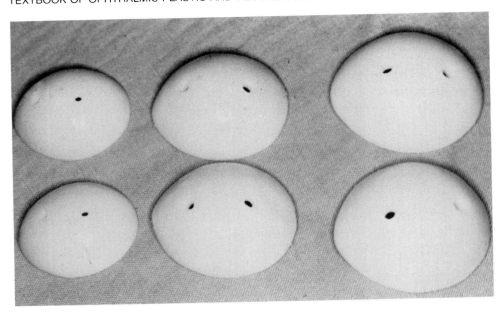

FIG. 12–4.   A variety of conformer sizes is available.

tion, enophthalmos, excessively deep superior sulcus, conjunctival shrinkage, contracted socket, laxity of the lower eyelid, and blepharoptosis of the upper eyelid.

Implant Extrusion. Extrusion may occur in the early postoperative period or develop gradually several years after surgery (Fig. 12–5). Early extrusion usually results from inadequate wound closure or infection.

Minor postoperative extrusions can be effectively man-

aged with scleral reinforcement after evisceration, or conjunctival and Tenon's reinforcement after enucleation. Placement of a scleral patch graft beneath a conjunctival-Tenon's lining may provide additional support.

After direct local infiltration with lidocaine 2% (Xylocaine), the edges of conjunctiva and Tenon's capsule (also sclera following evisceration) involved in the dehiscence are judiciously trimmed of friable or necrotic tissue. The implant is repositioned either within the scleral pouch (after evisceration) or beneath posterior

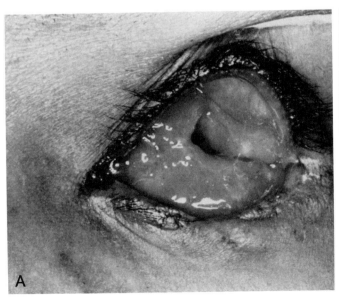
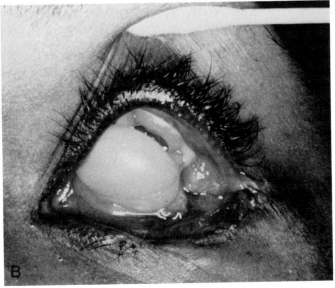

FIG. 12–5.   A, Early extrusion of enucleation implant, B, gradual increase in extrusion over time.

Tenon's capsule (after enucleation). If a small defect is encountered, it should be closed with interrupted 5-0 Vicryl mattress sutures. Following evisceration, defects in sclera and conjunctiva are closed independently in two layers. After enucleation, defects in Tenon's capsule and conjunctiva are similarly closed in two layers.

If a somewhat larger defect is encountered, a scleral patch may provide additional support (Fig. 12–6). The patch is fashioned from processed eyebank sclera irrigated in an antibiotic solution before placement. Once sutured in place with 5-0 Vicryl, the patch should be covered with conjunctiva (Fig. 12–7). A small conformer should be placed to maintain the fornices while minimizing stress on the suture lines.

More extensive extrusions require removal of the spherical implant, with later placement of a dermis fat graft as a secondary implant.

Extrusion and infection often coexist and are interdependent. A purulent infection necessitates removal of the implant and treatment with topical and systemic antibiotics as dictated by culture and sensitivity studies. Placing a drain may resolve an infection more rapidly. The volume of the orbit may be adequately filled by infection-induced collagenous tissue or by subsequent placement of a dermis fat graft as a secondary implant.

Dermis Fat Graft. Placement of a dermis fat graft is an excellent choice as a secondary implant following implant infection, or after extensive or delayed extrusion. It is also useful in severely contracted sockets because it provides both orbital volume and expansion of the conjunctival surface into the fornices. This procedure is applicable for enucleated and eviscerated sockets alike.

Before placing a dermis fat graft in the anophthalmic socket, any remaining orbital implant should be removed. In a suture line dehiscence, the wound edges should be freshened and trimmed of any nonviable tissue. In other cases, a 25 mm horizontal incision should be placed in the midportion of the socket. With blunt dissection, the socket should be opened anteriorly to afford subsequent graft positioning. Hemostasis is obtained with judicious electrocautery.

The donor graft is obtained from the lateral thigh near the buttock. This is in the region extending from the lateral iliac crest to the greater trochanter. After careful preparation, a dermatone is used to remove the epidermis, which should remain hinged on one side to facilitate later repositioning. A 25 mm circular or elliptical area of dermis is marked and incised to a depth of 25 mm in the fat layer. A circular or cylindrical plug of dermis with its subjacent fat completely attached is removed. This graft should have a diameter of 25 mm and a depth of 25 mm.

To give the donor site adequate strength, it should be closed in three layers: 4-0 Vicryl vertical mattress and 5-0 Vicryl horizontal mattress for the deeper layers, and 6-0 silk in an interrupted manner to close the overlying flap of epidermis.

Gloves should be changed and instruments resterilized before returning to the recipient socket. The periorbital area is again prepped. The dermis fat graft should be soaked in antibiotic solution and trimmed to fit the socket configuration. With the dermal surface uppermost, the dermis is sutured with 6-0 Vicryl to sclera in eviscerated

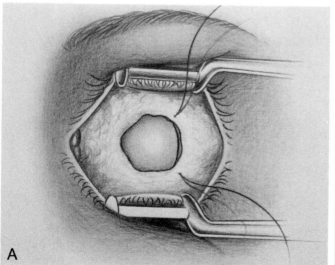 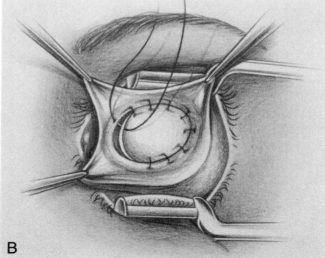

FIG. 12–6. A, Large socket defect will probably defy primary closure and will instead require a scleral patch, B.

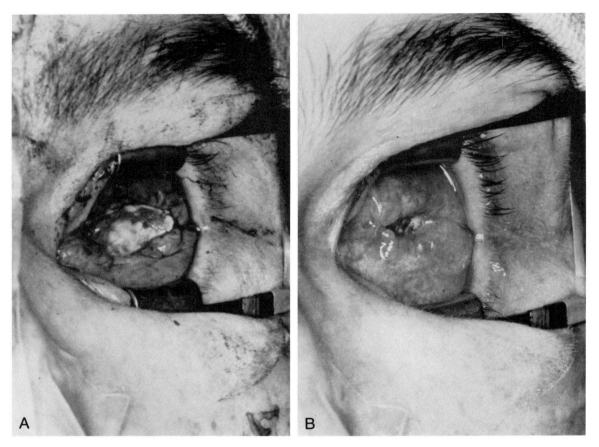

FIG. 12–7.   A, Scleral patch placed over extruding implant. B, Conjunctival covering over scleral patch.

sockets and to Tenon's capsule in enucleated sockets. If conjunctiva is abundant, it may be sutured over the dermis with a running 6-0 chromic catgut. If conjunctiva is deficient, it should not be used to cover the dermis. In these cases, the dermis repositions more conjunctiva at the fornices and provides for its expansion.

Anophthalmic Enophthalmos. When there is a disparity between the volume of the bony orbit and its contents, enophthalmos occurs. The principal cause is surgical anophthalmos after enucleation or evisceration. Coexistent orbital fractures may also contribute because orbital contents become outwardly displaced through bony defects, directly communicating with adjacent sinuses. Other contributions to enophthalmos include atrophy of orbital fat and muscle and gravity-induced factors.

Autogenous and homogenous implants of bone and cartilage have been used to correct this deformity. These are not recommended because they have the disadvantage of losing volume through atrophy and resorption, resulting in temporary improvement.

Various alloplastic materials have been used, including acrylic, Silastic, silicone, and Teflon. These implants are positioned subperiosteally in a manner similar to that of a blowout fracture repair through an infralash incision. The only difference is that here the implant is wedge-shaped, with the larger segment positioned posteriorly to enhance orbital volume and diminish enophthalmos (Figs. 12–8 through 12–10).

Anophthalmic Superior Sulcus Deformity. After enucleation or evisceration, an orbital volume deficit occurs. It may be minimized by the use of a large sphere (22 mm) at enucleation, but is not uniformly eliminated.

In 1967, the use of solid Pyrex beads was reported by Smith, Obear, and Leone. These were placed within a periosteal pocket fashioned at the superior portion of the orbital apex. The object of this procedure was to move the superior orbital contents forward to more normally fill in the sulcus.

This technique should not be performed in the presence of a seeing eye, or with a bony defect in the orbital

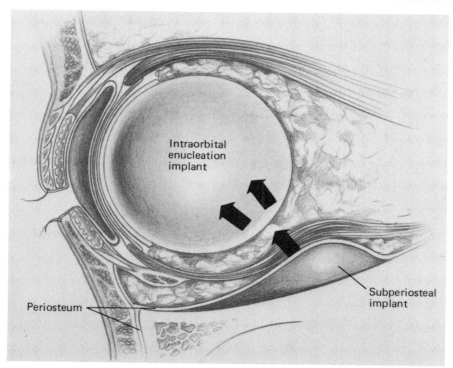

FIG. 12–8. Lateral view of an orbit depicting placement of subperiosteal wedge-shaped implant.

apex region. Retinal folds and edema have followed its use, obviating its applicaion in an eye with functional vision. Should a bony defect be suspected, preoperative orbital x-rays must be obtained to ensure that the apex is intact. Several instances of bead migration have been reported, subsequently obviating the placement of independent beads. From this technique evolved the approach currently in use, as described below.

Placement of Linked Teflon Beads at the Orbital Apex. A Mersilene suture can be used to link 25 to 30 5 mm

Teflon beads (Fig. 12–11). A minute drill hole is placed through each bead to afford its placement on the strand. Each prepared strand looks like a strand of miniature pearls with one end untied to allow the surgeon to remove excess beads.

Under general anesthesia, a 15 mm horizontal incision is made just lateral to the outer canthus overlying the lateral orbital rim (Fig. 12–12A). Using blunt and sharp dissection with Stevens scissors, the incision is carried through subcutaneous tissue and muscle to the periosteum at the lateral orbital rim (Fig. 12–12B). A 15 mm vertical incision is made through periosteum anterior and

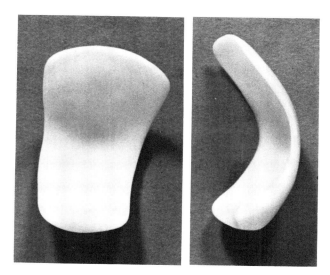

FIG. 12–9. Teflon sled-type implant.

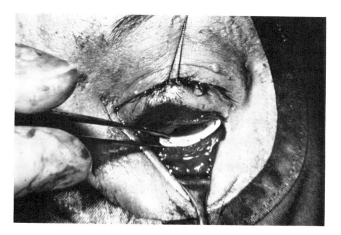

FIG. 12–10. Insertion of sled implant over the orbital floor.

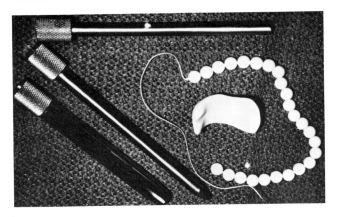

FIG. 12–11. Teflon beads photographed with three parts of the trochar inserter, along with a sled implant.

superior to the lateral orbital tubercle. The periosteum is undermined posteriorly toward the superior portion of the orbital apex (Fig. 12–12C). Periorbita separates easily from orbital bone. Excessive force is therefore not required and should not be used in this maneuver. The leading edge of the periosteal elevator should always remain in contact with bone so that the dissection remains in the subperiosteal space. The dissection should not extend beyond the oribital apex, to prevent injury to the supraorbital and infraorbital nerves.

After removal of the periosteal elevator, a specialized trochar inserter is placed through the dissection down to the level of the superior portion of the orbital apex (Fig. 12–12D). The stylet of the inserter is then withdrawn.

The sterilized linked Teflon beads should be soaked in an antibiotic solution before placement. They are then placed within the trochar introducer with the tied end at the lead. The plunger portion of the inserter is then positioned within the trochar. With gentle pressure on the plunger, the beads are inserted and distributed within the periosteal pocket as the trochar is gradually withdrawn. The number of beads used should be based on the extent of sulcus deformity. A slight intraoperative overcorrection is a desirable end point. It can be titrated intraoperatively by observing the superior sulcus as the beads are being positioned. Eighteen 5 mm beads are equivalent to 1 cc in volume. Most cases require 25 to 30 such linked beads. After placement, any unused beads are pulled off the strand and the end of the Mersilene suture is tied and secured.

Periosteum is closed with three interrupted 5-0 Vicryl sutures (Fig. 12–12E) followed by skin closure with running 7-0 silk (Fig. 12–12F). In addition to topical antibiotics, oral antibiotics are recommended postopera-

tively. Figures 12–13 and 12–14 show postoperative results.

Superior sulcus deformities can also be reduced with wedge-shaped orbital floor implants as described in the previous section. This mobilizes the enucleation sphere and orbital fat upwardly, filling the sulcus. Orbital floor implants have the additional advantage of applicability in cases with a sighted eye. The result is reduction of the sulcus deformity with minimal alteration of motility function.

Conjunctival Shrinkage and Contracture. Conjunctival shrinkage may result from extrusion of an evisceration or enucleation sphere. It may also follow burns (chemical, thermal, or radiation), trauma, infection, inflammation, and multiple surgical procedures, particularly following retinal surgery. Mild conjunctival shrinkage may make the fornices shallow, cause symblepharon, and result in limited socket contracture. Such changes may compromise prosthesis retention and require placement of a conjunctival or mucous membrane graft.

If the donor graft requirement is small, conjunctiva from the contralateral eye may be used and the procedure may be performed under local anesthesia. Most cases require larger grafts, necessitating the use of buccal mucosa (Fig. 12–15A) obtained under general anesthesia. The technique for harvesting these grafts is decribed in Chapter 2.

The area of socket contraction is incised with sharp Stevens scissors. Contributing cicatricial bands should be severed and hemostasis must be adequate.

The harvested graft should be trimmed to fit the recipient bed configuration and the corners secured with interrupted 6-0 chromic catgut sutures. The remainder of the graft is sutured with running 7-0 chromic catgut (Fig. 12–15B). A stent should be placed over the graft to inhibit contracture (Fig. 12–16A). Small silicone retinal sponges are excellent for this purpose. When the fornix is grafted, the stent should be anchored with several double-armed 4-0 silk sutures placed in a mattress fashion. Each suture end engages the stent, mucosal graft at the fornix, and periosteum at the orbital rim, before penetrating the eyelid to emerge through the overlying skin (Fig. 12–16B). At this point, the suture may be tied over a rubber bolster to minimize excoriation of the overlying skin. The sutures are removed after 2 to 3 weeks.

More severe socket contracture requires placement of a dermis fat graft. If an evisceration or enucleation implant remains, it should be removed before introduction of this graft. Dermis fat expands the fornices by extending the conjunctival surface and additionally contributes to socket volume as a secondary implant.

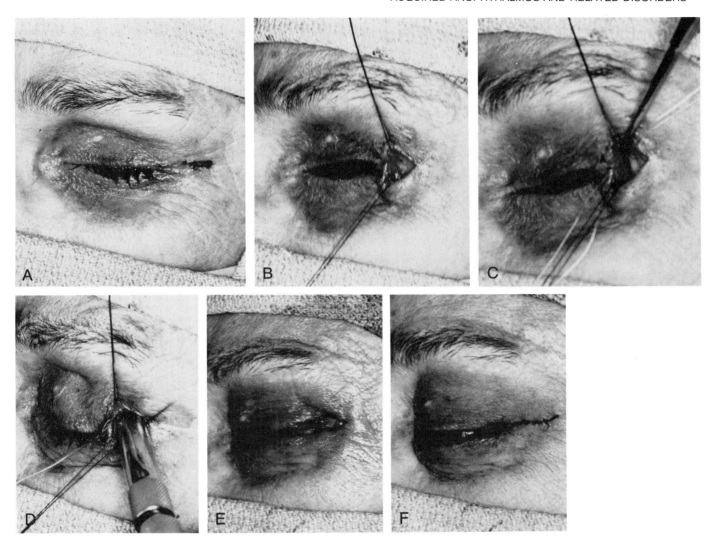

FIG. 12–12.   Placement of linked Teflon beads at orbital apex. A, Horizontal incision just lateral to outer canthal commissure. B, Periosteum exposed and C, opened. D, Trochar inserter is placed between periosteum and bone to the superolateral orbital apex. After bead placement, periosteum, E, and skin, F, are closed.

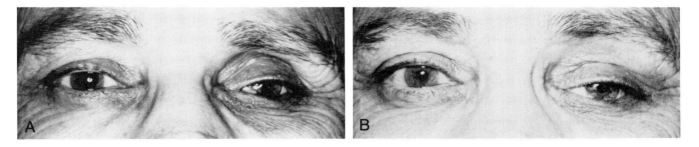

FIG. 12–13.   A, Enucleation-induced left superior sulcus deformity. B, Appearance after placement of linked Teflon beads at orbital apex.

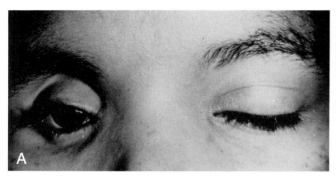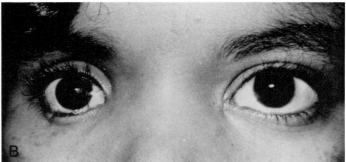

FIG. 12–14.   A, Enucleation-induced right superior sulcus deformity. B, Appearance after placement of linked Teflon beads at orbital apex.

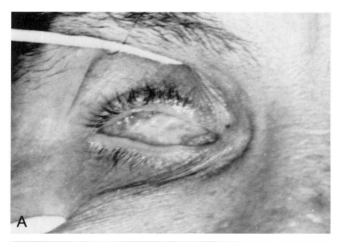

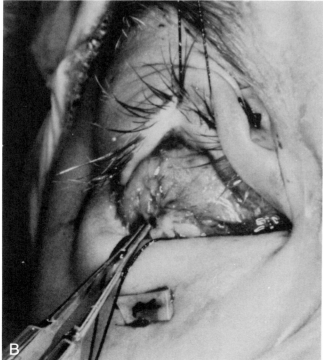

FIG. 12–15.   Contracted socket. A, Preoperative appearance. B, Treated with buccal mucous membrane graft, which is secured with chromic catgut sutures. This is further supported with mattress sutures extending through stents at the fornices, engaging periosteum at the orbital rims, emerging on the skin surface where the sutures are tied over bolsters.

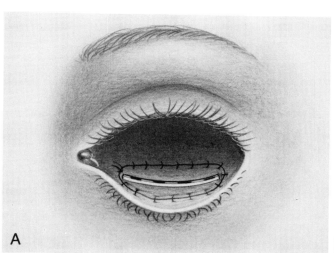

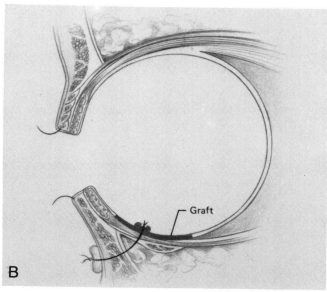

FIG. 12–16. A, Mucous membrane graft placed in contracted socket. Silicone retinal sponges may be used as a stent to inhibit contracture. B, Lateral view demonstrating anchorage of the stent to the fornix and periosteum at the orbital rim.

Eyelid Laxity. Evisceration and enucleation may cause lower eyelid laxity, which can be corrected by either a Bick procedure as described in Chapter 7 or a lateral canthal sling.

Lateral Canthal Sling. A lateral canthal sling is performed under local anesthesia. Following direct infiltration of lidocaine 2% (Xylocaine) into the lateral aspect of the lower eyelid and outer canthus, a lateral canthotomy is performed. Through the canthotomy the inferior crus of the lateral canthal tendon is disinserted from the lateral orbital rim. A flap of periosteum is fashioned on the anterior surface of the lateral orbital rim (Fig. 12–17A). This flap should be temporally based and positioned slightly higher than the lateral orbital tubercle.

The lower eyelid is pulled laterally to determine the point where it crosses over the lateral orbital rim. This is marked to denote the new lateral extent of the lower eyelid. A tongue of tarsus is fashioned at the temporal portion of the lower eyelid. This is accomplished by removing a small portion of eyelid margin, lashes, skin, orbicularis oculi muscle, and conjunctiva surrounding the lateral portion of tarsus. A 5-0 Vicryl suture is placed in a mattress fashion to join this tongue of tarsus to the periosteal flap (Fig. 12–17B). The skin is closed with running 7-0 silk sutures. This procedure elevates the outer canthus and horizontally tightens the lower eyelid.

An oversized prosthesis may cause mechanical ectropion, which readily responds to placement of tarsal rotation sutures, described in Chapter 7.

Blepharoptosis. If true blepharoptosis persists after optimal orbital reconstruction and prosthesis fitting, it should be corrected according to ordinary blepharoptosis indications and techniques (Fig. 12–18).

EXENTERATION

Orbital exenteration involves total removal of the orbital contents with partial or total removal of the eyelids. This mutilating operation is indicated only when the patient's life is threatened by a malignant neoplasm or infection within the orbit that cannot be cured or controlled by any less invasive modality. Most incurable cases should not undergo exenteration, although selected cases may benefit from diminution of tumor bulk and pain. The frequency of this procedure has been reduced because of advances made in radiotherapy, improved delivery of chemotherapeutic agents, and more effective treatment for life-threatening infections such as mucormycosis. Exenteration should never be based upon frozen section information. Instead, it should always be predicated upon findings from careful paraffin section analysis performed and reviewed preoperatively.

The purpose of exenteration is removal of the orbital contents and the pathologic process contained within *en bloc*. It is imperative to determine clearly the anatomic extent of the disease process. This may require orbital x-rays, CT studies, and angiography in indicated cases. Extension of a tumor beyond the orbit into the intra-

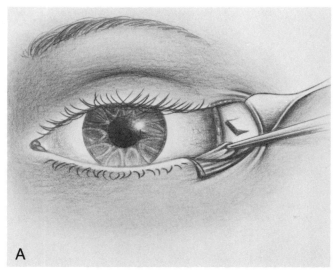
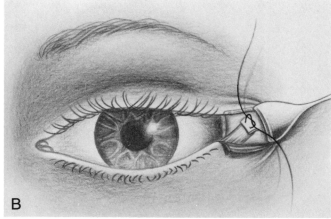

FIG. 12–17.   Lateral canthal sling. A, Through a lateral canthotomy, the inferior crus of the lateral canthal tendon is disinserted and a flap of periosteum is fashioned at the lateral orbital rim. B, A tongue of tarsus is fashioned at the temporal aspect of the lower eyelid and joined to the periosteal flap.

cranial compartment or sinus may require bone resection and surgical collaboration with a neurosurgeon or oto-laryngologist. Some vascular tumors may benefit from preoperative embolization to reduce intraoperative bleeding.

Before exenteration, patients should clearly understand their disease process and the therapeutic risks and alternatives. They should be informed of the extent of the resultant deformity and the process required toward its prosthetic rehabilitation. A review of clinical photographs of other exenteration patients with and without an external prosthesis can effectively communicate the anticipated postoperative result. Patients should be further informed that postoperative hypesthesia may extend from the cheek to the forehead.

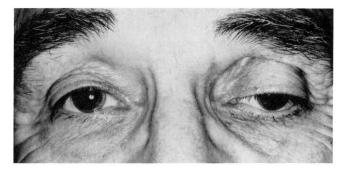

FIG. 12–18.   Following enucleation of the left globe, a true blepharoptosis developed from a dehiscence of the levator aponeurosis.

Under general anesthesia, the area of intended incision is marked with methylene blue. This should extend elliptically from the lower portion of the supraorbital rim below the brow hairline, through the inner and outer canthus overlying the medial and lateral orbital rims respectively, and over the upper portion of the infraorbital rim.

In total exenteration (eyelid tissue not spared) the eyelids may be joined by several 4-0 silk mattress sutures engaging the tarsal plates. Leaving these sutures long for upward traction facilitates surgical excision of the orbital contents. According to the marked lines, an incision is made with a #64 Beaver blade. The dissection is carried through subcutaneous tissue, muscle, and periosteum to bone (Fig. 12–19A). A periosteal elevator is used to separate periosteum, which is significantly less adherent on its periorbital surfaces (Fig. 12–19B). This dissection can be effectively extended to the orbital apex. Some resistance may be encountered at the trochlea and at the medial and lateral canthal tendons where periorbita is attached along suture lines.

At this point in the surgery, Metzenbaum scissors are directed back along the temporal orbital wall to sever the remaining apical stump of tissue as close to the bone as possible (Fig. 12–19C). The orbital contents are then removed and sent for histologic examination, while orbital bone is packed with pressure applied to control bleeding. Direct electrocautery with or without clamping is often required.

Careful examination of the remaining orbital bone

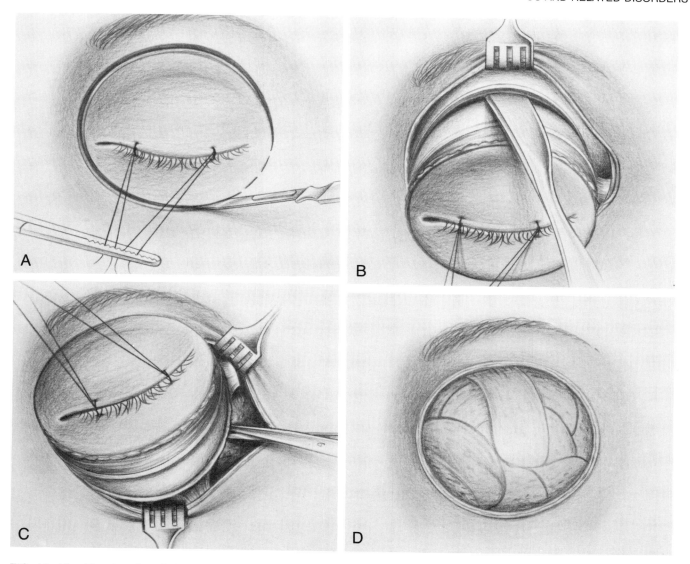

FIG. 12–19.   Exenteration. A, In a total exenteration, the eyelids may be joined by 4-0 silk mattress sutures. This facilitates traction. Elliptical incisions are made over the superior and inferior orbital rims, through the inner and outer canthi overlying the medial and lateral orbital rims. B, The dissection is carried through subcutaneous tissue, muscle, and periosteum to bone. C, Periosteum is separated from bone posteriorly and the apical orbital attachment is separated with Metzenbaum scissors. D, If the orbit is intended to heal through granulation, iodoform gauze is used as a pack.

should demonstrate no residual tumor or extension of tumor into adjacent sinuses. The presence of such tumor often requires extension of the surgical excision into these areas (extended exenteration). If the sinuses are inadvertently entered, a fistula may later form.

Most exenterated orbits are allowed to heal by granulation, and do not require skin grafting. If the orbit is intended to heal through granulation, a large iodoform gauze packing is secured within the orbit under moderate pressure (Fig. 12–19D).

If a split-thickness skin graft is used, it should be harvested from a hairless area of the inner thigh or abdomen with a dermatome. The size and depth of the dermatome should be preset to ensure a split thickness graft (0.006 in.) large enough to encompass the entire orbit.

The donor site should be adequately prepped with

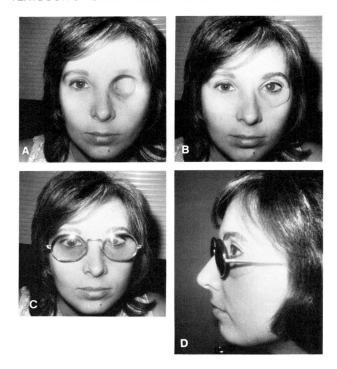

FIG. 12–20. A, Patient 6 weeks after exenteration for malignant fibrous histiocytoma of the intraorbital region. B, The same patient with Silastic prosthesis in place. C, Glasses provide effective camouflage for the prosthesis. D, Lateral view.

Betadine. Firm pressure must be maintained on the dermatome to maintain graft uniformity. As the graft emerges through the instrument, it is grasped with forceps to prevent scrolling or recycling within the blade. The resultant graft should be smooth and thin. An antibiotic ointment, Adaptic gauze, and a pressure dressing are applied to the donor site.

Skin grafts are contraindicated in cases of limited life expectancy, orbital infection, or anticipated postoperative radiotherapy.

The graft is kept moist with balanced salt solution until used. It should be rolled into a conical shape and placed within the orbit, ensuring that the epithelial surface is not touching bone. The graft is trimmed to fit the orbital dimension and secured with multiple 6-0 Vicryl sutures. Several fenestrations are made in the graft to afford adequate postoperative drainage. When orbital walls are removed, the exposed mucosal surfaces should not be covered with the graft. These areas later develop a mucosal covering of their own.

Large strips of Telfa imbricated with an antibiotic solution are placed within the graft cone. The dressing is further supported by a fluff dressing and 2-inch elastoplast secured with tincture of benzoin to maintain pressure between graft and bone postoperatively. This dressing may be left in place for 48 hours.

The socket will be sufficiently healed in 3 months to allow fitting of an external prosthetic device. Such a prosthesis must include a globe, eyelids, and in some cases orbital margins. Glasses may provide further camouflage (Fig. 12–20). Although not cosmetically perfect, such large prostheses are usually satisfactory and appreciated by patients who remember the life-threatening condition that required exenteration.

If the disease process is confined to the posterior orbit, a portion of the eyelids may be spared. In subtotal exenterations (anterior eyelid tissue spared), the entire lash margin of each eyelid is removed in a thin strip. The eyelid is split between the skin and orbicularis oculi muscle. Each eyelid is dissected distally anterior to the tarsus and orbital septum to the respective orbital rim. The tarsal plates are joined by several 4-0 silk mattress sutures, kept long for surgical traction. The dissection proceeds as for complete exenteration.

The spared eyelid skin is used for reconstruction. This tissue is used to line the bony defect and is secured with interrupted 6-0 Vicryl sutures. Although this does not provide enough skin to line the orbit entirely, the remainder will be filled in by tissue spreading and epithelialization.

BIBLIOGRAPHY

Baylis, H., and Shorr, N.: Correction of Problems of the Anophthalmic Socket. In McCord C.: Oculoplastic Surgery, New York, Raven Press 1981.

Bell, R.: Subperiostel glass bead deposition for plastic correction of enophthalmos. Ophthalmic Surg. 3:66–70, 1973.

Beyer, C.: The extruded implant. Trans. Am. Acad. Ophthalmol. Otolaryngol. 74:1311, 1970.

Beyer-Machule, C., and von Noorden, G.: Atlas of Ophthalmic Surgery. New York, Thieme-Stratton, 1985.

Callahan, M., and Callahan, A.: Ophthalmic Plastic and Orbital Surgery. Birmingham, Aesculapius, 1979.

Dryden, R., and Leibsohn, J.: Postenucleation Orbital Implant Extrusion. Arch. Ophthalmol. 96:2064, 1978.

Fraunfelder, F., and Wilson, R.: A New Approach for Intraocular Malignancy: the "No-touch" Enucleation. In Jakobiec, F: Ocular and Adnexal Tumors. Birmingham, Aesculapius, 1978.

Frueh, B., and Felker, G.: Baseball Implant. A method of secondary insertion of an orbital implant. Arch. Ophthalmol. 94:429, 1976.

Green, W., Maumenee, A., and Sanders, T.: Sympathetic uveitis following evisceration. Trans. Am. Acad. Ophthalmol. Otolaryngol. 76:625–644, 1972.

Guibor, P., and Smith, B.: Orbital glass-bead inserter. Trans. Am. Acad. Ophthalmol. Otolaryngol. 76:529, 1972.

Helveston, E.: Human bank scleral patch: for repair of exposed or extruded orbital implants. Arch. Ophthalmol. 82:83–85, 1969.

Helveston, E.: A scleral patch for exposed implantation. Trans. Am. Acad. Ophthalmol. Otolaryngol. 74:1307–1310, 1970.

Kennedy, R.: The effect of early enucleation on the orbit. Am. J. Ophthalmol. 60:277–306, 1965.

Kohn, R.: Mechanical ectropion repair utilizing tarsal rotation sutures. Ophthalmic Surg. 10:48, 1977.

Kohn, R., and Hepler, R.: Management of limited rhino-orbital mucormycosis without exenteration. Ophthalmology 92:1440, 1985.

McCord, C.: The extruding implant. Trans. Am. Acad. Ophthalmol. Otolaryngol. 81:587–590, 1976.

Putterman, A., and Scott, R.: Deep ocular socket reconstruction. Arch. Ophthalmol. 95:1221, 1977.

Rathbun, J., Beard, C., and Quickert, M.: Evaluation of 48 cases of orbital exenteration. Am. J. Ophthalmol. 72:191–199, 1971.

Reeh, M., Beyer, C., and Shannon, G.: Practical Ophthalmic Plastic and Reconstructive Surgery. Philadelphia, Lea and Febiger, 1976.

Smith, B., Obear, M., and Leone, C.: The correction of enopthalmos associated with anopthalmos by glass bead implantation. Am. J. Ophthalmol. 64:1088–1093, 1967.

Smith, B., and Petrelli, R.: Dermis-fat graft as a movable implant within the muscle cone. Am. J. Ophthalmol. 85:62–66, 1978.

Soll, D.: Correction of superior lid sulcus deformity with subperiosteal implants. Arch. Ophthalmol. 85:188–190, 1971.

Soll, D.: Insertion of secondary intraorbital implants. Arch. Ophthalmol. 89:214–216, 1973.

Soll, D.: Donor sclera in enucleation surgery. Arch. Ophthalmol. 92:494–495, 1974.

Soll, D.: The Anophthalmic Socket: In: Management of Complications in Ophthalmic Plastic Surgery, Birmingham, Aesculapius, 1976.

Soll, D.: The anophthalmic socket. Ophthalmology. 89:407–423, 1982.

Spivey, B., Allen, L., and Stewart, W.: Surgical correction of superior sulcus deformity occurring after enucleation. Am. J. Ophthalmol. 82:365, 1976.

Taiara, C., and Smith, B.: Correction of enophthalmos and deep supratarsal sulcus by posterior subperiosteal glass bead implantation. Br. J. Ophthalmol. 57:741–746, 1973.

Tenzel, R.: Treatment of lagophthalmos of the lower lid. Arch. Ophthalmol. 81:366–368, 1969.

13

LACRIMAL SYSTEM

Epiphora and dry eyes are the most prevalent functional disabilities attributable to the ocular adnexa. The causes of these conditions may be manifold and the treatment is often complex. Tearing is a very common symptom, elicited during even the most routine examinations. Further historical and clinical information should reveal the true source of epiphora.

Thorough knowledge of relevant lacrimal and nasal anatomy is essential in charting a proper evaluation and carrying it through a well-executed surgical correction. Conscientious postoperative follow-up is necessary to maintain a functional result.

The anatomy and physiology of the lacrimal secretory and drainage systems were reviewed in detail in Chapter 1. The secretory system (Fig. 13–1) consists of:

I. Basic secretors
   A. Mucin secretors
      1. Conjunctival goblet cells
      2. Crypts of Henle
      3. Glands of Manz
   B. Lacrimal Secretors
      1. Accessory lacrimal gland of Krause
      2. Accessory lacrimal gland of Wolfring
      3. Glands in the plica semilunaris
   C. Oil Secretors
      1. Meibomian glands
      2. Glands of Zeis and Moll
II. Reflex secretors
   A. Main lacrimal gland
   B. Exocrine glands other than those of the glands of Krause and Wolfring

EVALUATION OF THE LACRIMAL SECRETORY SYSTEM

Historical information should document the severity and duration of symptoms, along with the extent of functional impairment. Patients should relate whether the symptoms are unilateral or bilateral. Contributions from systemic disease (thyroid, collagen-vascular disease, arthritis, Riley Day syndrome) and ophthalmic disease should be explored. Allergic nasal disorders and previous nasal trauma or surgery may also contribute. Any topical or systemic medication in use should be discussed to ascertain whether a causal relationship exists.

The evaluation of epiphora must first differentiate nasolacrimal obstruction from hypersecretion, tear film disorders, and dry eye syndrome.

Hypersecretion may result from supranuclear, nuclear, and infranuclear central nervous system stimulation, as well as from direct and reflex stimulation of the lacrimal gland. Supranuclear stimulation of the lacrimal nucleus in the pons is triggered by emotion or other central nervous system factors. Infranuclear stimulation of the nervus intermedius may arise from tumors of the cerebellopontine angle. Misdirected cranial nerve VII fibers following Bell's palsy may yield a gustatory-lacrimal reflex ("crocodile tears").

Direct stimulation of the lacrimal gland may result from inflammation or tumor. This may variably cause increased or decreased tear production, depending on whether the effect is irritative or ablative. Reflex stimulation of the lacrimal gland is triggered by the ophthalmic division of the trigeminal (fifth) nerve. This stimulates the lacrimal nucleus toward a heightened lacrimal gland response by way of the seventh nerve. This process may be triggered by anterior segment disease, inflammation (allergy, conjunctivitis, keratitis, blepharitis, sinusitis), irritation (entropion, epiblepharon, trichiasis, distichiasis, blepharospasm, chalazion, molluscum contagiosum, papilloma, symblepharon), foreign body, uveitis, glaucoma, glaucoma medications, Graves' disease, or excessive retinal illumination. Extrinsic contributions to hypersecretion may be airborne particulate matter, wind, or fatigue.

These causes of hypersecretion should all be managed by treating the intrinsic cause or eliminating the extrinsic factor. Additional relief may be derived from the use of oral antihistamines or mild topical vasoconstrictor-astringent agents. Extirpation of the palpebral lobe of the lacrimal gland is not recommended because it will substitute a dry eye for a wet one, with resultant increased morbidity.

Pseudo-epiphora from a dry eye syndrome may activate the reflex arc between the fifth and seventh nerves

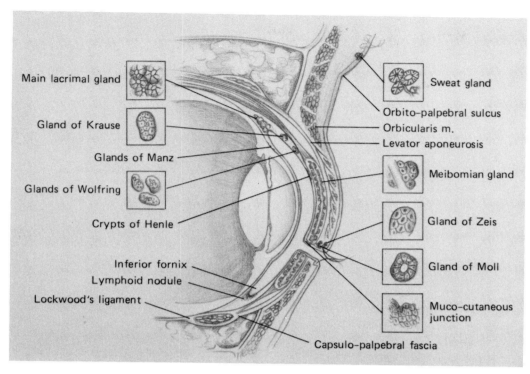

FIG. 13–1. Anatomy and histology of the components of the lacrimal secretory system.

to produce reflex tearing from the main lacrimal gland. The use of artificial tears obviates this reflex arc.

After hypersecretion is ruled out as a cause of tearing, the nasolacrimal system should be systematically evaluated. If an obstruction is present, its exact location and extent (partial or complete) must then be ascertained. A further assessment should be made defining the extent to which the symptoms interfere with the patient's daily function.

On slit lamp examination, the tear film should be observed for precipitates and break-up time. The use of either fluorescein or rose bengal provides additonal information. The tear meniscus should be quantified. Abnormalities suggest a tear film disorder as a cause of tearing.

placement in the fornix.) The extent of filter paper wetting from the notch is measured in millimeters after 5 minutes. The measurement is a reflection of the balance between tear production (both basic and reflex) and drainage.

If the paper is completely wet before 5 minutes, the time elapsed to produce complete wetting should be recorded. Normal median wetting approximates 15 mm, with a range of 10 to 30 mm. Excessive wetting suggests either hypersecretion or lacrimal obstruction. Less than 5 mm of wetting is abnormally low, suggesting a dry eye process. These patients often have corneal staining with fluorescein or rose bengal, and may demonstrate corneal filaments.

SCHIRMER #1 TEST

This study measures aggregate basic and reflex secretion. Patients should be in a dimly lit room to minimize reflex tearing from retinal stimulation. The Schirmer #1 Test is performed by placing a strip of filter paper in the inferior fornix near the outer canthus. (Specially prepared Schirmer strips are available composed of Whatman No. 41 paper, 35 mm long and 5 mm wide. A notch is located 5 mm from the end to facilitate bending for

BASIC SECRETION TEST

A few drops of topical anestheic solution are applied to the eye. This is followed by placing a cotton-tipped applicator stick moistened with 4% cocaine hydrochloride solution on the part of the conjunctiva where the filter paper is to be placed. The inferior fornix is dried with additional applicator sticks and the Schirmer paper (Whatman) is applied as described above. Room lights should be dimmed to eliminate tearing contributions from retinal stimulation. The extent of wetting is again recorded after 5 minutes.

In the basic secretion test, the anesthetic eliminates (or at least significantly reduces) the contribution from the reflex secretors, thereby quantifying the contribution from the basic secretors. If basic secretion is normal (approximating 10 mm), but the Schirmer #1 Test demonstrates rapid moistening in the presence of a patent lacrimal excretory system, hypersecretion from stimulation of the reflex secretors exists.

In patients with basic secretion of less than 3 mm, epiphora may be the result of induced reflex stimulation. Such dry eye conditions may respond to treatment with artificial tears.

SCHIRMER #2 TEST

When the Schirmer #1 test and basic secretion tests suggest a deficiency in reflex secretion, the Schirmer #2 test may distinguish a deficiency in reflex secretion from "fatigue block."

In this study, a few drops of topical anesthetic solution are applied to the eye. Schirmer paper is again placed in the inferior fornix near the outer canthus. The unanesthetized nasal mucosa in the area of the middle turbinate is irritated by a dry, cotton-tipped applicator stick. The extent of filter paper wetting from the notch is measured in millimeters after two minutes. This measurement should indicate the extent of reflex secretion.

No increase in the rate of wetting suggests a failure of reflex secretion. If the rate increases, the reflex secretors may be normal, but are not reacting due to a "fatigue block" involving the efferent nerve center, which mediates conjunctival afferent stimuli. The reflex secretors should return to normal function when the "fatigue" abates.

TEAR BREAK-UP TIME

Abnormalities of the mucin component of the tear film may have an adverse effect on corneal wetting. Pseudoepiphora may result and is measured by placing a small quantity of fluorescein on the superior bulbar conjunctiva. After several blinks, the patient is observed on the slit lamp with cobalt blue filter illumination. With the patient instructed to refrain from further blinking, the time for dry spots to appear on the cornea is noted. If the elapsed time is less than 10 seconds, it is considered abnormal. This condition should be treated with artificial tears.

EVALUATION OF THE LACRIMAL DRAINAGE SYSTEM

Although some cases may have an obvious cause and location of lacrimal obstruction and epiphora, most cases require further documentation. A dilated lacrimal sac that expresses purulent material through the punctum when digital pressure is applied to the sac heralds an obstruction of the nasolacrimal duct. Palpation of the lacrimal sac may also disclose dacryoliths, mucoceles, and tumors.

In most other situations, the location and extent (partial or complete) of lacrimal obstruction must be established through a combination of the following tests: dye disappearance test, Jones primary dye test, Jones secondary dye test, lacrimal irrigation, and dacryocystography. Lacrimal probing is not a useful diagnostic test, and its clinical applicability is restricted to cases of congenital nasolacrimal obstruction.

DYE DISAPPEARANCE TEST

One or two drops of fluorescein 2% are instilled into the inferior fornix of each eye. After two minutes, the extent of fluorescein retained in the tear meniscus, as well as any fluorescein epiphora tract is noted. An excessive meniscus or epiphora tract suggests a compromise of lacrimal drainage. Although the test is somewhat subjective, it is useful for comparative purposes in patients with unilateral symptoms.

JONES PRIMARY DYE TEST

Shrinking the nasal mucosa with topical cocaine 4% may facilitate the primary and secondary dye studies. Through a nasal speculum and under direct visualization with a head light, a small wire probe with a wisp of cotton covering its leading tip is inserted into the nose. It should extend to the level of the inferior meatus, below the inferior turbinate. The probe should extend approximately one inch into the the meatus, where it will come into contact with the inferior ostium of the nasolacrimal duct. An ordinary cotton-tipped applicator stick should not be used because it cannot extend adequately into the narrow meatus.

A drop of fluorescein 2% or equivalent is placed in the lower fornix (Fig. 13–2). Afer 5 minutes, the wire applicator is removed from the nose and the cotton tip is examined for the presence of fluorescein dye. In some cases, dye may also be recovered by simply occluding the opposite nostril and asking the patient to blow his

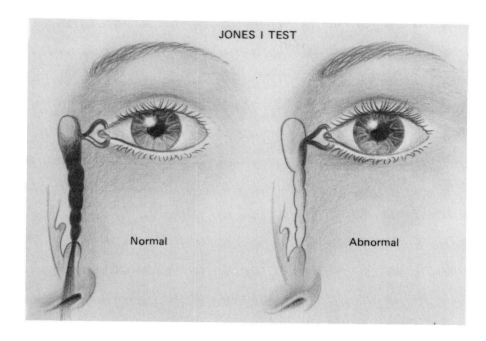

JONES I TEST

Normal   Abnormal

FIG. 13–2. Jones primary dye test. No dye recovery suggests a partial or complete obstruction.

nose into a tissue. The tissue is then checked for the presence of dye.

If dye is recovered by either method, the primary dye test is normal, signifying a patent and functional lacrimal drainage system. No further testing of the lacrimal drainage system is required. Such a result in the presence of epiphora suggests hypersecretion as the cause of tearing. If no dye is recovered, the primary dye test is abnormal, suggesting the presence of a partial or complete obstruction, or a diminished lacrimal pump. This requires further testing with the Jones Secondary Dye Test. Occasionally normal individuals will also demonstrate no dye recovery.

JONES SECONDARY DYE TEST

The secondary dye test is performed following an abnormal primary dye test. It differentiates partial from complete obstruction and provides an *estimate* of the site of blockage.

The conjunctival fornices should be irrigated to remove any residual fluorescein. Through a nasal speculum and under direct visualization with a head light, a second cotton-tipped wire probe is inserted into the inferior meatus. A lacrimal cannula is affixed to a 2 cc syringe and used to irrigate the ipsilateral canaliculi with saline. The cannula should be inserted through the lower punctum to the level of the common canaliculus (internal common punctum) (Fig. 13–3).

If irrigation fails to transmit fluid into the nose, a total obstruction is present. If irrigation transmits fluid con-

taining dye, a partial obstruction may be present at the level of the nasolacrimal duct. In this situation, fluid can sequester in the lacrimal sac, but can pass into the nose only under pressure. Fluid cannot pass into the nose under the normal conditions governed by the lacrimal pump mechanism alone. This result generally *suggests* the need for a dacryocystorhinostomy. If irrigation transmits clear fluid, a partial obstruction may be present at the level of the punctum or canaliculi. In this situation, fluid cannot sequester in the lacrimal sac and can pass into the nose only under pressure. This result generally *suggests* the need for a conjunctivo-dacryocystorhinostomy (Jones tube). The final choice of the procedure to recommend should be based on the extent of the patient's symptoms and the findings from the lacrimal irrigation test.

Secondary dye testing and the lacrimal irrigation test should not be performed in the presence of acute dacryocystitis. Irrigation in the presence of infection may significantly exacerbate the infectious process.

Primary and secondary dye testing do have some inherent inaccuracy. The results may be influenced by hyposecretion, functional block, eyelid malposition, disorders of the lacrimal pump, and lower eyelid laxity.

LACRIMAL IRRIGATION

The location of a complete obstruction can be precisely determined by lacrimal irrigation. This test is less effective, however, in distinguishing a partial obstruction from patency. The punctum is first expanded with a punc-

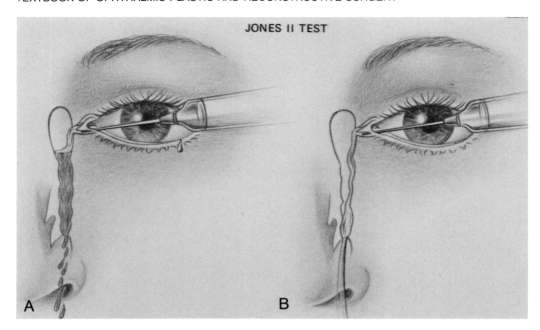

FIG. 13–3. Jones secondary dye test. No fluid recovery indicates a complete obstruction.
A. Dye recovery suggests partial obstruction at the level of the nasolacrimal duct. B. Clear
fluid recovery suggests partial obstruction at the level of the punctum or canaliculus.

tal dilator. In extreme punctal stenosis, the punctum may require dilatation using slit lamp visualization. Occasionally, the point of a 25-gauge needle may be necessary to enlarge the punctum to allow entrance of the dilator. After the punctum is dilated, a lacrimal irrigation cannula is used to irrigate the canaliculi with balanced salt solution or saline (Fig. 13–4). To provide accurate information, the cannula tip should be placed deep enough to enter the lacrimal sac, and 1 to 2 cc of fluid is injected. The patient should be asked to communicate whether this somewhat bitter and salty solution is felt in the nose or posterior pharynx (back of the throat), or tasted. During irrigation, an index finger should be placed over the lacrimal fossa to ascertain whether the lacrimal sac distends.

If a canaliculus is irrigated and the fluid comes directly back through that canaliculus without passing into the nose or dilating the lacrimal sac, a complete canalicular obstruction is present (Fig. 13–4A). A conjunctivo-dacryocystorhinostomy (Jones tube) is required to correct this condition.

If a canaliculus is irrigated and the fluid refluxes through the other canaliculus without passing into the nose or dilating the lacrimal sac, a complete common canalicular obstruction is present (Fig. 13–4B). In this situation, the lacrimal sac does not distend. A conjunctivo-dacryocystorhinostomy (Jones tube) or a common canalicular repair is required to correct this condition.

If a canaliculus is irrigated and the lacrimal sac distends without fluid passing into the nose, a complete nasolacrimal duct obstruction is present (Fig. 13–4C). This may be accompanied by reflux of fluid and/or pus back through one or both canaliculi. A dacryocystorhinostomy is required to correct this condition.

If a canaliculus is irrigated and fluid passes into the nasopharynx, a complete lacrimal obstruction is not present.

NASAL EXAMINATION

Before any consideration of surgery, the nose should be carefully examined with a nasal speculum and headlight (or indirect ophthalmoscope). Visualization may be facilitated by spraying the nose with cocaine, which provides vasoconstriction and anesthesia and should rule out the presence of a deviated septum, turbinate impaction, chronic rhinitis, sinusitis, nasal polyps, or carcinoma. Nasal septoplasty for a deviated septum, partial turbinectomy for a narrow inferior meatus, and polypectomy for polyps may reduce associated lacrimal symptoms in selected cases. Rhinitis and sinusitis contributions to tearing may be reduced by nasal decongestants.

DACRYOCYSTOGRAPHY

Dacryocystography is a safe and easy procedure usually using iophendylate (Pantopaque) as the contrast ma-

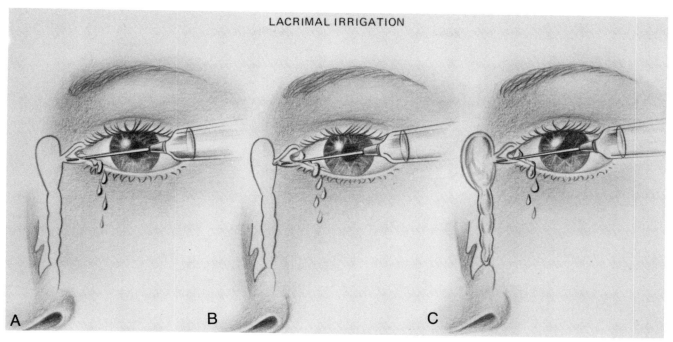

LACRIMAL IRRIGATION

FIG. 13–4. Lacrimal irrigation. A, If fluid refluxes through the canaliculus under irrigation without passing into the nose or dilating the lacrimal sac, a complete canalicular obstruction is present. B, If fluid refluxes through the other canaliculus without passing into the nose or dilating the lacrimal sac, a complete common canalicular obstruction is present. C, If the lacrimal sac distends without fluid passing into the nose, a complete nasolacrimal duct obstruction is present.

terial. The use of this iodinated compound is contraindicated in patients with allergic sensitivity to iodine. This procedure should also not be performed in the presence of active dacryocystitis.

In this study, the lower punctum is dilated and a lacrimal irrigation tip is used to irrigate the contrast material into the nose. In a normal lacrimal system, the material is evacuated from the lacrimal sac within 15 minutes (Fig. 13–5) and from the nasolacrimal duct within 15 to 30 minutes. Retention beyond 30 minutes suggests mechanical or functional blockage (Fig. 13–6). Spot films taken every few minutes yield precise anatomic information.

Although most cases do not require dacryocystography, in selected cases it may be useful in demonstrating localized stricture, partial obstruction, lacrimal diverticuli, fistulae, dacryoliths, and extrinsic or intrinsic tumors of the lacrimal drainage system.

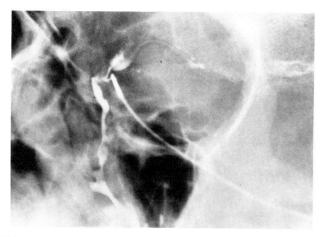

FIG. 13–5. A normal dacryocystogram demonstrating complete filling of the lacrimal drainage system and evacuation beginning within a few minutes following injection.

TREATMENT OF LACRIMAL OBSTRUCTION

Lacrimal production naturally diminishes over time, and the mere presence of an obstruction is not an indication for surgery. In cases involving partial or complete obstruction of the nasolacrimal system, surgical indications should be based on the extent of epiphora-related symptoms. The presence of intercurrent infection is an additional indication in some cases.

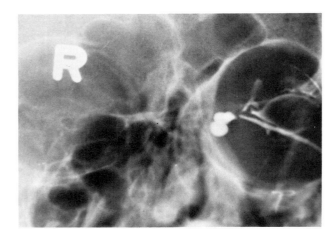

FIG. 13–6. Dacryocystogram revealing obstruction at the lower end of the lacrimal sac.

CONGENITAL ANOMALIES OF THE LACRIMAL DRAINAGE SYSTEM

CONGENITAL NASOLACRIMAL OBSTRUCTION

The most frequent congenital anomaly of the nasolacrimal system is dacryostenosis. It is common for neonates to present with nasolacrimal obstruction (5% of newborns). The nasolacrimal duct is the last portion of the lacrimal drainage system to develop and its nasal opening, the valve of Hasner, opens at approximately the time of birth. If this opening is delayed somewhat, an obstruction of the nasolacrimal duct will manifest. This condition is bilateral in one third of the cases. A small percentage of cases arises in newborns with extensive facial cleft anomalies. Such bony defects may pass through the nasolacrimal duct.

Symptoms and findings of congenital obstruction may include epiphora, purulent discharge, matting of the eye-lid margins, lacrimal sac enlargement, abscess, and/or dacryocutaneous fistula formation.

Lacrimal sac enlargement from dacryostenosis must be clearly distinguished from occasional cases of amniotocele or encephalocele. The latter presents as a bulge superior to the medial canthal tendon.

In most cases, the obstruction opens spontaneously during the first few months of life. Therefore, mild cases should be treated with topical antibiotics, nasolacrimal massage, and observation. Massage is performed by compressing the lacrimal sac from its apex (fundus) toward its junction with the nasolacrimal duct. If symptoms abate, no further treatment is required. If they persist, probing under general anesthesia may be performed at approximately 9 months of age, when the anesthetic risk is somewhat less. At this age, 90% of probings are successful. The presence of a purulent infection, abscess (Fig. 13–7), or fistula (Fig. 13–8), mandates earlier intervention. While office probing in a neonate may occasionally obviate the need for an anesthetic, it also increases the possibility of forming a false passage. Delayed probing after age 18 months has significantly less chance of success, and should therefore be combined with Quickert silicone intubation. After any probing failure, repeat probing should also be combined with silicone intubation.

Nasolacrimal Probing. Probing should conform to the anatomy of the lacrimal drainage system. On the involved side, both the upper and lower puncta are dilated with a punctal dilator (Fig. 13–9A). The upper canalicular system may be used for probing because its course facilitates the downward passage of the probe toward the inferior meatus. The lower canalicular system is used for irrigation because it more accurately represents the functional patency of the nasolacrimal system. If an obstruction of one canaliculus is encountered, the other must be used.

Lateral traction on the eyelid will straighten the can-

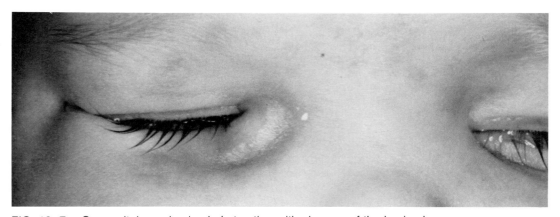

FIG. 13–7. Congenital nasolacrimal obstruction with abscess of the lacrimal sac.

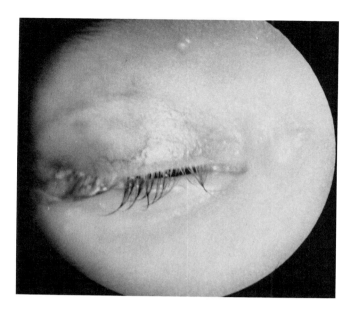

FIG. 13–8. Congenital nasolacrimal obstruction with dacryocutaneous fistula.

aliculus (Fig. 13–9B), aiding proper passage and minimizing the chance of false passage. A size 0 Bowman probe is passed vertically through the punctum and extended horizontally until bony resistance is felt. At this point, the probe is against the lateral wall of the nose, at the level of the lacrimal sac. The probe is next abruptly swung vertically in the direction of the first molar tooth (Fig. 13–9C). As the nasolacrimal duct is entered, grittiness is palpable and increased resistance is encountered. Steady and firm pressure with the probe usually opens the nasolacrimal duct obstruction at the valve of Hasner. If probe passage through the nasolacrimal duct is impeded by the inferior turbinate, the turbinate may be infractured toward the septum using the tip of a Freer elevator. A larger inferior meatus is thereby established.

To confirm patency, a second probe or hemostat is passed through the nares into the inferior meatus. A "metal upon metal" sensation confirms patency. The probe is then withdrawn. Confirmation of patency can also be determined by injecting a dilute fluorescein solution through the canaliculus using a lacrimal cannula. A small, clear-suction catheter tip is placed in the inferior meatus. As fluorescein is injected, it is observable within the suction tip if the system has been rendered patent.

Antibiotic drops are useful for the first week following probing. Although patency may now be established, epiphora and purulent reflux may persist for several days until the retained purulent material has been evacuated.

Failure to probe successfully may be the result of a false passage, aplasia of a portion of the nasolacrimal system, infection-induced scarring above the level of the valve of Hasner, or extrinsic obstruction of the valve of Hasner (nasal polyp, hypertrophic nasal mucosa, inferior turbinate).

Should symptoms persist despite successful probing, a repeat probing may be performed 1 to 2 months later. Should this also fail, the next probing should be performed placing Quickert silicone tubing at the same time to maintain the patency of the nasolacrimal duct and allow epithelialization. Obstruction from a contiguous inferior turbinate may be managed by infracturing this structure medially to provide more room.

Some children with congenital nasolacrimal obstruction may present for evaluation and treatment at an older age. The success of simple probing diminishes after 1 year of age. Therefore, children 18 months of age or older with congenital obstruction should be probed in conjunction with Quickert silicone intubation as a primary procedure.

Quickert Silicone Intubation. Quickert silicone intubation is useful in a multitude of surgical circumstances: failed or delayed nasolacrimal probing, punctal aplasia, punctal stenosis, focal canalicular stenosis canaliculitis, after removal of canalicular calculi, canalicular laceration, dacryocystorhinostomy, and obstruction of the internal common punctum.

This procedure can be performed either under local or general anesthesia. The latter may provide significantly more comfort to the patient. On the involved side, both puncta are expanded with punctal dilators. The Jackson version (Storz) of the Quickert intubation system is suitable, with its swaged-on, malleable, hollow probes connected by a length of silicone tubing. Each probe is sequentially passed through the nasolacrimal system and recovered in the inferior meatus (Fig. 13–10A). Lubricating the junction between tubing and probe lessens the chance of disconnection during passage. The method of passing the probes is identical to that of lacrimal probing as previously described. The probes may be externalized using either a grooved director or by simply grasping the leading edge of the probe with a hemostat and withdrawing (Fig. 13–10B). If the probe is impeded by the inferior turbinate, this structure may be infractured with a Freer elevator (Fig. 13–11).

Following their passage, the probes are cut free of the silicone tubing. The tubing should be tied with multiple square knots at the external nares (Fig. 13–10C). As the silicone is slippery and tends to untie, I make seven such knots. These knots may be further secured by crimping with several interrupted 4-0 silk sutures. The tubing is further anchored to the lateral wall of the nasal ala with an additional 4-0 silk suture. This facilitates later removal and inhibits tube migration toward the lacrimal sac. Re-

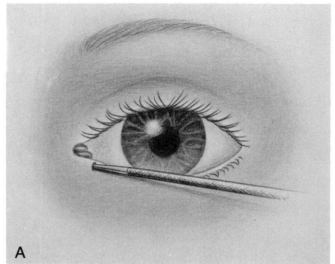

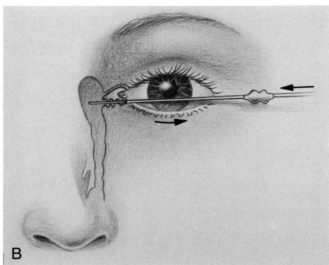

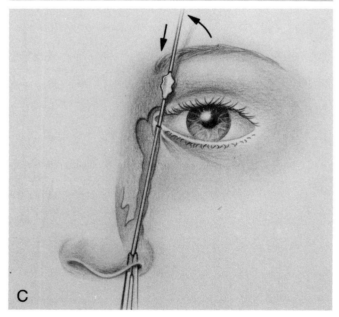

FIG. 13–9. Nasolacrimal probing. A, Puncta dilated with a punctal dilator. B, Probing with a Bowman probe. This is facilitated with lateral traction on the eyelid. C, The probe is rotated vertically in the direction of the first molar tooth. Firm pressure should open the obstructed nasolacrimal duct.

dundant tubing should be excised several millimeters beyond the knots. The loop of tubing at the inner canthus should be left flat and snug at the canthus, without undue tension on the puncta.

Quickert tubes rarely become infected. Should infection occur, however, the tube should be removed and replaced when infection subsides. If the tube is too tight, it may cheese-wire the puncta. If this occurs, the tube should be removed and replaced with one that is less taut.

The tube may occasionally loop toward the globe. In most cases, the tubing can be repositioned by pulling the nasal end downward or "walking" the canthal end toward each punctum with forceps. Should the knot pro-

lapse into the lacrimal sac, it may be repositioned by the technique described by Burns. He passes a second set of swaged-on tubing through either the lower or upper canalicular system. The second tubing must be looped around the first tubing. As the second set of probes is withdrawn from the nose, its tubing reposits the primary tubing at the ala. The secondary tubing is then cut and discarded. The primary tubing is again sutured to the lateral wall of the nasal ala.

Quickert silicone tubes may be left in place from several days to many months, depending on their purpose. They are removed by simply grasping and pulling the nasal end while cutting the inner canthal segment. The material should never be cut if it cannot be directly

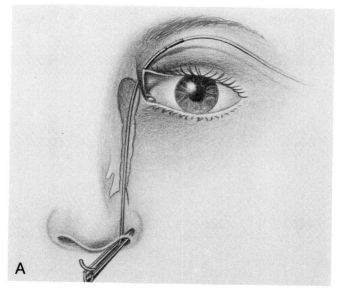

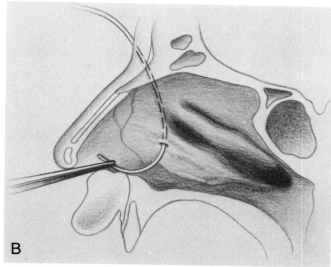

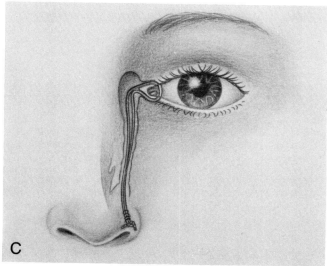

FIG. 13–10. Quickert silicone intubation. A, Each probe is sequentially passed through the nasolacrimal system. B, The probes are externalized by either using a grooved director or grasping them with a hemostat. C, After passage, the probes are discarded and the tubing is tied with multiple square knots and further secured with 4-0 silk sutures.

externalized through the nose. Otherwise, it could fall into the posterior pharynx and lodge in the respiratory passages.

Anomalies of the puncta and canaliculi may include complete aplasia, partial stenosis, and reduplication. Punctal stenosis is managed in the manner described for punctal/focal canalicular stenosis. Some cases of punctal reduplication are associated with canalicular reduplication, and in others the extra puncta lead to a blind passage. Reduplication requires no treatment.

PUNCTAL APLASIA

If only the upper punctum is absent, symptoms are usually minimal and no treatment is required. If the

lower punctum is absent and the child has significant epiphora, the condition should be surgically corrected. In most cases where the puncta and/or canaliculi are absent, the nasolacrimal sac is also absent. These cases require conjunctivorhinostomy (Jones tube) during adolescence. Yet, some cases of punctal aplasia may have the remainder of the lacrimal drainage system intact. The only way to ascertain the extent of aplasia is through surgical exploration.

Under general anesthesia, a vertical stab incision is made at the lacrimal papilla. In some cases, the incision may readily unite with a patent canalicular system. If it does, Quickert silicone tubing should be passed to maintain the patency of the punctum and encourage epithelialization. The tubing may be removed after 3 months.

If the stab incision does not communicate with the

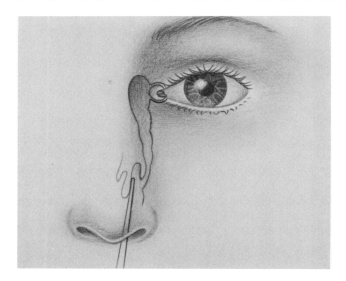

FIG. 13–11. The inferior turbinate may be infractured to provide more room at the meatus.

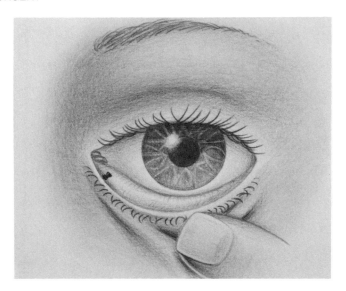

FIG. 13–12. Punctal expansion provided by a three-snip procedure.

canaliculus, the lacrimal sac should be opened with a dacryocystorhinostomy incision (see section on dacryocystorhinostomy, later in this chapter). A size 0 Bowman probe is passed in a retrograde manner through the canalicular and punctal areas. Over the probe, the punctum and canaliculus may be slit along the conjunctival surface of the eyelid margin. Quickert tubing should be passed to cannulate the system. The lacrimal sac is closed with interrupted 7-0 chromic catgut and the incision is closed in two layers. The tubing may be removed after 3 months. If this procedure fails, a later conjunctivorhinostomy (Jones tube) will be required.

ACQUIRED LACRIMAL OBSTRUCTION

PUNCTAL STENOSIS AND FOCAL CANALICULAR STENOSIS

The punctum and focal areas of the canaliculus may become stenotic from a variety of causes. These include topical medications: epinephrine, echothiophate iodide (phosphylene iodide), idoxuridine (IDU); infections: trachoma, vaccinia, herpes simplex, herpes zoster, varicella; inflammation: ocular pemphigoid, chronic cicatricial conjunctivitis, Stevens-Johnson syndrome, severe allergy; burns: thermal, chemical, radiation; systemic chemotherapy; and direct trauma. Early elimination of causal factors may obviate further dysfunction.

In symptomatic acquired punctal stenosis, the three-snip procedure is indicated (Fig. 13–12). Under local anesthesia, the punctum is dilated. One blade of Stevens

scissors is inserted into the vertical portion of the canaliculus to the level of the ampulla. The other blade of the scissors rests on the conjunctival surface. With the scissors tip directed slightly laterally, the first snip is made. A similar second snip is made with the scissors directed somewhat medially. The incisions are joined at their base with the third snip, thereby excising the inner wall of the vertical portion of the canaliculus (along with subjacent tarsus and conjunctiva). This creates a keystone-shaped canalicular opening. Judicious electrocautery applied to the walls of the incised vertical canaliculus helps to enlarge the opening and maintain the desired gap. Quickert tubing is placed for 6 weeks to ensure the enlarged opening remains patent.

In symptomatic acquired focal canalicular stenosis, Quickert silicone intubation may prove curative. If it fails, a conjunctivo-dacryocystorhinostomy (Jones tube) is required.

PUNCTAL ECTROPION

Punctal ectropion is managed surgically by either an infracanalicular tarsoconjunctival spindle excision or Byron Smith's lazy T procedure. The latter is simply a combination of infracanalicular tarsoconjunctival spindle excision with an adjacent horizontal eyelid shortening. Both procedures are described in Chapter 7. Cases of punctal ectropion secondary to medial canthal tendon laxity may be corrected by simply plicating the superficial head of the tendon.

DIMINISHED LACRIMAL PUMP

Significant diminution of the lacrimal pump occurs from facial nerve paralysis. A qualitative diminution of the pump may also occur in the absence of paralytic ectropion. In such cases, a flaccid eyelid does not maintain its normal tight continuity with the globe. Patients further demonstrate diminution of orbicularis oculi tone, which diminishes the function of the lacrimal pump. On examination, lower eyelids do not spring back as briskly as normal. Patients may be improved with horizontal eyelid shortening as in the Bick procedure, which reduces tear accumulation by increasing the arc of eyelid contact with the globe.

CANALICULITIS

Canaliculitis is a relatively uncommon inflammatory condition of the canaliculus. Its etiology is usually infectious (Actinomyces israelii), and may also variably be of bacterial, viral (Herpes simplex, Herpes zoster), or chlamydial (Trachoma) origin. Canalicular calculi may also be present.

Canaliculitis is manifested by epiphora, inflammation of the canaliculus and overlying tissue, discharge with pressure over the canaliculus, and papillary conjunctivitis. The punctum may at times be hypertrophic or stenotic. These infections usually respond slowly to topical (Erythromycin or Bacitracin) and systemic antibiotics combined with vigorous moist heat. A canaliculotomy with removal of intracanalicular debris and silicone intubation may be required in resistant cases.

CANALICULAR CALCULI

Calculi may form in the canaliculi from lacrimal stagnation with or without superimposed fungal infection. This is further predisposed by canalicular dilatation.

Canalicular calculi are removed by a canaliculotomy. A horizontal skin incision is carried through the orbicularis oculi muscle fibers to the canalicular mucosa. The mucosa is incised and the calculi are removed. A small curette may be passed to ensure that no other concretions persist. Quickert silicone tubing is passed and the canaliculus is closed with 9-0 nylon sutures under the operating microscope. These sutures should be tied external to the canalicular lumen to ensure patency. The overlying tissue is closed in two layers.

CANALICULAR LACERATION

In medial eyelid lacerations physicians should have a high index of suspicion for a coexistent canalicular laceration (Figs. 13–13 and 13–14). The canalicular structures are so fragile that a nearby laceration often extends into the canaliculus. Traumatic disruption of either a lower or an upper canaliculus requires microsurgical reconstruction. Although gravity makes the lower canaliculus the more important structure, the upper canaliculus is also significant in transporting tears through the lacrimal drainage system. Therefore, an upper canaliculus should never be willingly sacrificed.

Canalicular repair is based on (1) bridging the defect with an effective splint that can remain in place for six to twelve weeks and (2) suturing the torn canalicular ends with fine nylon sutures. The stent serves to maintain the contiguity of the sutured canalicular ends following surgery. This also encourages epithelial mucosa to bridge the defect.

Under general anesthesia, an operating microscope is used to identify the cut ends of the canaliculus. Injecting a fluorescein solution through the intact punctum while compressing the lacrimal sac may help to identify the cut proximal end of the canaliculus. Fluorescein will be seen extravasating.

At the outset of the procedure, a stent must be positioned to bridge the defect between the torn canalicular

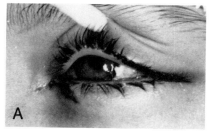
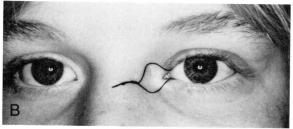

FIG. 13–13. Left lower canalicular laceration. A, Preoperative appearance. B, Postoperative appearance after cannulation with 4-0 silk suture and canalicular anastomosis with 9-0 nylon sutures.

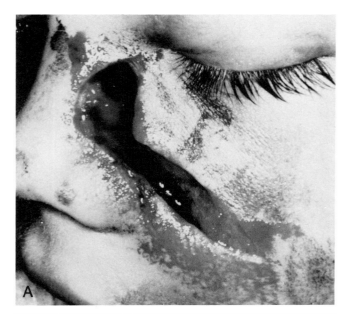

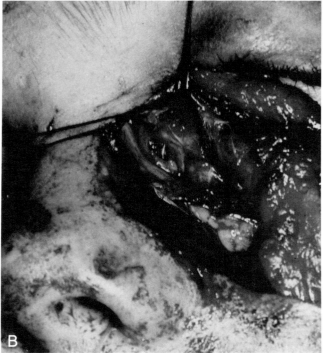

FIG. 13–14. Left lacrimal sac laceration. A, Superficial appearance. B, Enhanced exposure of depth of wound demonstrating a large laceration of the lacrimal sac.

ends. If both ends are identifiable, Quickert tubing with swaged-on probes is used as the stent (Fig. 13–15A). If only the tarsal (punctal) end of the canalicular laceration is identifiable, a *blunt* pigtail probe may be used to pass a 4-0 silk suture as the stent. In this technique, one end of the probe is used to cannulate the intact punctum and canaliculus, emerging through the cut proximal end of the severed canaliculus. The passage must conform to the normal anatomy of the canalicular system. Some pressure may be required to facilitate passage beyond the medial canthal tendon, while not forcing the instrument. This should prevent a false passage in the process. The operating microscope will confirm whether the probe emerges from the cut proximal end of the canaliculus or from a false passage. If the passage was correct, a 4-0 silk suture without attached needle is placed through the eyelet opening at the tip of the probe. Placement may be facilitated by stiffening the suture with bone wax. One end of this suture becomes properly positioned within the canalicular system as the probe is gently withdrawn.

The other end of the pigtail probe is used to cannulate the punctum adjacent to the severed canaliculus, emerging through the cut distal end. Once positioning is microscopically confirmed, the other end of the 4-0 silk suture (without needle) is placed through the eyelet opening of the probe. This portion of the suture becomes properly positioned as the probe is again gently withdrawn. Once the canaliculi are completely encircled with this suture, the suture is shortened and tied in a small loop at the inner canthus.

Irrespective of the cannulation method, the next step is suturing the severed canalicular ends using an operating microscope. If the laceration is gaping and under some tension, it may be necessary to place a 4-0 silk traction suture near the severed ends of the canaliculus. Tying this suture should diminish suture tension for the anastomosis, without interfering with visualization of the severed canalicular ends.

Three 9-0 nylon sutures are used to join corresponding edges of the severed canaliculus (Fig. 13–15B). Each suture should be positioned approximately 120 degrees apart around the canalicular circumference. Care must be taken to ensure that each suture passage is direct, without looping around the stent. The sutures should be placed to allow the knots to be tied outside the canalicular lumen. Once the canaliculus is joined, the wound is closed in two layers: interrupted 6-0 Vicryl for the subcutaneous layer and running 7-0 silk for the skin (Fig. 13–15C).

Either stent is allowed to remain for 6 to 12 weeks. If the canalicular anastomosis is optimal, 6 weeks is usually adequate, whereas 12 weeks may be necessary to facil-

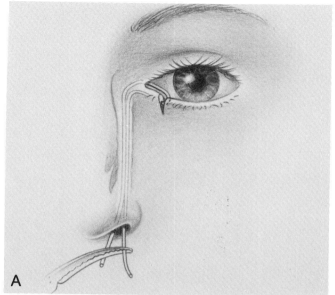

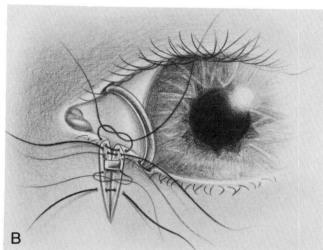

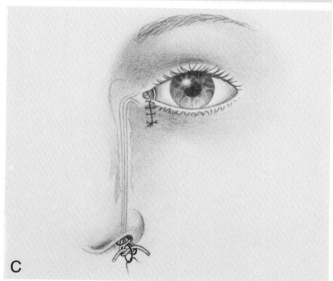

FIG. 13–15. Canalicular laceration repair. A, Before canalicular suture placement, it is imperative that the lacrimal system be cannulated. B, Three 9-0 nylon sutures join the severed canaliculus. C, The wound is closed in two layers.

itate epithelialization if the anastomosis is suboptimal. Quickert tubing is removed by grasping the tied end with forceps through the external nares at the same time as the inner canthal loop is cut with scissors. This material should never be cut if it cannot be directly externalized through the nose. If 4-0 silk was used as the stent material, it is removed by cutting the inner canthal loop and simply pulling the suture out.

If both canaliculi are lacerated, it may be difficult to identify the severed ends. In this case, a pigtail probe technique is of no use. Quickert intubation may be useful if all severed ends are identifiable. If not identifiable, the lacrimal sac may have to be opened to allow retrograde probing and identification of the canalicular com-

ponents. Once this is done, the reconstruction proceeds as previously described.

ACQUIRED NASOLACRIMAL DUCT OBSTRUCTION

Acquired nasolacrimal duct obstruction usually occurs at the lower portion of the lacrimal sac or at the junction of the nasolacrimal duct with the lacrimal sac. In cases of medial orbital fracture, the obstruction of the duct occurs within the bony canal.

Patients typically present with epiphora and a dilated lacrimal sac (Figs. 13–16 and 13–17) that will reflux

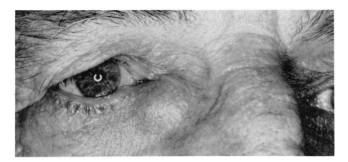

FIG. 13–16.   Right nasolacrimal duct obstruction with the body of the lacrimal sac dilated.

either clear or purulent material with digital pressure placed upon the sac. Obstructions may intermittently present with a purulent dacryocystitis, which may sometimes extend into an orbital cellulitis. Streptococcus, staphylococcus, and pneumococcus are frequently isolated. Such infections usually respond to management with systemic and topical antibiotics as dictated by culture and sensitivity studies, along with vigorous moist heat applied to the infected area. Antihistamines and nasal decongestants may also be beneficial in some cases. Although this treatment clears the acute infection, the underlying obstruction persists and should be surgically

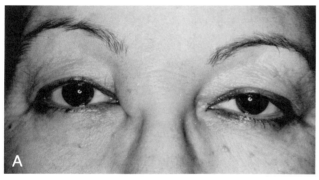

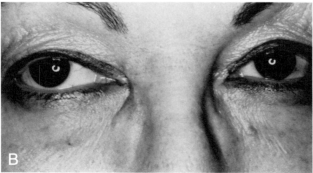

FIG. 13–17.   A, Preoperative appearance of a patient with right nasolacrimal duct obstruction with a dilated lacrimal sac fundus. B, Postoperative appearance.

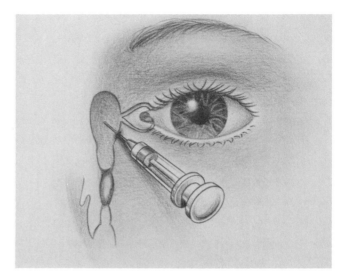

FIG. 13–18.   Percutaneous decompression of a lacrimal sac abscess may provide purulent material for culture and also afford clinical improvement.

corrected. Surgery may proceed once the infection has cleared. Further surgical delay may cause recurrent infections which may compromise subsequent surgery with excessive scar tissue.

Obstructions of the nasolacrimal duct or lower segment of the lacrimal sac must be corrected by a procedure that bypasses the blockage. This is achieved through a dacryocystorhinostomy designed to create a broad anastomosis between the nasal cavity and the lacrimal sac.

Ideally, a dacryocystorhinostomy should not be performed during an acute infection. Surgery with an active infection increases intraoperative bleeding and the likelihood of postoperative infection. Additionally, the mucous membrane flaps are much more friable and hold sutures with less reliability. If the obstruction-induced infection does not abate after proper medical management, however, the surgeon may have to proceed.

If an abscess of the lacrimal sac develops, antibiotics and heat are relatively ineffective. In such cases, an 18-gauge needle may be used for percutaneous decompression (Fig. 13–18). This needle aspirates some of the pus, which may then be sent for culture and sensitivity studies. The remainder of the pus may be milked out through the needle track with pressure from applicator sticks. The track also affords subsequent drainage, while not causing a fistula or the trauma that would follow a larger incision and drainage procedure.

Dacryocystitis rarely develops into cellulitis. If it does, hospitalization is required, with intensive intravenous and topical antibiotics and moist heat around the clock.

Dacryocystorhinostomy. This operation is used to create

an anastomosis (internal fistula) between the lacrimal sac and the nasal mucosa. A fiberoptic headlight greatly assists visualization during dacryocystorhinostomy. Under general anesthesia, the ipsilateral middle meatus of the nose is packed with 4% cocaine. Umbilical tape is suitable for this packing, which shrinks the mucosa at the meatus and affords hemostasis. The intended incision line is marked with methylene blue at the inner canthus (Fig. 13–19A). This line should extend for 15 to 20 mm in a curvilinear direction just medial to the medial orbital rim. The apex of the marks should extend approximately 3 mm above the level of the inner canthal angle. Subjacent to this mark, 2% lidocaine (Xylocaine) with epinephrine (1:200,000) is infiltrated to afford additional hemostasis. Either the cocaine or epinephrine, or both, may be deleted if contraindicated by hypertensive or cardiac-related factors.

According to the marked line, an incision is made with a #64 Beaver blade. Blunt dissection with Stevens scissors is used to extend the dissection through orbicularis oculi muscle (Fig. 13–19B) to periosteum anterior to the anterior lacrimal crest. Applicator sticks are useful in further exposing periosteum. The angular vessels can usually be retracted out of the field of dissection (Fig. 13–19C). Any appreciable bleeding, including that from the angular vessels, should be directly cauterized. Suction may be intermittently required to enhance visualization. Either a self-retaining lacrimal retractor or multiple 4-0 silk traction sutures are used to expose periosteum and the anterior lacrimal crest.

Periosteum is opened vertically with a #64 Beaver blade just anterior to the anterior lacrimal crest (Fig. 13–19D). A periosteal elevator is used to separate periosteum from bone posteriorly. The superficial head of the medial canthal tendon may be partially disinserted to facilitate the dissection. At the anterior lacrimal crest, the bone abruptly curves posteriorly. Here the elevator must gently remain in contact with the bone. This allows the lacrimal sac (with overlying periosteum) to be reflected laterally out of the lacrimal fossa without damaging the sac. Too much pressure on the bone may cause an unintentional fracture, damaging the important subjacent nasal mucosa.

Before the drill is used, the nasal pack should be removed so that the nasal mucosa will not be damaged by being sandwiched between pack and bone. The bony opening is made in a grinding manner, using fine burr tips on a Hall air drill (Fig. 13–19E). A periosteal elevator or retractor is used to protect the adjacent lacrimal sac and medial portion of the globe. The osteotomy should be centered at the anterior lacrimal crest, extending both anteriorly and posteriorly within the lacrimal fossa (Fig. 13–19F). This opening should not extend superiorly be-

yond the medial canthal tendon to avoid penetration of the cribriform plate and resultant cerebrospinal fluid leak. The ethmoidal air cells should also not be entered. As the bone is being thinned, visualization is facilitated by intermittent saline irrigation with a bulb syringe, along with intermittent suction. This also avoids thermal damage to surrounding tissues.

Once a small, full-thickness bony opening has been achieved, a muscle hook is passed through this hole to separate and protect the subjacent nasal mucosa. The bony opening is further enlarged with a Kerrison punch or Takahashi forceps (Fig. 13–19G). The final opening should approximate the size of a thumbnail (15 mm × 15 mm) (Fig. 13–19H). The larger the bony opening, the more nasal mucosa will be mobilized to contribute to the flaps.

The exposed nasal mucosa should be slit vertically through its entire length with a #12 Bard Parker blade. This creates an anterior and posterior mucosal flap. Relaxing "H" cuts may be made at the extremities of these flaps to facilitate mobilization. Bleeding at this point may be controlled with direct pressure, thrombin, or an epinephrine pack (unless medically contraindicated). Visualization may be improved by placing a second suction tip intranasally at the middle meatus. Care must be taken to ensure that suction does not injure the nearby nasal mucosa flaps. Then 6-0 Vicryl sutures on half-circle spatula lacrimal needles are carefully passed through the central edge of each flap for later use and to facilitate later identification.

A Bowman probe is then introduced into the canaliculus and lacrimal sac. The sac with its periosteal covering is identified as it is tented by the probe (Fig. 13–19I). With the probe as a guide, a corresponding vertical incision is made in the medial wall of the lacrimal sac with a #12 Bard Parker blade. This opening should extend from the fundus of the sac to the nasolacrimal duct and must penetrate both the mucosa and its periosteal covering. As an anterior and posterior flap of the lacrimal sac is thus being fashioned, it exposes the leading end of the Bowman probe. The probe is withdrawn and relaxing "H" cuts may be made in the extremities of these flaps. Any dacryoliths (composed of sloughed epithelium, lipid, and/or calcium) or purulent material should be removed from the lacrimal sac at this time.

The 6-0 Vicryl suture secured to the posterior flap of nasal mucosa is passed through the central edge of the posterior lacrimal sac flap, tied, and cut. Several additional 6-0 Vicryl sutures are additionally positioned to further secure and widen the posterior flap anastomosis (Fig. 13–19J).

Quickert tubing with two swaged-on probes is then placed (Fig. 13–19K). Its initial pass positions the probes

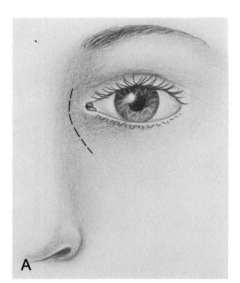

FIG. 13–19. Dacryocystorhinostomy. A, The incision line is marked with methylene blue. B, After incision, the dissection is carried through the orbicularis oculi muscle, C, down to periosteum anterior to the anterior lacrimal crest. D, Periosteum is opened vertically. E, The initial bone opening is made with a drill using a small burr tip. A periosteal elevator or retractor should be placed to protect the adjacent lacrimal sac and medial portion of the globe.

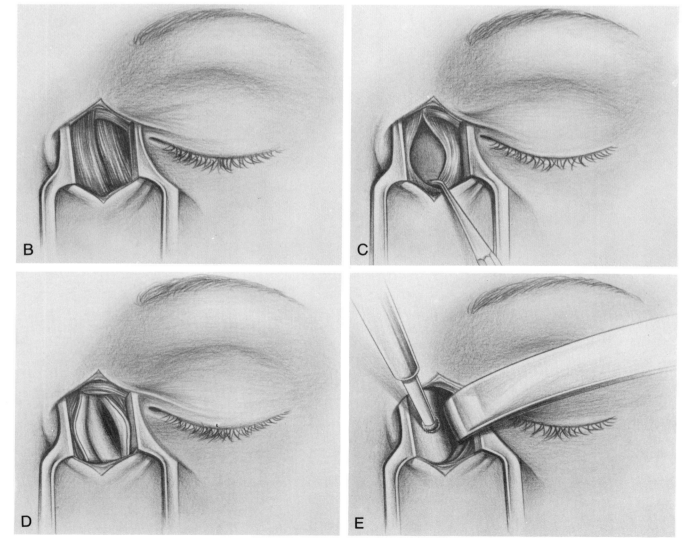

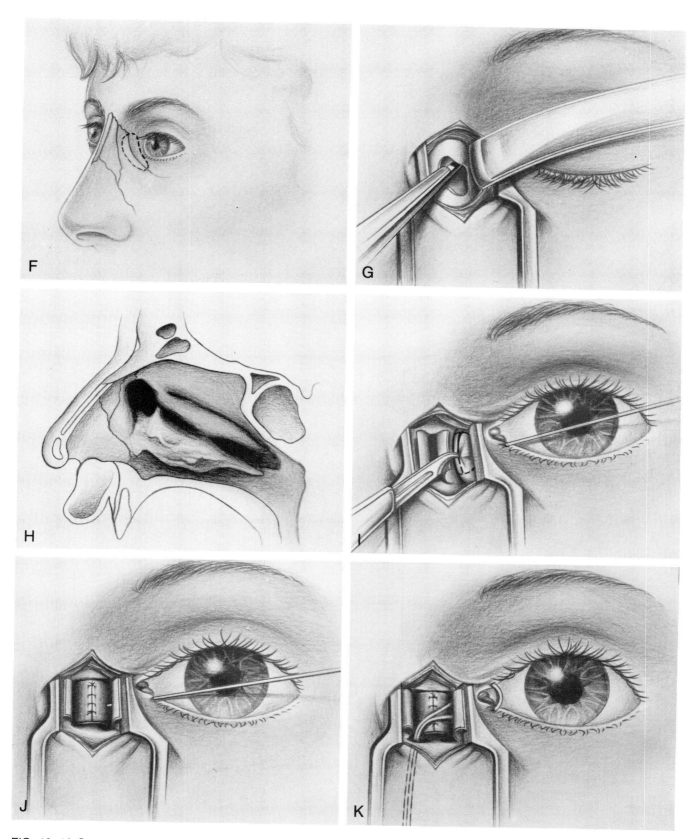

FIG. 13–19 Cont.   F, The osteotomy is centered at the anterior lacrimal crest, extending both anteriorly and posteriorly within the lacrimal fossa. G, The bony opening may be enlarged with Kerrison punch or Takahashi forceps. H, Bony opening at the middle meatus as seen from an intranasal perspective. I, The lacrimal sac with its periosteal covering is identified with a Bowman probe and its medial wall is incised with a #12 Bard Parker blade. J, Multiple 6-0 Vicryl sutures are used to join the posterior nasal mucosa and lacrimal sac flaps. K, Quickert tubing is passed anterior to the united posterior flap.

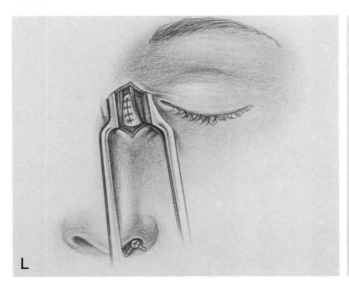

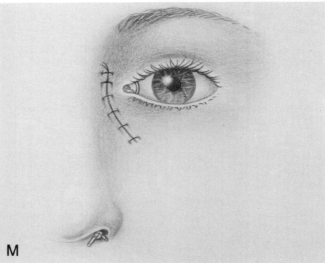

FIG. 13–19 Cont.   L, Multiple 6-0 Vicryl sutures are used to join the anterior nasal mucosa and lacrimal sac flaps. M, The wound is closed in two layers and the Quickert tubing is secured in the usual manner.

anterior to the conjoined posterior flaps. A hemostat is then passed up through the nose until it appears above the posterior flaps. The Quickert probes are sequentially fed into the hemostat and pulled out through the external nares. The probes are removed and the Quickert tubing is tied at the nares, secured with a 4-0 silk suture, and anchored to the nasal ala. This silicone tubing keeps the anterior and posterior flaps separate, and also discourages cicatricial closure of the bony osteum.

The 6-0 Vicryl suture attached to the anterior flap of nasal mucosa is passed through the central edge of anterior lacrimal sac flap, tied, and cut. Several additional 6-0 Vicryl sutures are additionally positioned to further secure and widen the anterior flap anastomosis (Fig. 13–19L).

The retractor or traction sutures are removed and the wound is closed in two layers. The subcutaneous layer is secured with 5-0 Vicryl mattress sutures, and the skin is closed with running 7-0 silk sutures (Fig. 13–19M). Antibiotic ointment is applied to the suture line and a folded gauze 2 × 2 is placed over the inner canthus. A small "moustache" dressing may be applied to absorb any subsequent epistaxis.

When the "moustache" dressing is removed on the first postoperative day, attention must be focused on not disrupting the tied end of Quickert tubing. Skin sutures are removed in six days. The tubing is removed six weeks postoperatively as previously described.

Postoperative irrigation of the nasolacrimal system is required only if symptoms persist or recur. Probing is contraindicated after surgery because it may injure the flaps.

Failure of dacryocystorhinostomy to relieve symptoms may result from an improper choice of procedure or operative failure. Such failure is attributable to a variety of causes. Inadequate union of the mucosal flaps or subsequent closure of the bony window may be corrected with Quickert silicone intubation. Should this not be possible, or prove inadequate, a repeat dacryocystorhinostomy involving revision of the flaps or enlargement of the bony osteum is required. Excessive scar tissue and bone overgrowth impinging upon the anastomosis should also be removed. Obstruction from the middle turbinate may compromise the result in some cases. This may be managed by surgically infracturing the turbinate, affording more room at the osteum (see Fig. 13–11). Excessive hemorrhage is readily managed intraoperatively and is rarely a postoperative problem. The extensive vascular supply to the lacrimal fossa area renders infection uncommon despite the flora normally found in the nose.

A set of Jones tubes should always be available during revisions. This allows a surgical alternative (conjunctivo-dacryocystorhinostomy) if an adequate revision proves impossible.

OBSTRUCTION OF THE COMMON CANALICULUS OR THE INTERNAL COMMON PUNCTUM

An obstruction of the common canaliculus or the internal common punctum must be surgically corrected through a dacryocystorhinostomy incision. After the lacrimal probe is positioned in the canaliculus. The pouting tip of the probe is noted in the area of the obstructed common punctum. This overlying tissue may be excised with sharp Stevens scissors or a Beyer trephine 5 mm in diameter (Fig. 13–20). If the lacrimal sac is not obstructed, a bony opening is not required as dacryocystorhinostomy flaps are not necessary. The lacrimal system is simply intubated with Quickert tubing to keep the common canaliculus or the internal common punctum open postoperatively. The lacrimal sac is closed with 6-0 Vicryl and the wound is closed in two layers. The tubing may be removed in 6 to 12 weeks. If either the lacrimal sac or nasolacrimal duct is obstructed, the operation proceeds as in dacryocystorhinostomy with Quickert intubation.

ACQUIRED CANALICULAR OR LACRIMAL SAC OBSTRUCTION

A conjunctivo-dacryocystorhinostomy may be performed in a symptomatic patient with obstruction of the canaliculi or a significant portion of the lacrimal sac. This is also indicated in dacryocystorhinostomy failure that is not amenable to surgical revision. The Jones tube is used to facilitate conjunctivo-dacryocystorhinostomy.

Conjunctivo-dacryocystorhinostomy. The goal of this procedure is to establish a channel for tear flow directly between the lacrimal lacus and the middle meatus of the nose. This procedure is identical to that of a dacryocystorhinostomy, with the addition of several steps involving insertion of a Jones pyrex glass tube (Fig. 13–21). Pyrex is an ideal choice of material because it provides capillary attraction, does not easily occlude, and is minimally irritating to surrounding tissue.

Excellent Jones tube sets are available from either William Cox (The Cox System, Eye Foundation Hospital, Birmingham, Alabama) (see Fig. 13–22) or Gunther Weiss (Portland, Oregon). These sets contain multiple tubes ranging in length from 11 mm to 30 mm, in 1 mm increments, along with insertion probes and sleeves. Each tube has an upper collar 3 to 4 mm in diameter and a slight lower flare. Relatively complete sets should be available and sterilized for each case to afford a choice of tube length for any given case and clinical situation.

Once the posterior flaps have been completely joined, an eyelid speculum is placed. The caruncle is excised to provide an area in which to position the tube collar in the lacrimal lacus. This also prevents later obstruction of the tube osteum. The sharp trochar inserter provided with these sets is used to create the canal in which the tube will be positioned (Fig. 13–21G). This instrument is inserted into the lacrimal lacus 2 to 3 mm posterior to the cutaneous margin of the medial canthal angle. The trochar tip is advanced toward the dacryocystorhinostomy opening and should emerge just anterior to the posterior flaps. This positioning must be precise. From the nasal perspective, it is anterior to the body of the middle turbinate in the area of the middle meatus. A portion of the turbinate may occasionally need to be resected if it interferes with the path of the needle. The trochar is removed and sharp Stevens scissors are placed in its path (Fig. 13–21H). Opening the scissors gently expands the path somewhat. The path should allow room for Jones tube insertion, without being excessively large so that the tube displaces nasally.

The scissors are removed and the guide rod provided with the Jones tube set is placed in the channel, extending from the inner canthus to the middle meatus. A Jones tube is placed over the guide rod (Fig. 13–21I). An ideal size to start with is a 17 mm tube. The Teflon sleeve "pusher" is placed over the tube and used to push

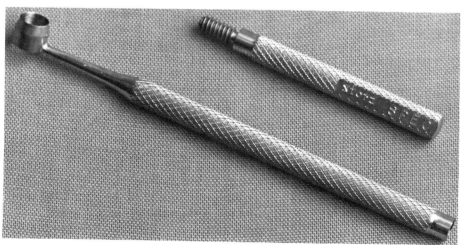

FIG. 13–20. The 5 mm Beyer lacrimal trephine.

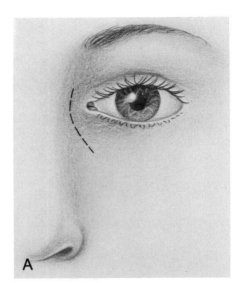

FIG. 13–21. Conjunctivo-dacryocystorhinostomy. A, The incision line is marked with methylene blue. B, Following incision, the dissection is carried through the orbicularis oculi muscle, C, down to periosteum anterior to the anterior lacrimal crest. D, Periosteum is opened vertically. E, The initial bone opening is made with a drill using a small burr tip. A periosteal elevator or retractor should be placed to protect the adjacent lacrimal sac and medial portion of the globe.

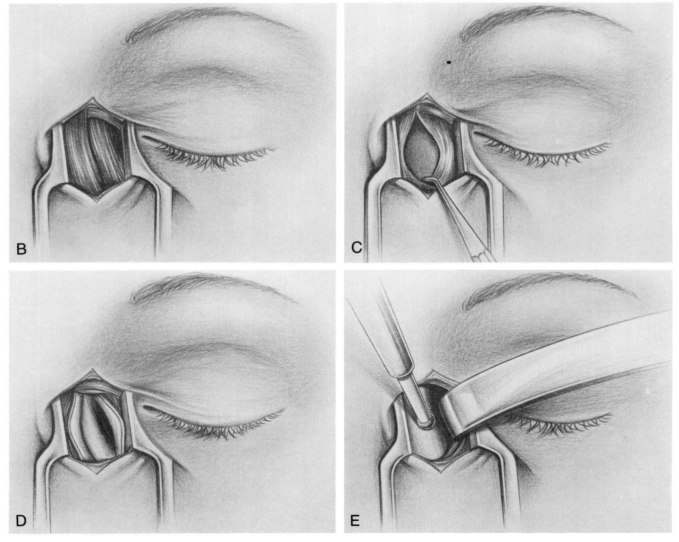

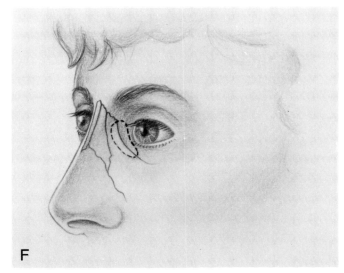

F

FIG. 13–21 Cont.   F, The bony opening may be enlarged with Kerrison punch or Takahashi forceps. G, Posterior flaps are isolated and united as in dacryocystorhinostomy. The caruncle is excised. A lacrimal trochar is inserted into the lacrimal lacus 2 to 3 mm posterior to the cutaneous margin of the medial canthus, emerging anterior to these flaps. H, Sharp Stevens scissors replace the trochar and are used to expand the path for subsequent Jones tube passage. I, A guide rod is substituted for the Stevens scissors. An appropriately sized Jones tube is placed over the guide rod and gently pushed into proper position. J, Jones pyrex tube in place.

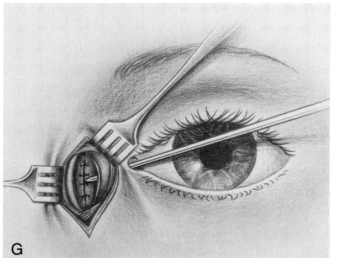

G

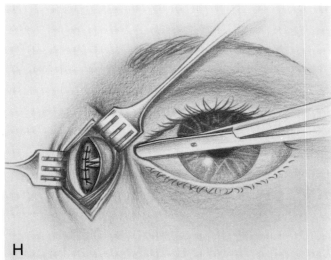

H

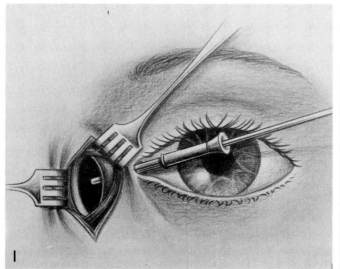

I

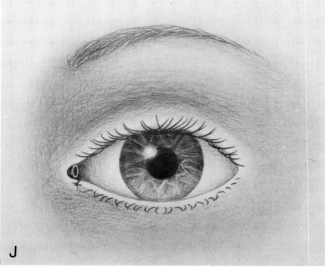

J

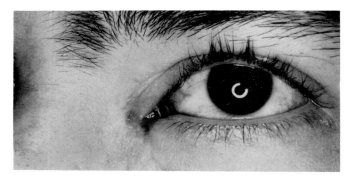

FIG. 13–22.   A properly positioned Jones tube.

the Jones tube in position. Mild to firm pressure may be required. When properly positioned, the tube should have its lip contiguous with the tissue just posterior to the cutaneous margin of the inner canthal commissure (Fig. 13–21J). Its nasal end should extend sufficiently into the middle meatus without abutting upon the nasal septum. If the tube is impeded by the middle turbinate, the turbinate should be removed with a Kerrison punch.

Proper positioning of the Jones tube is essential (Fig. 13–22). If it is too horizontal, tears will not drain properly. Once the tube appears to be of proper length and position, the guide rod is removed. The tube should be irrigated to confirm that it has been functionally placed. This is done by placing a suction tip near the tube's nasal end within the meatus. Balanced salt solution is irrigated into the lacrimal lacus. If the irrigant is copiously suctioned through the tube, tube placement should be correct. If the tube is of incorrect length, it should be replaced by one of a different length. This is performed by reinserting the guide rod through the positioned tube, removing the tube while retaining the rod in the surgically created channel. A tube of different size is then placed as described. Tubes may need to be interchanged several times to ensure proper length and function.

Once the tube is correct and correctly positioned, the guide rod is removed and anterior flaps are sutured over the tube. The incision is closed as for a dacryocystorhinostomy. Sterile antibiotic ointment is placed on the suture line daily.

Postoperatively, the Jones tube must be irrigated on several occasions to ensure its function. If function is suboptimal, the middle meatus should be directly visualized to ensure that the tube is long enough to extend into the middle meatus, but not so long that it touches the nasal septum. The skin sutures are removed on the the sixth postoperative day.

Patients should be instructed to avoid blowing the nose or sneezing too vigorously after surgery. If they do, they must place a fingertip at the medial canthal angle to

further stabilize the tube. Postoperative swelling and cicatrization may require a tube of different length from that required at surgery. The surgeon should be prepared to change tubes in the office, using the guide rod and sleeve as previously described.

Jones tubes may become intermittently obstructed by mucus or debris. Patients can open the lumen by blowing a small jet of air through the tube while compressing the inner canthal angle.

Postoperatively, the tube may become partially or completely lined by epithelium after several years. This occurrence should not be relied upon, however, and the tube should not be removed unless required due to infection or excessive irritation.

Conjunctival hyperplasia or granuloma formation may occasionally partially or completely cover the opening of the tube. This tissue must be surgically excised. Conjunctival tissue may then be carefully united around the tube just below the collar.

If the tube becomes partially displaced toward the globe, it can be repositioned in the office using the positioning probe and sleeve. Lateral extension may also result from a fibroblastic response at the bony opening, which may force the tube laterally. This extension is corrected by surgically removing the fibroblastic tissue within the nose and enlarging the nasal osteum.

If the tube extrudes completely, it should be reinserted with the probe and sleeve as soon as possible, before the epithelial channel closes.

Conjunctivo-dacryocystorhinostomy surgery requires prolonged follow-up and, in some cases, frequent manipulation of the tube. Such surgery in a child is usually best deferred until an adequate level of cooperation is achievable.

LACRIMAL FISTULA

Lacrimal fistulas may follow nasolacrimal obstruction proximal (medial) to the lacrimal sac. They are simply epithelial extensions of the lacrimal sac. Fistulas may be excised at the same time as the underlying obstruction is surgically corrected. Unless the etiology is treated, excision of fistula alone will lead to recurrent fistulization or dacryocystitis.

TUMORS OF THE LACRIMAL DRAINAGE SYSTEM

Tumors of the nasolacrimal system are uncommon. They may range from benign processes (squamous papilloma, dermoid, hemangioma, cyst), through more aggressive infiltrates (lymphoma, amyloid), to life-threatening malignancies (papillary squamous cell carcinoma, (Fig. 13–23), epidermoid carcinoma).

Benign tumors and infiltrates are managed by simple tumor exision and dacryocystorhinostomy. Malignancies are aggressive and may be multicentric. They require wide local excision, with removal of subjacent bone in indicated cases. If this proves curative, a later conjunctivorhinostomy (Jones tube) will re-establish lacrimal function.

Dacryocystectomy. The primary indication for dacryocystectomy is a lacrimal sac tumor. It may also be useful for some elderly patients with dacryocystitis for whom the longer and more invasive dacryocystorhinostomy is medically contraindicated. The goal of dacryocystectomy is to excise the entire lacrimal sac, along with the adjacent portions of nasolacrimal duct and canaliculi.

Dacryocystectomy is performed under local anesthesia. The incision site is marked as for a dacryocystorhinostomy. Subjacent to the marking, local anesthetic is infiltrated. The dissection is similar to that in a dacryocystorhinostomy, and is carried to the lacrimal fossa, where the lacrimal sac is fully exposed. A small Babcock clamp is used to grasp the sac within its periosteal lining. The sac is completely excised, along with adjacent portions of nasolacrimal duct and canaliculi (Fig. 13–24). The wound is then closed in two layers as in dacryocystorhinostomy.

TREATMENT OF DRY EYE SYNDROME

Congenital absence of the lacrimal gland (congenital alacrima) is rare. A quantitative diminution may result from age-induced fibrocytic changes within the reflex secretors. A dry eye may also be a component of familial dysautonomia (Riley-Day syndrome), Sjögren's syndrome, Mikulicz's disease, ocular pemphigoid, Stevens-Johnson syndrome, xerophthalmia, and certain collagen-vascular diseases (rheumatoid arthritis, giant cell arteritis, systemic lupus erythematosis, scleroderma, and polyarteritis nodosa). Oral decongestants and topical cycloplegic agents (atropine, scopolamine) may also significantly reduce tear production.

Some patients with dry eye syndrome may paradoxically present with subjective symptoms of epiphora. This is the result of a dry cornea stimulating reflex tearing (often an abortive attempt at reflex tearing).

Any underlying medical etiology should be adequately treated and predisposing medications discontinued, if possible. Maximum medical treatment for dry eye conditions and keratitis sicca include Liquifilm Forte every one to two hours during the daytime, along with Lacri-Lube ointment at bedtime. Desiccation may be further minimized by placing a moisture chamber over the involved globe. A room humidifier adds moisture to the air and lessens the opportunity for further nocturnal drying.

Some cases may also benefit from punctal occlusion. Before permanent surgical occlusion is performed, temporary occlusion may be placed to determine the effectiveness of this approach. This procedure is performed either with a punctal plug, placement of a temporary occlusive punctal suture, or limited diathermy. These methods are completely reversible.

If permanent occlusion proves efficacious, it may be performed by excision of the punctum and distal canal-

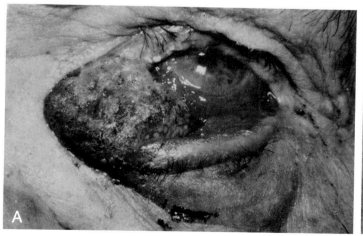
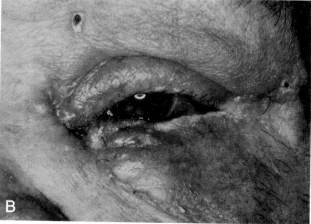

FIG. 13–23.   A, Papillary squamous cell carcinoma of the canaliculus and lacrimal sac. B, Appearance following wide local excision (including subjacent bony walls) and reconstruction. Published with permission from Kohn, R., Nosfinger, K., and Freedman, S.: Rapid recurrence of papillary squamous cell carcinoma of the canaliculus. Am. J. Ophthalmol. 92:363–367, 1981.

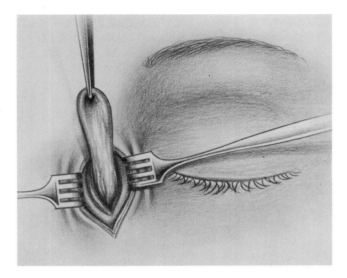

FIG. 13–24. Dacryocystectomy with the lacrimal sac exposed through a dacryocystorhinostomy incision. The sac may be grasped with a small Babcock clamp and excised with Stevens scissors using blunt and sharp dissection.

iculus, closing tissue with 6-0 silk. More vigorous diathermy may also affect a permanent closure.

DACRYOADENITIS

Dacryoadenitis represents an inflammatory or infiltrative enlargement of the lacrimal gland. If associated with swelling of the salivary gland, it may be part of Mikulicz's disease. Dacryoadenitis presents as unilateral rapid enlargement of the lacrimal gland (particularly the palpebral lobe) with associated erythema, pain, tenderness, and swelling. The subjacent conjunctiva may be chemotic and preauricular lymphadenopathy may coexist. Proptosis may be present in some cases of infiltrative origin.

Inflammatory causes include sarcoidosis, pseudotumor, and Sjögren's syndrome. Infiltrative causes include lymphoma, benign lymphoid hyperplasia, leukemia, multiple myeloma, and macroglobulinemia. Infectious causes may be bacterial (staphylococcus, streptococcus, gonococcus, syphilis, tuberculosis, leprosy), viral (mumps, measles, mononucleosis, herpes zoster, herpes simplex, influenza), fungal, parasitic, and chlamydial (trachoma).

Differentiation between dacryoadenitis and neoplasm may necessitate hematologic studies, CT scanning, ultrasound, and/or diagnostic biopsy.

Management is directed toward the underlying cause: antibiotics for infection, oral steroids for pseudotumor and sarcoidosis, radiation therapy for lymphoma and be-

nign lymphoid hyperplasia, and surgical excision and/or chemotherapy for malignancy.

BIBLIOGRAPHY

Anderson, R., and Edwards, J.: Indications, complications and results with silicone stents. Ophthalmology 86:1474–1487, 1979.

Baylis, H., and Axelrod, R.: Repair of the lacerated canaliculus. Ophthalmology 84:1271, 1978.

Berlin, A., Roth, B., and Rich, L.: Lacrimal system dacryoliths. Ophthalmology 11:435–436, 1980.

Beyer, C.: A modified lacrimal probe. Arch. Ophthalmol. 92:157, 1974.

Callahan, M., and Callahan, A.: Ophthalmic Plastic and Orbital Surgery. Birmingham, Aesculapius, 1979.

Cox, C.: A technique for conjunctivo-dacryocystorhinostomy. Am. J. Ophthalmol. 72:931, 1971.

Crawford, J.: Intubation of obstructions in the lacrimal system. Can. J. Ophthalmol. 12:289, 1977.

Demant, E., and Hurwitz, J.: Canaliculitis: a review of 12 cases. Can. J. Ophthalmol. 15:73, 1980.

Doane, M.: Interaction of eyelids and tears in corneal wetting and the normal human eyeblink. Am. J. Ophthalmol. 89:507–516, 1980.

Doane, M.: Blinking and the mechanics of the lacrimal drainage system. Ophthalmology 88:844–851, 1981.

Dortzbach, R., France, T., Kushner, B., and Gonnering R.: Silicone intubation for obstruction of the nasolacrimal duct in children. Am. J. Ophthalmol. 94:585–590, 1982.

Doucet, T., and Hurwitz, J.: Canaliculodacryocystorhinostomy in the management of unsuccessful lacrimal surgery. Arch. Ophthalmol. 100:619–621, 1982.

Doucet, T., and Hurwitz, J.: Canaliculodacryocystorhinostomy in the treatment of canalicular obstruction. Arch. Ophthalmol. 100:306–309, 1982.

Durso, F., Hand, S., Ellis, F., and Helveston, E.: Silicone intubation in children with nasolacrimal obstruction. J. Pediatr. Ophthalmol. Strabismus 17:389–393, 1980.

Farris, R., Stuchell, R., and Mandel, I.: Basal and reflex human tear analysis I and II. Ophthalmology 88:852–862, 1981.

Flanagan, J., and Stokes, D.: Lacrimal Sac Tumors. Trans. Am. Acad. Ophthalmol. Otolaryngol. 85:1282–1287, 1978.

Goldberg, A., and Hurwitz, J.: Congenital abnormalities of lacrimal drainage: management of difficult cases. Can. J. Ophthalmol. Otolaryngol. 14:106–109, 1979.

Hurwitz, J.: Treatment of canalicular obstructions. Can. J. Ophthalmol. 17:13, 1982.

Hurwitz, J.: The slit canaliculus. Ophthalmic Surg. 13:572, 1982.

Iliff, C.: A simplified dacryocystorhinostomy. Arch. Ophthalmol. 85:856, 1971.

Jackson, S.: A new probe for silicone intubation of the lacrimal drainage system. Ophthalmic Surg. 588–590, 1980.

Jones, L.: Epiphora. II. Its relation to the anatomic structures and surgery of the medial canthal region. Am. J. Ophthalmol. 43:203–212, 1957.

Jones, L.: An anatomical approach to problems of the eyelids and lacrimal apparatus. Arch. Ophthalmol. 66:111–124, 1961.

Jones, L.: The cure of epiphora due to canalicular disorders, trauma, and surgical failures on the lacrimal passages. Trans. Am. Acad. Ophthalmol. Otolaryngol. 66:506, 1962.

Jones, L: Conjunctivodacryocystorhinostomy. Am. J. Ophthalmol. 59:733, 1965.

Jones, L.: The lacrimal secretory system and its treatment. Am. J. Ophthalmol. 62:47, 1966.

Jones, L., and Linn, M.: The diagnosis of the causes of epiphora. Am. J. Ophthalmol. 67:751, 1969.

Jones, L: Anatomy of the tear system. Int. Ophthalmol. Clin. 13:3–22, 1973.

Jones, L., Marquis, M., and Vincent, N.: Lacrimal function. Am. J. Ophthalmol. 73:658–659, 1975.

Jones, L., and Wobig, J.: Surgery of the Eyelids and Lacrimal System. Birmingham, Aesculapius, 1976.

Jones, L., and Wobig, J.: Newer concepts of tear duct and eyelid anatomy and treatment. Trans. Am. Acad. Ophthalmol. Otolaryngol. 83:603–616, 1977.

Katowitz, J.: Silicone tubing in canalicular obstruction. Arch. Ophthalmol. 91:456–462, 1974.

Kohn, R., Ramano, P., and Puklin, J.: Lacrimal obstruction after migration of orbital implant. Am. J. Ophthalmol. 82:934–936, 1976.

Kohn, R., Nofsinger, K., and Freedman, S.: Rapid recurrence of papillary squamous cell carcinoma of the canaliculus. Am. J. Ophthalmol. 92:363–367, 1981.

Kraft, S., and Crawford, J.: Silicone tube intubation in disorders of the lacrimal system in children. Am. J. Ophthalmol. 94:290–299, 1982.

Kushner, B.: Congenital nasolacrimal system obstruction. Arch. Ophthalmol. 100:597–600, 1982.

Linberg, J., Anderson, R., and Bumsted, R., and Barreras, R.: Study of intranasal osteum external dacryocystorhinostomy. Arch. Ophthalmol. 100:1758–1762, 1982.

Older, J.: Routine use of a silicone stent in dacryocystorhinostomy. Ophthalmic Surg. 13:911–915, 1982.

Pashby, R., and Rathbun, J.: Silicone tube intubation of the lacrimal drainage system. Arch. Ophthalmol. 97:1318–1322, 1979.

Putterman, A.: Reconstruction of absent lacrimal puncta. Ophthalmolic Surg. 10:20–24, 1979.

Quickert, M., and Dryden, R.: Probes for intubation in lacrimal drainage. Trans. Am. Acad. Ophthalmol. Otolaryngol. 74:431–433, 1970.

Reeh, M., Beyer, C., and Shannon, G.: Practical Ophthalmic Plastic and Reconstructive Surgery. Philadelphia, Lea and Febiger, 1976.

Ryan, S., and Font, F.: Primary epithelial neoplasms of the lacrimal sac. Am. J. Ophthalmol. 76:73–88, 1973.

Saunders, D., Shannon, G., and Flanagan, J.: The effectiveness of the pigtail probe method of repairing canalicular lacerations. Ophthalmic Surg. 9:33, 1978.

Sevel, D.: Development of congenital abnormalaities of the nasolacrimal apparatus. J. Pediatr. Ophthalmol. Strabismus 18:13–19, 1981.

Tenzel, R.: Canaliculodacryocystorhinostomy. Arch. Ophthalmol. 84:765, 1970.

Walter, W.: The use of the pigtail probe for silicone intubation of the injured canaliculus. Ophthalmic. Surg. 13:488–492, 1982.

Weinberg, R., Sartoris, M., Buerger, G., and Novak, J.: Fusobacterium in presumed actinomyces canaliculitis. Am. J. Ophthalmol. 84:371–374, 1977.

Worst, J.: Method for reconstructing torn lacrimal canaliculus. Am. J. Ophthalmol. 53:520, 1962.

14

ESSENTIAL BLEPHAROSPASM

Essential blepharospasm is a relatively uncommon condition in which the eyelids close due to involuntary contractions of the orbicularis oculi muscle. It is a bilateral focal dystonia that begins with intermittent mild involuntary eyelid twitches. It may progress unremittingly toward constant forceful orbicularis oculi muscle contracture and functional blindness. Affected patients may, therefore, demonstrate a wide range of manifestations: mild to severe, intermittent or constant.

The contraction may involve other muscles innervated by the seventh nerve (Meige syndrome), including the lower face, mouth, lips, jaw, neck, or soft palate. Benign essential blepharospasm may, in fact, represent an atypical form of Meige syndrome. Brow ptosis, dermatochalasis, levator aponeurosis and lateral canthus defects may result. Blepharospasm affects both sexes, but is more frequent in females. Onset may range from the fourth to eighth decade, peaking in the fifth and sixth decades. No etiology has yet been defined, although a dysfunction of the basal ganglia is suspected.

Patients with essential blepharospasm are most troubled with spasm-induced vision loss, particularly associated with driving, reading, or social interaction. If the symptoms are intermittent clinical corroboration may be difficult or delayed. The spasm is not present during sleep (or under general anesthesia).

Diagnosis of blepharospasm is based on a compatible history, directly observing the spasm, and excluding irritative causes that may secondarily induce blepharospasm (entropion, trichiasis, distichiasis, blepharitis, corneal erosion, keratitis, conjunctivitis, keratoconjunctivitis sicca, foreign body, iritis, medications, and posterior fossa tumors). It is essential to note the severity, symmetry, and location of the periorbital muscles that are involuntarily contracting, along with contributions from other facial muscles, particularly the orbicularis oris.

Essential blepharospasm should be distinguished from hemifacial spasm. The latter is a unilateral seventh-nerve dysfunction manifested by intermittent involuntary unsynchronous contraction of facial muscles to a milder degree than blepharospasm and involving only one side of the face. It may persist during sleep. Although usually idiopathic, hemifacial spasm may result from compression of the facial nerve in the cerebellopontine angle by either a blood vessel loop or tumor (acoustic neuroma, meningioma, cholesteatoma). Neurosurgical decompression of this nerve resolves hemifacial spasm in 80% of cases when compression is the cause.

Preoperatively, it is imperative to rule out any extrinsic irritative cause of blepharospasm as previously noted.

ANATOMY OF THE SEVENTH NERVE

To effectively manage blepharospasm, the clinician must be knowledgeable of seventh nerve anatomy and appreciate the variable course that its external branches may take over the face.

The trunk of the seventh nerve emerges from the stylomastoid foramen, sending off an occipital branch and a branch to the stylohyoid muscle and posterior belly of the digastric muscle. The nerve then moves forward and laterally through the retromandibular fossa and into the posterior aspect of the parotid gland, lying between its inner lobe and larger outer lobe. The nerve then fans over the face in a defined but somewhat variable distribution. An auricular branch, if present, is the most superiorly positioned. It is followed by the branch to the frontalis muscle. Directly below this are the 2 or 3 branches to the corrugator and orbicularis oculi muscles. The branch to the nasal ala and upper lip may variably innervate the orbicularis oculi muscle and the corner of the mouth. It is this branch that most commonly impairs the result in facial nerve avulsion surgery. Maintenance of this branch may cause residual blepharospasm; severance of it may cause drooping of the angle of the mouth. Recurrent nerve branches may variably be present.

TREATMENT OF BLEPHAROSPASM

Oral medications used to treat blepharospasm in the past include tetrabenazine, clonazepam, lorazepam, diazepam, baclofen, trihexyphenidyl (Artane), haloperidol, acetamidobenzoate (deanol), amantadine, meprobamate, lithium, diphenylhydantoin, levodopa, and other anti-parkinsonian agents. These have rarely been of benefit. Psychiatric counseling, hypnosis, biofeedback, alcohol injection, percutaneous thermolysis of the facial nerve, and acupuncture have not proven beneficial in disassociating blepharospasm from stressful triggering factors. Neurologic consultation, however, may be useful in identifying rare cases with coexistent neurologic disease.

Two surgical procedures are available for the treatment of blepharospasm: (1) avulsion of the nerve supply to the eyelid protractors and (2) excision of the eyelid protractors combined with brow lift. Of the two operations, the latter has been more successful and has resulted in fewer complications. Both operations, though, have a somewhat limited risk/benefit ratio and are now used infrequently due to the availability of Botulinum toxin (Oculinum) for injection. This less-invasive technique has demonstrated comparable clinical effectiveness with far fewer complications than its two surgical counterparts. These three approaches will be discussed in order of historical development.

Selective Avulsion of Facial Nerve (Reynolds Procedure). This procedure is performed under general anesthesia. Muscle relaxants such as curare should not be used because they will impede neural transmission, which is essential to the surgical identification of the facial nerve and its branches. Coexistent use of local anesthetics would likewise impair this identification.

As the condition is bilateral, both sides should be treated in the same operation (only the affected side should be operated upon in cases of hemifacial spasm not amenable to neurosurgical correction). The area of intended incision is marked with methylene blue, placed approximately 2.5 cm anterior to the external auditory meatus and extended vertically approximately 3.5 cm. The incision is extended through the skin and subcutaneous tissue to the level of the parotid gland. Parotid fascia is incised and the gland is entered with careful blunt dissection. Keeping the scissors in a horizontal plane avoids excessively deep penetration into the gland. The use of cotton-tipped applicator sticks rather than scissors may prove less traumatic as the facial nerve and its branches are approached. Hemostasis is essential in this highly vascular area. Cautery may cause facial contracture from its effect on the nearby facial nerve branches. Once the facial nerve is identified, it is imperative to recall that location of branches varies considerably among patients and between the two sides in each patient.

The upper branches generally extend forward and upward, innervating the frontalis and corrugator muscles. The middle branches extend forward, innervating the

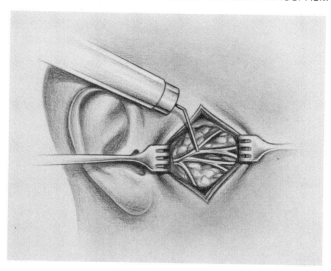

FIG. 14–1. Exposure of facial nerve branches through the parotid gland in the Reynolds procedure. Nerve stimulation helps to identify functional distribution.

orbicularis oculi and mid facial muscles. The lower branches extend forward and downward, innervating the orbicularis oris muscle. Branch identification is confirmed by use of a neurosurgical nerve stimulator (Fig. 14–1). The muscles served by the nerve being stimulated will contract selectively. Once a branch is found, the dissection is carried proximally to locate the other facial nerve branches. The branches (and recurrent branches) serving the eyelids and mouth should all be identified in this manner. Repeated neural stimulation should be avoided because it may induce muscle fatigue, which may result in inaccurate identification.

Once the branches are identified, they are further exposed by careful dissection. All branches (and recurrent branches) that innervate the orbicularis oculi muscle should be avulsed. Only in cases where frontalis muscle is contributing to the spasm should its branches be removed. All branches (and recurrent branches) that innervate the mouth should be left intact.

In avulsing the appropriate facial nerve branches, a tantalum clip is placed on the proximal end on the nerve branch (Fig. 14–2). The branch is severed just distal to the clip. Cauterizing the nerve stumps and folding the clipped end back toward the ear will help discourage nerve regeneration. A hemostat then engages the severed distal end of the nerve. The branch is removed in as long a segment as possible by pulling its nerve endings out of the muscle fiber synapses using a second hemostat in a hand-over-hand manner. After avulsion of these branches, the nerve trunk should again be stimulated to ensure that all branches innervating the orbicularis oculi

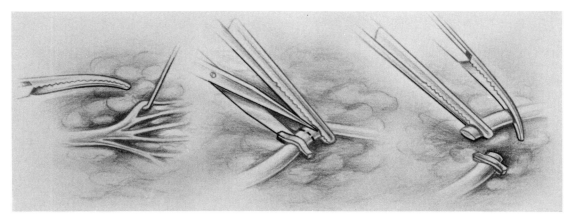

FIG. 14–2. Once the appropriate facial nerve branches are identified for avulsion, a tantalum clip is placed on the proximal end. The branch is severed distal to the clip. The clipped end is cauterized and folded back toward the ear. A hemostat is used to engage and avulse the distal end.

muscle have been removed and that all branches innervating the orbicularis oris have been left undisturbed.

The subcutaneous tissue is closed with vertical and horizontal mattress sutures of 4-0 and 5-0 Vicryl respectively. Excessive preauricular skin may be excised at this time. Skin is reapproximated with running 6-0 silk sutures. Drains are rarely required, although a pressure dressing for 24 to 48 hours postoperatively may optimize hemostasis. Oral antibiotics may be useful in minimizing postoperative infections. The skin sutures are removed 1 week postoperatively.

If appreciable blepharospasm remains or significant asymmetry manifests in the immediate postoperative period, early reoperation should be considered. The tantalum clips may aid in reidentifying nerve branches. In reoperation, it is again imperative that the orbicularis oris be spared.

Complications. The most common complication of facial nerve avulsion is delayed recurrence, which occurs in 50% of cases during the first 2 years after surgery. This may sometimes be associated with aberrant regeneration of the facial nerve. Should appreciable spasm return months or years later, further facial nerve surgery is not recommnded. Cicatricial tissue makes identification of nerve branches difficult and also makes unintentional nerve breakage more likely. In delayed recurrence, an alternative treatment should be used.

Facial numbness and paresthesia are common after nerve avulsion surgery, as is significant diminution of facial expression. Paralytic ectropion of the lower eyelids may occur in approximately 10% of cases and lateral canthal tendon laxity may become more manifest. If significant, ectropion and laxity can be corrected by a Bick horizontal eyelid shortening procedure. Postoperative

lagophthalmos and corneal exposure are usually limited. Despite careful selection of nerve branches for avulsion, brow ptosis or droop of the angle of the mouth may occur in some cases. Dermatochalasis and true blepharoptosis may be exacerbated from this procedure. Parotid-cutaneous fistulas have been reported in 12% of cases, but these are usually self-limited. A persisent fistula should respond to simple excision of the fistula tract.

Eyelid Protractor Excision Combined with Brow Lift (Anderson's Procedure). This procedure is designed to weaken the eyelid protractors and strengthen the retractors. It has four surgical components: (1) browplasty and blepharoplasty incisions with meticulous extirpation of all protracting muscles of the eyelids, including orbital orbicularis oculi, procerus, corrugator superciliaris, pretarsal and preseptal orbicularis; (2) removal of facial nerves in the postorbicular fascia of the eyelid and lateral canthal region; (3) brow elevation with fixation to frontalis muscle; (4) levator aponeurosis repair and/or lateral canthal tendon plication in patients found to have such coexistent defects.

In this operation, it is impossible to remove all orbicularis oculi muscle fibers. Postoperatively, the nerves attempt to regenerate (at times anomalously) and the remaining muscle hypertrophies. Therefore, the surgical result is proportional to the meticulousness of removal of this muscle and the facial nerve segments lying in the postorbicular fascia.

This procedure may be performed under local anesthesia. The elliptical incision site is bilaterally marked at that position where the brow is ptotic. The lower limb of the intended incision site is marked at the upper border of the brow hairline. This is essential to camouflage the scar postoperatively. With the patient sitting up to demonstrate the full extent of brow ptosis, the distance of this line to its desired position overlying the supraorbital rim is measured. The patient returns to a reclining position. The upper limb of the intended incision is marked 5 mm higher than the measured distance to allow for postoperative tissue stretching. Marks on both brows are compared to ensure symmetry. Subjacent to this, local anesthetic is infiltrated.

According to the marked lines, a skin incision may be made with a #64 Beaver blade. To minimize hair loss, this incision should be parallel to the hair follicles. The incision is carried through the subcutaneous tissue down to the level of the frontalis muscle. Redundant skin, subcutaneous tissue, and muscle outlined by the incision are excised.

Extending downward from this incision, the tissue overlying the anterior surface of the orbicularis oculi muscle is dissected to expose the orbicularis oculi from the region of the frontalis muscle superiorly to the region of the eyelid crease inferiorly. This segment of orbicularis oculi muscle is excised, along with the corrugator superciliaris. Undermining medially between the two brow incisions allows exposure and excision of the procerus muscle. Throughout this operation, hemostasis must be meticulous. The brow incision is closed in three layers using 4-0 Vicryl sutures in a vertical mattress fashion, 5-0 Vicryl sutures in a horizontal mattress fashion, and running 6-0 silk sutures to reapproximate the skin. In this closure, establishing fixation to the frontalis muscle is essential.

A second incision site is marked in the upper eyelid as for a blepharoplasty. The lower border is marked at the location of the desired eyelid crease. The upper border is marked according to the degree of cutaneous laxity. Subjacent to this, additional local anesthetic is infiltrated. According to these lines, a skin incision should be made with a #64 Beaver blade. Using blunt and sharp dissection with Stevens scissors, the pretarsal and preseptal portions of the orbicularis oculi muscle are exposed from the superficial head of the medial canthal tendon to the lateral canthal tendon. The orbicularis oculi muscle is severed from its superior attachments and its undersurface is dissected free inferiorly, medially, and laterally. A small segment of the lowermost portion of the pretarsal orbicularis oculi muscle should remain to protect the lash follicles, while the remainder of the orbicularis oculi muscle is removed.

Through the lateral portion of the lid crease incision, the fascia lateral to the lateral orbital rim is excised. This excision should include some orbicularis oculi muscle fibers from the lower eyelid and branches of the seventh cranial nerve entering this area and extending into the

temporal aspect of the lower eyelid. A drain is placed in this lateral area because it is the most gravitationally dependent area of the surgical dissection.

Coexistent blepharoptosis can be corrected at this point of the procedure using either levator resection or aponeurotic dehiscence repair techniques, depending on the etiology of the blepharoptosis (see Chapter 5). Likewise, laxity of the lateral canthal tendon can be eliminated through plication with 4-0 Vicryl or Supramid sutures.

Any additional excessive skin may be conservatively excised from the upper aspect of the eyelid crease incision. To accurately quantify this, eyelid skin should never be removed until the brow incision is closed. The upper eyelid skin is closed with three interrupted 6-0 silk sutures and a running 7-0 silk suture. Supratarsal fixation can be used to ensure an ideal postoperative eyelid crease and to take up any residual dermatochalasis. This is done by joining the skin edges with an intervening pass through the superficial fibers of the levator aponeurosis just above the tarsal border.

Despite excision of all orbicularis oculi fibers from the upper eyelid, the upper eyelids blink normally because of force from the lower lids transmitted through the outer canthus, which acts as a fulcrum.

This operation usually obviates the need for removal of lower eyelid orbicularis oculi muscle. In severe cases of blepharospasm or in hemifacial spasm, removal of this muscle from the lower eyelids may be necessary. It is performed after administration of additional local infiltrative anesthesia through an infralash lower eyelid blepharoplasty incision. The superficial portions of the pretarsal and preseptal orbicularis oculi muscles are excised from the lower eyelid. The uppermost pretarsal orbicularis and the deeper aspect of both the pretarsal and preseptal segments are spared to preserve the lash follicles and avoid ectropion, respectively. Excess lower eyelid skin is removed as per lower blepharoplasty technique. The skin incision is closed with running 7-0 silk sutures. A firm dressing is applied to all surgical sites and oral antibiotics may optionally be given. The sutures are removed 1 week postoperatively.

Complications. Complications of this operation include partial recurrence of blepharospasm (22%), which may later necessitate removal of additional orbicularis fibers, particularly from the lower eyelid and brow. Other sequelae may include exposure keratitis, corneal erosion, areas of skin necrosis, areas of forehead hypesthesia, periorbital edema, and transient lymphedema.

Botulinum A Toxin Injection. Clostridium botulinum produces six distinct toxins: A, B, C, D, E, and F. Botulinum toxin inhibits conduction in peripheral nerves by

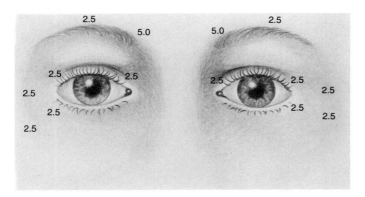

FIG. 14–3. Currently recommended Botulinum toxin (Oculinum) unit dose and distribution for initial injection.

means of presynaptic blockade, preventing release of acetylcholine by disrupting calcium ion metabolism in the nerve terminal. It does not affect the electrical excitability or the conductivity of nerve or muscle. The induced muscle paralysis is reversible, with no resultant damage to the nerve or muscle. Systemic absorption is minimal because of its rapid and tenacious binding.

Botulinum A toxin for the treatment of blepharospasm (or strabismus) is currently being investigated under strict Federal Drug Administration jurisdiction and research protocol procedure. Each patient entering this study is apprised of the experimental nature of this treatment, along with the risks and benefits of this and alternative therapeutic approaches. An informed consent form must be signed.

The botulinum injections are carried out under sterile conditions with careful attention paid to the protocol, including proscribed disposal of the toxin. It is administered in a tuberculin syringe through a 30-gauge needle. In the initial phase of the study, 12.5 units of botulinum toxin were administered to each side, 2.5 units at each of five injection sites. Experience has now led the protocol to a higher initial dose, 20 units (using a solution of 2.5 units/0.1 mL) to each side according to the distribution shown in Figure 14–3. The injections are given subcutaneously, without local anesthetic. To minimize post-treatment blepharoptosis, no injection is given in the central aspect of the upper eyelids. No injection is given in the central or medial aspect of the lower eyelid to avoid ectropion, epiphora, and corneal exposure. Follow-up examinations are done at 2 days, 1 week, and then every 1 to 2 months. Most patients require multiple treatments.

Doses at or above 20 units to each side appear to delay recurrence. The usual interval between injections is 10 to 12 weeks. If the spasm-free interval after injection is less than 3 months, the dosage may be increased by 50% on subsequent injections, usually until blepharoptosis begins to occur as a limiting side effect.

Botulinum toxin (Oculinum) has been used on over 7000 cases of blepharospasm in over 50 centers. Preliminary data indicate transient but significant effectiveness. Most patients note relief from blepharospasm symptoms for 6 to 12 weeks after injection. When blepharospasm returns, most patients request reinjection, which results in a comparable clinical response. Reduction in the effectiveness of subsequent injections has occurred only when the reinjections were given too early. The therapeutic results have been somewhat less encouraging when applied to Meige syndrome.

Complications. Complications from periorbital infiltration of botulinum toxin have all been mild, well tolerated, and resolved over 2 to 4 weeks. These transient effects have included keratitis sicca, superficial punctate keratopathy from diminished blinking, lagophthalmos from orbicularis oculi muscle paralysis, tearing and blurred vision, blepharoptosis and vertical diplopia from diffusion of the toxin to adjacent muscles, brow ptosis, and ectropion. Blepharoptosis occurs with higher doses and limits dose escalation. Corneal exposure symptoms are minimized by the use of artificial tears and lubricating ointments. The frequency of complications appears higher in patients who have had previous eyelid surgery.

Oculinum injection is safe, simple, repeatable, and effective in temporarily ameliorating the symptoms of blepharospasm. Because it is less invasive than either facial nerve avulsion or proceptor excision and has much less morbidity and comparable therapeutic benefit, botulinum toxin A (Oculinum) must currently be considered the treatment of choice for essential blepharospasm.

BIBLIOGRAPHY

Callahan, M, and Callahan, A.: Ophthalmic Plastic and Orbital Surgery. Birmingham, Aesculapius, 1979.

Dortzbach, R.: Complications and surgery for blepharospasm, Am. J. Ophthalmol. 75:142–147, 1973.

Dresner, S., Gauthier, S., and Codere, F.: Essential blepharospasm and the Meige syndrome (letter). Arch. Ophthalmol. 102:1268, 1984.

Frueh, B., Callahan, A., and Dortzbach, R.: A profile of patients with intractable blepharospasm. Trans. Am. Acad. Ophthalmol. Otolaryngol. 81:591–594, 1976.

Frueh, B., Callahan, A., and Dortzbach, R.: The effects of differential section of the seventh nerve on patients with intractable blepharospasm. Trans. Am. Acad. Ophthalmol. Otolaryngol. 81:595–602, 1976.

Frueh, B.: Intractable Blepharospasm. In Stewart, W.: Ophthalmic Plastic Reconstructive Surgery. San Francisco, American Academy of Ophthalmology, 1984.

Frueh, B., Felt, D., Wojno, T., and Musch, D.: Treatment of blepharospasm with botulinum toxin. A preliminary report. Arch. Ophthalmol. 102:1464, 1984.

Gillum, W., and Anderson, R.: Blepharospasm surgery, an anatomical approach. Arch. Ophthalmol. 99:1056–1062, 1981.

Harvey, H.: Resection of the facial nerve for blepharospasm. Arch. Ophthalmol. 86:178–181, 1971.

Janetta, P.: The cause of hemifacial spasm: Definitive microsurgical treatment at the brainstem. Trans. Amer. Acad. Ophthalmol. Otolaryngol. 80:319, 1975.

Jankovic, J., Havins, W., and Wilkins, R.: Blinking and blepharospasm: mechanism, diagnosis, and management. JAMA 248:3160–3164, 1982.

Jankovic, J., and Ford, J.: Blepharospasm and or facial-cervical dystonia: clinical and pharmacological findings in 100 patients. Ann. Neurol. 13:402–411, 1983.

Jankovic, J., and Orman, J.: Blepharospasm. Demographic and clinical survey of 250 patients. Ann. Ophthalmol. 16:371, 1984.

McCord, C., Coles, W., and Shore, J.: Treatment of Essential Blepharospasm. Comparison of facial nerve avulsion and eyebrow-eyelid muscle stripping procedure. Arch. Ophthalmol. 102:226–268, 1984.

Meige, H.: Les convulsions de la face, une forme clinique de convulsion faciale, bilaterale et medicale. Rev. Neurol. (Paris) 10:437–443, 1910.

Putterman, A., and Friedman, E.: Isolation of the facial nerve trunk in treatment of essential blepharospasm. Ophthalmic Surg. 3:60–64, 1972.

Reynolds, D., Smith, J., and Walsh, T.: Differential section of the facial nerve for blepharospasm. Trans. Am. Acad. Ophthalmol. Otolaryngol. 71:655–664, 1967.

Scott, A., Rosenbaum, A., and Collins, C.: Pharmacologic weakening of extraocular muscles. Invest. Ophthalmol. Vis. Sci. 12:924, 1973.

Scott, A., Kennedy, R., and Stubbs, H.: Botulinum A toxin injection as a treatment for blepharospasm. Arch. Ophthalmol. 103:347–350, 1985.

Shorr, N., Seiff, S., and Kopelman, J.: The use of botulinum toxin in blepharospasm. Am. J. Ophthalmol. 99:542–546, 1985.

Tsoy, E., Buckley, E., and Dutton, J.: Treatment of blepharospasm with botulinum toxin. Am. J. Ophthalmol. 99:176–179, 1985.

Weingarten, C., and Putterman, A.: Management of patients with essential blepharospasm. Ear Nose Throat J. 55:183–188, 1976.

15

ORBITAL TUMORS

JAMES ORCUTT, M.D.

Kronlein revolutionized the management of orbital tumors in 1888, when he described a lateral approach to the orbit. The diagnosis and management of orbital disease progressed slowly over the next 60 years, causing Benedict to state in 1949, "It is seldom that one can make a diagnosis of any particular type of orbital tumor from clinical evidence alone . . . when all methods of differentiation have been utilized the surgeon must decide whether exploration of the orbit is necessary." The imprecision of diagnosis and limited surgical capabilities were also noted by Foster, leading him in 1950 to state "Orbital surgery is . . . in fact, not, from the ophthalmic point of view, a gentleman's operation." Negative or positive contrast orbitography, orbital thermography, and orbitometry were short-lived attempts toward improvement in diagnosis.

The forerunner of this text by Reeh, Beyer, and Shannon was written at the beginning of the recent evolution in orbital diagnosis and treatment. Eleven pages were devoted to orbital diagnosis and surgery; four of these pages involved exenteration. Diagnostic developments include orbital venography, skull radiographs, and ultrasonography. These studies are used mostly now as confirmatory tests, having been replaced by CT scanning. Surgical improvements include microscopic surgery, lasers, better instrumentation, and hypotensive anesthesia.

The future will bring additional technology to orbital diagnosis and therapy. Lasers will probably continue to increase in usefulness for managing orbital tumors. Fiberoptic endoscopy of the orbit will aid our ability to diagnose and treat orbital tumors. Improvements in CT scanning and MRI techniques, along with improvements in software, will increase the precision of diagnosis. MRI spectrometry may eventually lead to tissue diagnosis by radiologic techniques. The use of monoclonal antibodies for tissue diagnosis is already a reality, and will continue to expand. Cytotoxic agents coupled to tissue specific antibodies may provide effective therapy for neoplasia.

This chapter is divided into the following four sections: (1) orbital diagnosis, (2) orbital treatment modalities, (3) surgical approaches to the orbit, and (4) a review of common orbital diseases and their management. Thyroid ophthalmopathy was covered in a separate chapter.

ORBITAL DIAGNOSIS

Most orbital diagnoses can be made based on historical and physical signs alone. If not, differential diagnosis can be narrowed so that appropriate diagnostic tests can be ordered. All patients with orbital disease deserve a complete eye examination including refraction and fundoscopy. The following comments concern specific portions of the examination directed toward orbital diagnosis. This mnemonic is offered to simplify orbital evaluation:

S Symptoms
I Innervation (sensory and motor)
M Muscle involvement
P Progression
L Location (globe displacement and palpation)
E External signs

SYMPTOMS

The important symptoms to be elicited from the patient are pain, visual loss, and associated systemic disease.

Pain. Pain is uncommon in orbital disease. Painful orbital diseases include orbital inflammatory pseudotumor, malignant lacrimal gland tumors, orbital hemorrhage, and orbital cellulitis. Less frequently painful are invasive nasopharyngeal carcinomas, sarcomas, metastatic orbital tumors, and arteriovenous fistulae or malformations. In contrast, most orbital diseases, including thyroid eye disease, basal cell carcinoma, and pleomorphic adenomas of the lacrimal gland, are rarely painful.

The pain history should be specific. Five characteristic types of orbital pain may be elicited. The first is commonly described as deep, boring, constant pain directly behind the eye. Such severe pain is common in orbital pseudotumor, malignant lacrimal gland tumors, orbital hemorrhage, and orbital cellulitis.

The second type of orbital pain occurs with ocular movement and is generally mild to moderate. Such pain may be associated with optic neuritis, orbital myositis, and anterior sinusitis.

The third type of pain occurs with palpation (tenderness). Responsible lesions commonly include inflamed leaking dermoid cysts, mucoceles, and pyoceles.

Ocular pain is the fourth type. Examples of ocular pain include the foreign body pain induced by corneal abrasion, the photophobia of uveitis, and the asthenopic symptoms associated with accommodative spasm.

The fifth type of orbital pain is referred from another site. Irritation of a sensory nerve anywhere along its course from the nucleus to receptor will be referred to the area of the sensory nerve endings. Referred pain is one of the most common causes of orbital pain. Headaches comprise the largest group of referred pain syndromes. The pain is usually described as located around or in the general vicinity of the eye. The patient commonly localizes the pain with the open hand held over the eye and forehead. Migraine, cluster headache, Raeder's paratrigeminal neuralgia, and tension headache are commonly referred to the orbital area.

Orbital and ocular referred pain can also be caused by irritation of the ophthalmic division of the trigeminal nerve anywhere along its intracranial or intraorbital route. Irritation of the spinal tract of the trigeminal nucleus may occur due to its close association at the C2 level with the greater occipital nerve. Occipital neuralgia or cervical spasm can, therefore, be referred to the orbit. Most intracranial tumors do not cause pain, with the notable exception of invasive nasopharyngeal carcinomas. The referred orbital pain of intracranial aneurysms is caused by stimulation of a recurrent plexus of nerves to the dura which is derived from the ophthalmic division of the trigeminal nerve. Masses within the cavernous sinus or orbital apex may also lead to referred orbital pain. Examples include the painful ophthalmoplegias (Tolosa-Hunt), intracavernous aneurysms or meningiomas, and invasive nasopharyngeal carcinomas.

Vision Loss. Vision loss in relation to other orbital findings, especially proptosis, can be valuable in the differential diagnosis of orbital tumors. Marked vision loss with low grade proptosis leads one to consider optic nerve glioma or nerve sheath meningioma. Long-standing marked proptosis without visual loss in the adult should bring to mind the likelihood of cavernous hemangioma or neurilemmoma. Acquired unilateral hyperopia, with or without choroidal folds, can be idiopathic, but more commonly is related to intraconal tumors reducing the axial length of the eye.

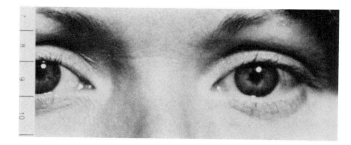

FIG. 15–1. Measurement of palpebral fissures. Palpebral fissure measurements are taken along the midpupillary line from lower to upper eyelid margins. (See text for details.)

Associated Systemic Disease. The presence of associated systemic disease may aid in the diagnosis of orbital tumors. Symptoms associated with common sources of metastatic tumors should be elicited. Females should be asked about breast lumps, prior breast surgery, previous mammograms, and the date of the most recent breast examination. Males should be asked about smoking, pulmonary symptoms, hemoptysis, and weight loss to determine the likelihood of lung carcinoma. The patient should be questioned about the presence of soft palate vascular masses when considering orbital varices, cutaneous capillary hemangiomas in the presence of a suspected orbital capillary hemangioma in a young child, evidence of neurofibromatosis in a patient with an optic nerve glioma, or sinusitis with secondary orbital cellulitis.

INNERVATION

Motor. Defects in motor innervation to the orbit may result in either ophthalmoplegia or blepharoptosis. Restrictive ophthalmoplegia must be differentiated from neurogenic ophthalmoplegia. Differential tests are discussed in a later section. Ductions are estimated between 0 to 4+ in each cardinal gaze direction. Vergences are stated with the nonparetic eye fixating (primary deviation) and the paretic eye fixating (secondary deviation). Phorias and tropias are quantified with prisms. Palpebral fissures are measured in the midpupillary line between the upper and lower eyelid margins with the eye in primary position (Fig. 15–1). Levator function is measured by asking the patient to look down while placing his thumb to stabilize the brow and fixate the frontalis muscle (Fig. 15–2A). Care must be taken to push directly inward on the frontalis muscle. The patient is then directed to look up, and the excursion of the eyelid margin is measured with a ruler (Fig. 15–2B).

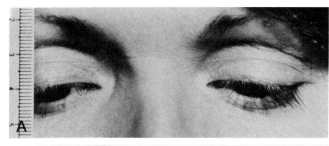

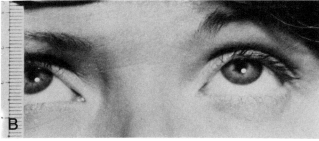

FIG. 15–2. Measurement of levator function. A, Levator function is measured by asking the patient to look down. B, The patient is then directed to look up and the excursion of the upper eyelid margin is measured. (See text for details.)

Sensory. Sensory defects caused by orbital tumors can include visual acuity loss, visual field loss, or trigeminal hypesthesia. The localization of orbital tumors is often aided by associated sensory losses. A complete eye examination with visual acuity, manifest refraction, pupillary examination for a relative afferent pupillary defect, visual field, and ophthalmoscopy of the optic nerve are mandatory to rule out optic nerve involvement. Sensory damage to the trigeminal nerve may be detected by examining cutaneous and corneal sensation.

MUSCLE INVOLVEMENT

Restrictive ophthalmoplegia must be differentiated from neurogenic ophthalmoplegia. Several examination methods are available: forced ductions, elevation of intraocular pressure in the restricted field of gaze, and saccadic velocity in the field of unrestricted gaze.

Forced Ductions. Forced ductions are performed by anesthetizing the insertion of the rectus muscle opposite the restricted field of movement with 4% cocaine. A pledget or a cotton-tip applicator soaked with anesthetic is placed over the muscle insertion for several minutes, then removed. The patient is asked to look into the limited field of movement. The insertion is grasped with medium sized toothed forceps and an attempt is made to pull the globe into the limited field of gaze. The ophthalmoplegia is probably neurogenic if the globe can be pulled easily into the restricted field (negative forced duction). Inability or difficulty in moving the globe into the restricted field of movement implies a restrictive ophthalmoplegia (positive forced duction). The examiner must be careful not to retroplace the globe while performing forced ductions as this may lead to false negative conclusions.

A device for performing forced ductions using suction through a scleral contact lens has been described (Fig. 15–3A). The scleral contact is placed over the globe after application of local anesthetic drops, suction is applied, and the handle is used to move the globe (Fig. 15–3B). The device is simple to use and eliminates the patient's fear of having the globe grasped with forceps. The suction duction device is useful in performing forward traction tests in patients with previous orbital fractures.

Eyelid forced ductions can also be performed. The upper lashes are grasped and the eyelid pulled inferiorly.

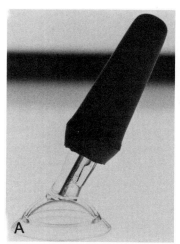

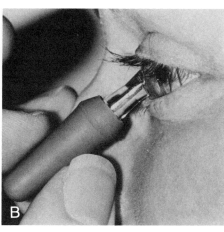

FIG. 15–3. A, The appearance of the suction-duction device. B, The device in place. (See text for details.) (Ocular Instruments, Inc., Bellevue, Washington, 98009).

Restrictive lesions in the superior orbit or thyroid eyelid retraction produce restrictive eyelid ductions.

Gaze-Induced Elevation of Intraocular Pressure. Elevation of intraocular pressure over 4 mm Hg. when attempting to move the eye into a limited field of gaze has been suggested as a means of diagnosing restrictive ophthalmoplegia. Intraocular pressure measurements are taken in primary position and while moving the eye into a position of limited movement. Contraction of the antagonist rectus muscle against a restricted muscle retroplaces the globe slightly into the orbital fat and squeezes the globe against the restricted muscle, thus transiently increasing the intraocular pressure. A neurogenically weak muscle would not be able to move the eye and thus could not increase the intraocular pressure.

Conversely, the examiner must be aware of artifactual elevations of intraocular pressure in restrictive orbitopathies, such as thyroid eye disease. The inferior rectus is commonly enlarged and restricts movement into superior or even primary gaze. The intraocular pressure in thyroid patients should, therefore, be taken in slight downgaze.

Saccadic Velocity. A paretic rectus muscle cannot generate full velocity saccadic eye movements. A normal rectus muscle limited by a restrictive process can generate normal saccadic movements in a gaze position where the restriction is not present. For example, a globe restricted in abduction due to thyroid eye disease involving the medial rectus muscle would have normal abducting saccades when the globe began in an adducted position.

PROGRESSION

Progression of an orbital tumor can be determined retrospectively from the history or prospectively by following the patient clinically. Progression can be classified as acute, chronic or intermittent.

Acute. Acute progression of orbital tumors may occur over days to weeks. Examples include inflammatory orbital pseudotumor, rhabdomyosarcoma, tumors metastatic to the orbit, and malignant lacrimal gland tumors. Explosive proptosis may occur over minutes to hours, e.g., in orbital hemorrhage or cellulitis.

Chronic. Chronic signs and symptoms of progressive orbital tumors may occur over months to years. Cavernous hemangiomas, neurilemmomas, neurofibromas, meningiomas, optic nerve gliomas, pleomorphic adenomas of the lacrimal gland (benign mixed tumors) and dermoid cysts commonly present with chronic progression.

Intermittent. Intermittent signs and symptoms of orbital disease are helpful in diagnosis. Orbital varices may increase proptosis with valsalva or a head-down position. Lymphangiomas of the orbit may increase in size along with a generalized lymphadenopathy. Gaze-evoked vision loss has been described with cavernous hemangiomas, nerve sheath meningiomas, optic nerve gliomas, and an orbital osteoma.

LOCATION

Location of a mass in the orbit can be assessed by palpation, globe retroplacement, and globe displacement. The importance of tumor location lies in differential diagnosis and surgical approach planning. A mass in any of the four quadrants may displace the globe in the opposite direction. An example is a sinus mucocele with a palpable mass in the supranasal quadrant and displacement down and out with minimal proptosis. Intraconal masses are not palpable, but may limit globe retroplacement. They usually result in axial proptosis. Axial proptosis implies forward proptosis and lateral displacement along the center line of the orbit. For each 2.5 mm of forward displacement, there should be an equivalent 1 mm of lateral displacement (Fig. 15–4). An example would be an intraconal cavernous hemangioma producing axial proptosis with decreased retroplacement (Fig. 15–24). The location of common anterior orbital tumors is shown in Fig. 15–5.

Pseudoproptosis must be recognized to eliminate unnecessary diagnostic procedures and surgery. Globe asymmetry (high myopia or microphthalmos), orbital asymmetry, blepharoptosis, eyelid retraction, or contralateral enophthalmos must be ruled out (Fig. 15–29).

Palpation. Orbital masses in the anterior orbit can often be palpated through the eyelid. The patient should not look away from the area being palpated because this tenses the orbital septum, reducing the ability to palpate an underlying mass. The examiner should simultaneously palpate the normal orbit to detect asymmetry. Palpation under general anesthesia may provide additional information. An expanding mass behind the orbital septum may displace and compress orbital fat or the lacrimal gland ahead of the lesion, giving a false impression that the lesion may be more superficial than it is. Masses in each quadrant of the orbit have their own characteristic etiologies (Fig. 15–5).

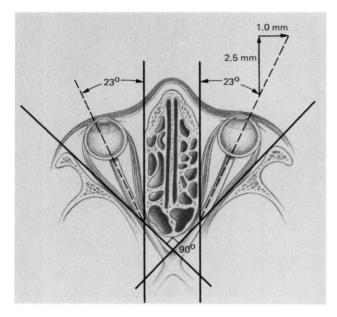

FIG. 15–4. Axial proptosis. The center line of the orbit extends along a line 23 degrees from the sagittal plane. A mass behind the globe would push the globe along the center line, resulting in 1 mm lateral displacement of the globe for every 2.5 mm of forward displacement (axial proptosis).

Globe Retroplacement. Globe retroplacement has been measured in the past by orbitography, but this was discontinued with the advent of modern radiologic techniques. Qualitative comparison of globe retroplacement with the normal eye can aid in the diagnosis of masses in the posterior orbit. The sensitivity of the method is limited and results should not be overinterpreted. Precise techniques to measure globe retroplacement or orbital compliance have been developed. Orbital compliance may not be extremely useful in orbital differential diagnosis, but may be valuable in following patients with orbital masses and also predicting which patients with thyroid eye disease are at risk of developing optic neuropathy.

Globe Displacement. Globe displacement must be measured in all three axes. The presence of anterior displacement is determined by looking over the patient's brow and noting relative proptosis compared to the normal globe. The forehead is used as a baseline (Fig. 15–6). Quantification of anterior displacement requires the use of an exophthalmometer. The Hertel exophthalmometer foot plates are placed over the lateral orbital rims (Fig. 15–7A). The distance between the lateral walls can be read from the scale on the handle. The globe should be in primary position while measurements are taken. This can be assured by the examiner sitting directly in front of the patient and closing his right eye. The patient is instructed to look at the examiner's left eye, and the scale reading corresponding to the corneal apex seen in the mirror is read and recorded for the patient's right eye (Fig. 15–7B). The procedure is reversed to measure the left eye. The scale readings are recorded, as well as the distance of the corneal apices anterior to the lateral orbital rims. The Ludde exophthalmometer may also be used to measure the distance of the corneal apex anterior to the lateral orbital rim (Fig. 15–8). The patient must be directed to look straight ahead while measurements are obtained. Parallax is avoided by aligning the marks on opposite sides of the exophthalmometer. The normal range in caucasians is less than 21 mm and less than 2 mm of asymmetry.

Preparatory to measuring horizontal displacement, one must place a mark in the center of the nasal bridge.

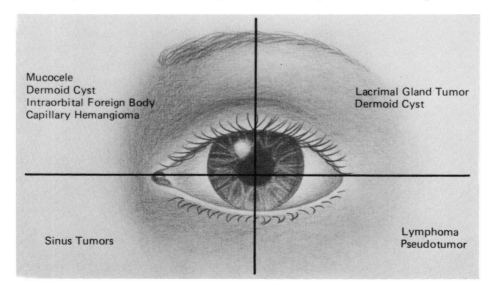

FIG. 15–5. Anterior orbital tumors occur most commonly, but not exclusively, in the quadrants shown.

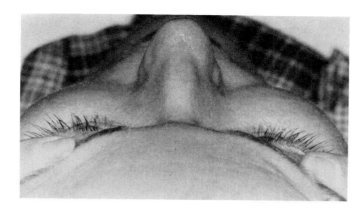

FIG. 15–6. Qualitative determination of proptosis. Unilateral proptosis or enophthalmos is estimated relative to the normal eye using the forehead as a reference.

A straight-edge rule is placed from the right to the left lateral canthus. Any mark on the rule can be placed under the nasal mark and the distance from the mark to the medial limbus recorded for each eye (Fig. 15–9). The globe should be in primary position, which can be guaranteed by first performing a cross-cover test to rule out a strabismic deviation and by having the patient look directly ahead into the examiner's open eye as described for exophthalmometry.

Vertical deviation can only be estimated. A straight edge is placed from the right to the left lateral canthus.

The deviation of the pupil center above or below this line is estimated in millimeters relative to the normal eye (Fig. 15–9).

EXTERNAL SIGNS

Many ocular, periorbital, and systemic diseases may involve the orbit. Examples of ocular findings helpful in diagnosis of orbital disease include the salmon-colored elevated conjunctival lesion of lymphoma, uveitis asso-

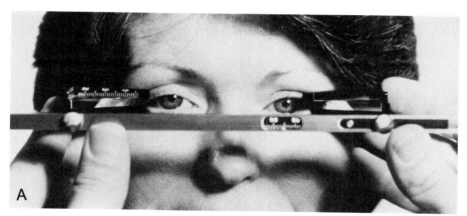

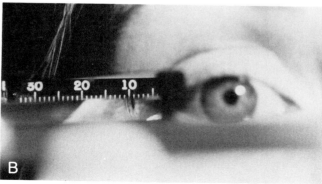

FIG. 15–7. Hertel exophthalmometry. A, Placement of the exophthalmometer. B, The distance from the lateral orbital rim to the corneal apex is read from the mirror. (See text for details.)

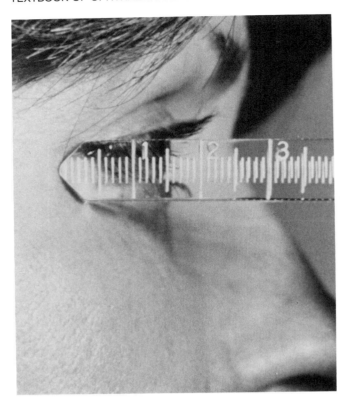

FIG. 15–8. Ludde exophthalmometry. The exophthalmometer notch is placed over the lateral orbital rim and readings are taken from the patient's side. (See text for details.)

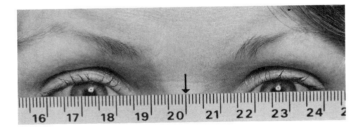

FIG. 15–9. Measurement of horizontal and vertical globe displacement. Horizontal displacement is measured from the midline to the nasal limbus. Vertical displacement is estimated from the deviation of the pupil from the straight edge relative to the normal eye. (See text for details.)

TABLE 15–1. Opticociliary Shunt Vessels

1. Optic nerve sheath meningioma
2. Central retinal vein occlusion
3. Optic nerve glioma
4. Optic nerve sarcoid
5. Craniosynostosis
6. Congenital
7. Papilledema

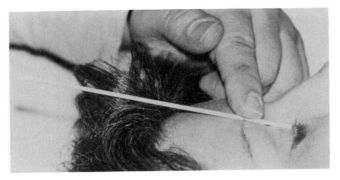

FIG. 15–10. Magnification of globe pulsation. The patient's eyes are closed and the end of a cotton-tipped applicator is placed over the eyelid in the region of the corneal apex. The applicator is held over the brow, which acts as a fulcrum. Small movements of the globe are translated into larger movements of the tip of the cotton applicator.

ciated with orbital inflammatory disease, opticociliary shunt vessels (Table 15–1, Fig. 15–30), optic atrophy associated with orbital compressive lesions, optic nerve dysplasia associated with encephaloceles, and choroidal folds associated with increased orbital mass effect.

Globe pulsation should be evaluated. Pulsation of the globe is most easily determined either subjectively by the patient reporting oscillopsia with each heartbeat or objectively by noting globe movement with each heartbeat when viewed from the side. Subtle pulsation may be magnified by use of a cotton-tipped applicator held on the brow (Fig. 15–10) or noting more shifting of the mires using Goldman applanation tonometry than would be expected from the normal ocular pulse. Globe pulsation may be present with or without an orbital bruit (Table 15–2). An orbital bruit is best examined by placing the stethoscope bell over the closed eyelids and having the patient gently open the eyelids. This technique reduces the muscle contraction noise generated if the eyelids are held closed. Pulsation associated with a bruit is usually vascular in nature, while pulsation without a bruit is generally due to transmission of cerebral spinal fluid pulsations through a bony dehiscence.

Eyelid position is determined by inspection as well as

TABLE 15–2. Globe Pulsation

1. Associated with an orbital bruit
   a. Carotid cavernous fistula
   b. Dural fistula
   c. Arteriovenous malformations
2. Unassociated with an orbital bruit
   a. Neurofibromatosis
   b. Removal of the orbital roof
   c. Trauma
   d. Encephalocele
   e. Chronic hydrocephalus
   f. Metastatic orbital tumors

TABLE 15–3. Eyelid Retraction

1. Thyroid eye disease
2. Contralateral ptosis
3. Aberrant 3rd nerve regeneration
4. Parkinson's disease
5. Bell's palsy
6. Posterior commissure lesions
7. Meningitis
8. Hypokalemic periodic paralysis
9. Large filtering blebs
10. Superior cul-de-sac lymphoma

by measurements of eyelid fissure opening and levator function. Lower and upper eyelid retraction are commonly associated with thyroid ophthalmopathy and other disorders (Table 15–3). Periorbital findings associated with orbital disease include eyelid erythema associated with orbital pseudotumor or cellulitis, facial asymmetry secondary to lymphangioma, and an S-shaped eyelid associated with lesions in the lacrimal fossa.

It is important not to overlook the opportunity to gain additional diagnostic information from systemic examination. Examples include systemic findings of neurofibromatosis, such as café-au-lait spots or cutaneous neurofibromas, palate vascular anomalies associated with orbital varices, thyroid acropathy associated with thyroid ophthalmopathy, or orbital cellulitis associated with sinusitis.

The SIMPLE approach described above has been made even SIMPLER with the advent of modern radiologic techniques:

S Symptoms
I Innervation
M Muscle involvement
P Progression
L Location
E External findings
R Radiology

RADIOLOGY

Orbital radiologic evaluation includes skull roentgenograms, orbital venography, hypocycloidal tomography, computerized tomographic scanning (CT), and magnetic resonance imaging (MRI). Skull roentgenograms are useful in some disorders such as metallic intraorbital foreign bodies, sinusitis, orbital fractures, enlargement of the optic canal, and evaluation of bone erosion or remodeling. Soft tissue is difficult to evaluate with conventional skull roentgenographic techniques. The most useful views are the Caldwell, Waters, lateral and optic foramen. The Caldwell projection places the petrous pyramids just below the inferior orbital rim, achieving the

best view of orbital structures. The Waters view enables one to view the maxillary and ethmoid sinuses as well as the inferior orbital floor without obstruction by the petrous bones.

Orbital venography is used to evaluate vascular lesions of the orbit. The examination requires contrast injection into a frontal vein, which may be difficult, and prior orbital surgery may make the study uninterpretable. The test is performed by placing a tourniquet around the head below the hairline. The frontal vein is entered percutaneously with a butterfly needle. The tourniquet is removed and 10 cc of dye is injected while the patient occludes the angular veins with his fingers. An AP skull roentgenogram shows the superior ophthalmic vein in both orbits in a M-shaped pattern. Abnormal filling or displacement of the normal pattern indicates orbital pathology. CT scanning has, for the most part, replaced venography.

Hypocycloidal tomography is useful to delineate an orbital fracture and define the optic canal. A properly positioned CT scan can demonstrate fractures and the optic canal equally well, and has largely replaced orbital tomography.

CT scanning is the most useful orbital radiologic evaluation. Axial, coronal, and off-axis sagittal views are essential. Thin (1.5 mm) overlapping sections provide good detail and allow adequate resolution during reconstruction. Normal orbital structures as seen on CT scan are shown in Fig. 15–11. Correct positioning aids evaluation. The head should be positioned so that the lens and posterior clinoid tips are on the same axial scan, ensuring that the scan demonstrates the full length of the optic canal. Coronal scans are best obtained directly rather than reconstructed. Off-axis sagittal scans should pass along the length of the optic nerve.

The magnetic resonance image is generated by the nuclear resonance (NMR) signal arising from the tissue slice being studied. Producing the NMR signal requires that the patient be surrounded by a strong magnetic field within which weaker radio frequency impulses are sent into the tissue being studied. Polarized nuclei then emit a weak signal as they become unpolarized. The MRI image is produced from these weakly emitted signals. Hydrogen is most responsible for emitting these signals. Therefore, tissues with high water content, such as fat, will emit the strongest signal and appear whiter on the MRI image. Tissues with low water content, such as bone, will emit only a very weak signal and appear black on the scan (Fig. 15–12). Varying the radio frequency can alter the return signal and produce scans of varying intensity (T_1 and T_2 weighting). Bone and flowing blood, however, always appear black.

Advantages of the MRI scan include an ability to pro-

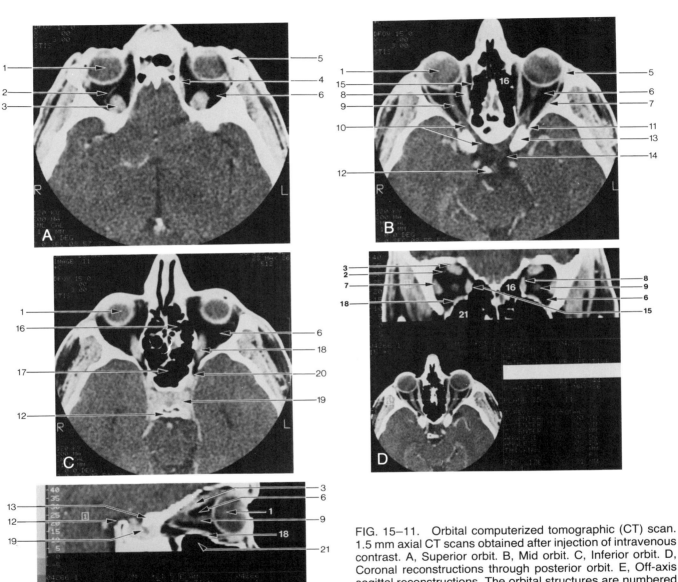

FIG. 15–11. Orbital computerized tomographic (CT) scan. 1.5 mm axial CT scans obtained after injection of intravenous contrast. A, Superior orbit. B, Mid orbit. C, Inferior orbit. D, Coronal reconstructions through posterior orbit. E, Off-axis sagittal reconstructions. The orbital structures are numbered as follows: 1. Vitreous cavity and lens. 2. Superior ophthalmic vein. 3. Superior rectus and levator muscles. 4. Superior oblique muscle. 5. Lacrimal gland. 6. Orbital fat. 7. Lateral rectus muscle. 8. Medial rectus muscle. 9. Optic nerve. 10. Optic canal. 11. Superior orbital fissure. 12. Posterior clinoid process. 13. Anterior clinoid process. 14. Pituitary fossa. 15. Lamina papyracea of the ethmoid sinus. 16. Ethmoid sinus. 17. Sphenoid sinus. 18. Inferior rectus muscle. 19. Cavernous sinus. 20. Inferior orbital fissure. 21. Maxillary sinus.

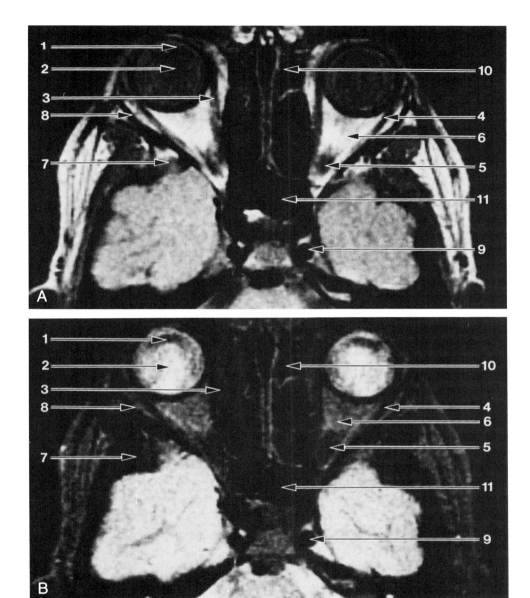

FIG. 15–12. Orbital magnetic resonance imaging (MRI). Magnetic resonance imaging scans obtained in the axial plane through the midline of the orbit. A, T_1-weighted scan. B, T_2-weighted scan. The orbital structures shown are as follows: 1. Lens. 2. Vitreous cavity. 3. Medial rectus muscle. 4. Lateral rectus muscle. 5. Inferior rectus muscle. 6. Orbital fat. 7. Greater wing of the sphenoid bone. 8. Lateral orbital wall. 9. Carotid artery. 10. Ethmoid sinus. 11. Sphenoid sinus.

duce sections in any plane, avoidance of radiation or contrast injection, and elimination of bone artifact. Disadvantages include narrow magnet aperture, claustrophobia, inability to perform the study in the presence of a magnetic foreign body, the increased scan times required (5 to 8 min. per slice compared to 5 to 10 sec. per slice for CT), and relatively poor detail. The last two disadvantages may well be eliminated with the use of stronger magnets, surface coils, and additional software. MRI spectrophotometry may eventually provide an exciting tool to probe tissue constituents nonsurgically.

TREATMENT MODALITIES

Three modalities are available to the physician for managing orbital tumors: surgery, medical management, or no treatment. Risks and benefits are associated with each option. A thorough discussion with the patient is required to portray the implications, risks, and goals of suggested treatment and alternatives.

SURGERY

The risks of orbital surgery include vision loss, diplopia, and tumor spread. Benefits include pathogenic diagnosis, possible cure, and prevention of visual deterioration. Planning orbital surgery requires information about the location of the mass, the nature of the mass, and the goal of surgery. Location and nature of the mass can be inferred from the orbital examination and diagnostic imaging. The goal of surgery can be incisional biopsy, excisional biopsy, drainage, or decompression. Table 15–4 relates the location and nature of the mass and the goal of surgery to the available surgical approaches.

Combined surgical approaches can be used in unusual circumstances, e.g., combination of a lateral and anterior orbital approach for excision of medial apex masses. Consultation from other surgical disciplines may be required for an adequate approach to some orbital masses.

MEDICAL MANAGEMENT

Risks of medical management include drug side effects, lack of biopsy confirmation, and disease progres-

sion. Benefits include avoidance of surgical risk, simplicity, and patient acceptance. Medical management may include corticosteroid therapy, antibiotics, chemotherapy, and radiotherapy. Table 15–5 relates medical treatments to common orbital disorders.

NONTREATMENT

Observation of orbital disease avoids the risks of surgical or medical treatment, but incurs the risks of lack of biopsy confirmation and disease progression. Nontreatment of orbital disease may be appropriate in some benign, nonprogressive, or slowly progressive orbital lesions without significant morbidity. Vascular anomalies, neurofibromas, cavernous hemangiomas, capillary hemangiomas, blow-out fractures, optic nerve sheath meningiomas, and gliomas may be followed without therapy in selected cases. Self-limited inflammatory lesions such as thyroid eye disease and orbital pseudotumor may be followed without treatment if significant morbidity does not develop. The ongoing choice of nontreatment is difficult, both for the patient and the physician. The patient wants "something done" and the physician is anxious about possible progression of the disease without attempts at control. The physician can take the credit for cure if he institutes therapy on a self-limited disease. He must, however, also assume responsibility for the complications associated with treatment of a disease which would have resolved or not progressed to any significant

TABLE 15–4.   Surgical Management of Orbital Tumors

Location in Orbit	Nature of Lesion	Goal of Surgery	Surgical Approach	Example
Anterior	Localized	Excision	Anterior orbitotomy	Dermoid
		Biopsy	Anterior orbitotomy	Pseudotumor
Anterior	Diffuse	Biopsy	Anterior orbitotomy	Lymphoma
		Drainage	Anterior orbitotomy	Abscess
Posterior	Localized	Excision or biopsy	Medial anterior orbitotomy	Medial mass
			Lateral orbitotomy	Lateral mass
Posterior	Diffuse	Biopsy	Anterior orbitotomy	Pseudotumor
			Lateral orbitotomy	Metastases
			Needle biopsy	Metastases
Optic nerve	Mass	Excision biopsy	Transcranial	Glioma
			Fine needle	Meningioma
			Lateral orbitotomy	Glioma
	Increased CSF pressure	Decompression	Medial anterior orbitotomy	Benign intracranial hypertension (BIH)
Extensive	Malignant	Excision	Exenteration	Basal cell carcinoma (BCC)
Lacrimal fossa mass	Malignant	Biopsy	Anterior orbitotomy	Adenoid cystic carcinoma
	Benign	Excision	Lateral orbitotomy	Pleomorphic adenoma

TABLE 15–5. Medical Management of Orbital Tumors

Treatment	Orbital Disorder	Alternative Therapy
Steroid	Pseudotumor	None (follow-up) Radiation Chemotherapy
	Thyroid eye disease	None (follow-up) Radiation Chemotherapy Decompression
Antibiotics	Cellulitis	—
	Abscess	Drainage
Chemotherapy	Neoplasms	Radiation
	Pseudotumor	Steroids Radiation None (follow-up)
Radiation	Pseudotumor	Steroids None (follow-up) Chemotherapy
	Thyroid eye disease	None (follow-up) Steroids Decompression
	Neoplasms	Chemotherapy

sequelae without treatment. If he elects not to treat, the patient must be followed closely. Should any finding or symptom deviate from those expected for the disorder being followed, the decision must be reconsidered.

SURGICAL APPROACHES TO THE ORBIT

Orbital surgery should be contemplated only when an honest assessment of the risk-benefit ratio is favorable. Important in the assessment is the experience of the surgeon. Surgeons should undertake orbital surgery only when they feel that their experience is adequate to perform such surgery.

Adequate instrumentation is required to perform orbital surgery. An operating headlight is beneficial for illumination. The magnification of the operating microscope is useful for dissecting some orbital tumors. A retinal cryoprobe can be used to freeze onto and manipulate orbital tumors (Fig. 15–14E). Orbital retractors, brain retractors, bipolar cautery, sagittal saw, drills, rongeurs, periosteal elevators, and bone wax are required for adequate exposure and hemostasis. A heated scalpel for skin incisions may be helpful in reducing bleeding. Hypotensive anesthesia will reduce hemorrhages, and self-retaining suction devices can clear blood from the field.

Anterior orbitotomies can be performed with infiltration anesthesia combined with nerve blocks. A combination of 2% lidocaine with epinephrine provides adequate anesthesia and hemostasis. See the section in Chapter 2 concerning local anesthesia for ophthalmic plastic surgery.

A close working relationship with the ocular pathologist is also important to avoid incorrect tissue handling and to extract the maximum information from the biopsy. Frozen sections are not usually useful in either diagnosis or required to determine adequacy of biopsy, but can be extremely helpful for selecting appropriate tissue fixatives and checking for clear margins. Special immunocytochemical markers are becoming more available for tissue diagnosis for which special fixatives are required. Tissue may, therefore, need to be processed in several fixatives at the time of surgery.

ANTERIOR ORBITOTOMY

Anterior orbitotomies can be performed using one of several possible incisions (Fig. 15–13). The transseptal approach (Figs. 15–13A and 15–14) is useful for biopsy of anterior orbital masses (Table 15–4). The approach will be described for the upper eyelid; however, a similar approach can be performed in the lower eyelid. The incision is placed through the eyelid crease (Fig. 15–14A). The crease should be measured before surgery and marked before injection of local anesthesia. The incision is carried through skin and orbicularis muscle (Fig. 15–14B). The orbital septum is localized by pressure on the lower eyelid, bulging the preaponeurotic fat under the septum. An incision is then made vertically through the septum, resulting in prolapse of the preaponeurotic fat (Fig. 15–14C). The septum can then be opened hor-

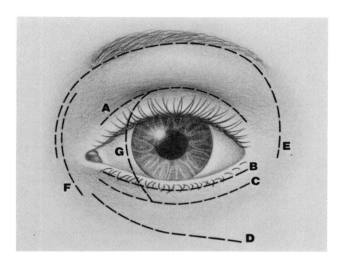

FIG. 15–13.   Anterior orbitotomy incisions. A, Upper eyelid crease incision. B, Subciliary incision. C, Lower eyelid crease incision. D, Lower orbital rim incision. E, Orbital rim incision. F, Medial incision. G, Transconjunctival incision.

izontally, exposing the preaponeurotic space (Fig. 15–14D). Exposure and hemostasis can be enhanced with the use of 3-0 silk traction sutures placed through the skin and orbicularis (Fig. 15–14E). A mass present in this space can be either excised or biopsied. The incision is closed with interrupted or running 6-0 silk or nylon skin sutures (Fig. 15–14F). Closure of the septum is generally not required. A drain may be placed if any risk of postoperative hemorrhage is present or if an abscess requires drainage (Fig. 15–14G).

Alternatives to the transseptal approach include the subciliary incision (Fig. 15–13B) and the transconjunctival approach (Fig. 15–13G). A subciliary incision may produce a more pleasing cosmetic result in the lower eyelid, but is associated with a higher incidence of cicatricial ectropion. The incision is made 3 mm below the lower eyelid margin and parallel to the margin. Skin and orbicularis are incised, followed by dissection inferiorly, remaining anterior to the orbital septum. An incision through the orbital septum then provides access to the anterior orbit. Exposure can be improved with the use of 3-0 silk traction sutures through the wound edges. The transconjunctival incision (Fig. 15–13G) has also been advocated for approaching the anterior orbit. Lesions lying on the orbital side of the eyelid retractors may be approached by way of the transconjunctival incision. The transconjunctival approach is made through a limbal peritomy with wide relaxing incisions in the quadrant overlying the mass. A combined flap of conjunctiva and Tenon's capsule is elevated and retracted with sutures. An intraconal mass can be approached after disinsertion of a rectus muscle from the globe and the exploration continued posteriorly by incising the posterior Tenon's capsule. Closure of the wound is performed by reattachment of the extraocular muscle tendon to its insertion with a 5-0 absorbable suture. The conjunctiva is closed with interrupted 6-0 plain catgut sutures. The transconjunctival approach produces less scarring, but exposure is reduced.

The extraperiorbital space can be reached by incisions lying 3 to 5 mm outside the orbital rim (Fig. 15–13E). The incision is carried down through skin, orbicularis, and periosteum to the bone. A periosteal elevator is then used to elevate the periosteum from the bone, exposing the extraperiorbital space. The extraperiorbital space is a potential space that can be easily opened once the periosteum is released from its attachment at the orbital rim. Exposure can be enhanced by the use of 4-0 silk traction sutures placed through the periorbita. Lesions lying in the extraperiorbital space can then be removed or a biopsy obtained. This is also an excellent approach to the orbital floor for repair of blow-out fractures. Masses lying against the periosteum on the orbital side can be biopsied by forming a trap-door incision through the periorbita. The periosteum is closed with interrupted absorbable sutures such as 4-0 chromic catgut. A drain may be placed if necessary. The skin is closed with interrupted 6-0 silk or subcuticular running 6-0 nylon.

Alternative incisions to reach the extraperiosteal space include the subciliary incision (Fig. 15–13B) or the eyelid crease incision (Fig. 15–13C). The subciliary incision is placed 3 mm below and parallel to the eyelid margin. Skin and orbicularis are incised and the dissection is carried downward anterior to the orbital septum. When the orbital rim is reached, an incision is made through the periorbita and the surgery continued as described for the orbital rim incision. The eyelid crease incision is performed as described under anterior orbitotomy (Figs. 15–13A and 15–13C). On reaching the septum, the incision is carried inferiorly to the orbital rim, where the periorbita is opened. The remainder of the procedure is carried out as described for the extraperiorbital approach.

The lower orbital rim incision (Fig. 15–13D) is less cosmetically acceptable than the subciliary incision and may result in persistent eyelid edema if the lateral third of the incision is carried upward. The orbital rim incision, however, provides better exposure with less risk of cicatricial ectropion than the subciliary incision.

LOWER EYELID SWINGING FLAP

The lower eyelid swinging flap (Fig. 15–15) has been advocated as a combination of the transconjunctival and

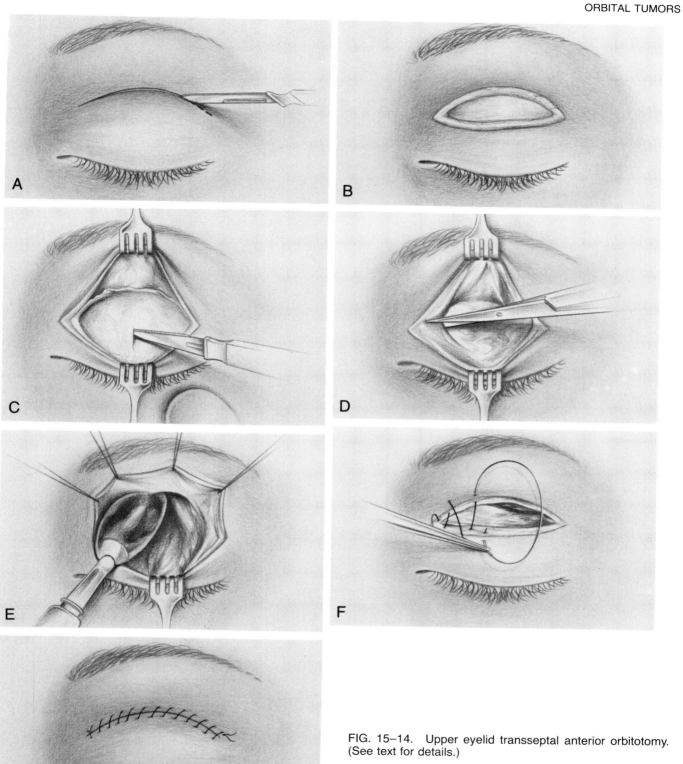

FIG. 15–14. Upper eyelid transseptal anterior orbitotomy. (See text for details.)

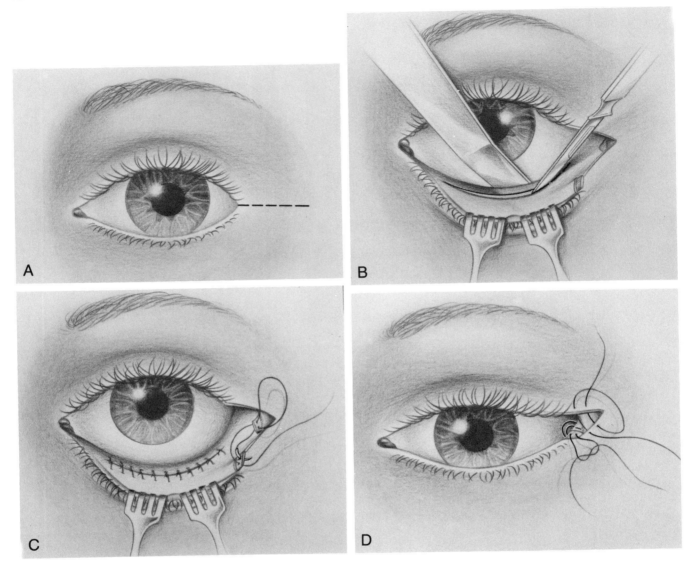

FIG. 15–15. Lower eyelid swinging flap. (See text for details.)

anterior approaches to access the inferior orbit. An extended lateral canthotomy (Fig. 15–15A) is followed by cantholysis of the lower lateral canthal tendon. The incision is then extended through the inferior fornix and lower eyelid retractors into the anterior orbital space (Fig. 15–15B). The incision can be carried inferiorly to the orbital rim to approach the orbital floor or more posteriorly to the extraconal space. Exposure is obtained with malleable retractors. Closure is performed by reapproximation of the conjunctiva with interrupted or running 5-0 chromic catgut sutures (Fig. 15–15C). Closure of the conjunctiva reapproximates the retractors to the tarsal plate, therefore eliminating the necessity of direct

retractor closure. The lower lateral canthal tendon is closed with a double armed 5-0 Mersilene or Polydek suture placed through the inferior canthal tendon and brought out through the lateral tarsal plate and tied (Figs. 15–15C and 15–15D). The cut ends of the sutures can be rounded and shortened by heating with thermal cautery. Such rounding prevents the suture from untying. The skin is closed with interrupted 6-0 silk or nylon sutures, paying attention to reforming the lateral canthal angle (Fig. 15–15D).

The lower eyelid swinging flap is especially helpful in approaching the inferior anterior orbit. The exposure is excellent, the incision is cosmetically acceptable, and the risk of cicatricial ectropion is lower than with a subciliary approach. The disadvantage is the presence of orbital fat in the operative field.

LATERAL ORBITOTOMY

The lateral approach to the orbit provides access to the middle and posterior thirds of the orbit (Fig. 15–16). The head is rotated opposite the side of the incision. A plastic self-adhesive drape is placed over the incision site. The plastic sheet provides a sterile surface as well as a means of keeping the eyelids closed.

An incision is made in an S-shaped curvilinear fashion from the brow to the superior border of the zygomatic arch (Fig. 15–16A). A 3 to 4 mm scratch at right angles to the incision will help later in matching the skin edges. The superior portion of the incision may be placed just below the brow, thus eliminating the need to shave the brow. The total length of the incision is usually 4 to 5 cm. The incision is carried through skin and underlying facial musculature to the level of the temporalis fascia (Fig. 15–16B). The fascia is exposed into the temporalis fossa and anteriorly over the lateral orbital rim. Traction sutures, of 3-0 silk, are useful for retracting the skin-muscle flap and for hemostasis. Periosteum is incised with a #15 Bard-Parker blade beginning at the superior rim and continuing along the lateral orbital wall until the zygomatic arch is reached (Fig. 15–16B). The incision should lie 3 to 4 mm outside the lateral orbital rim to make periosteal elevation and closure easier. The incision is then directed posteriorly along the zygomatic arch. Exposure can be improved with the use of Desmarres retractors placed over the skin-muscle flap. A periosteal elevator is used to detach the periosteum at the lateral orbital rim (Fig. 15–16C). The posterior periosteum is elevated until the posterior border of the frontal process of the zygomatic bone is reached. Periosteum divides at this point to envelop the temporalis muscle. The periosteum is released from the frontal process of the zygomatic bone with a #15 Bard-Parker blade. The temporalis muscle can then be displaced out of the temporalis fossa using gauze packing forced into the temporalis fossa (Fig. 15–16C). The gauze packing also provides hemostasis if left in position while the surgeon's attention is directed to the orbital periosteum. A relaxing incision is placed into the superior periosteum, as in Figure 15–16B, but directed cephalad, for 5 to 6 mm. This incision will allow freedom of movement of the periosteal flaps.

Orbital periosteum (periorbita) is detached from the orbital rim with a periosteal elevator (Fig. 15–16C). Care must be taken not to open the periorbita, especially if

one is removing a pleomorphic adenoma of the lacrimal gland. The periorbita is easily separable from the orbital wall once it has been released from the orbital rim. The lateral canthal tendon must be released from the orbital tubercle, which lies just inside the lateral orbital rim. Retraction of the periorbita exposes the lateral orbital rim, which must next be removed.

The initial bone cut is placed just superior to the zygomaticofrontal suture. The lower saw cut is placed at the level of the superior border of the zygomatic arch. Before the saw cuts are made, holes are drilled 2 to 3 mm above and below each saw cut and approximately 3 to 4 mm from the orbital rim to permit later suturing of the bone fragment in place. The holes are made with an air-driven drill using a 2 mm twist bit (Fig. 15–16D). The orbital contents are protected with a malleable retractor placed between the periorbita and the lateral orbital wall while drilling as well as cutting. A sagittal saw is used to incise the bone to a depth of approximately 2 cm or until membranous bone is reached (Fig. 15–16E). A relaxing cut may be placed at the base of the bone fragment to make removal easier. The lateral wall is then grasped with a bone clamp and fractured outward. The bone fragment is removed and placed in saline. Membranous bone is removed with rongeurs from the lateral wall until diploic bone of the greater wall of the sphenoid is reached. Hemostasis is achieved with bone wax. Removal of the membranous posterior lateral wall also leaves an opening in the wall, through which any postoperative hemorrhage may escape into the temporalis fossa.

A T-shaped incision through periorbita allows access to the orbit (Fig. 15–16F). The vertical portion of the T overlies the lateral rectus muscle and the horizontal portion is parallel to and approximately 5 mm posterior to the lateral orbital rim. Exposure of masses within the orbit is achieved with malleable retractors or retractors specifically designed for orbital retraction. The lateral rectus muscle should be isolated and tagged, using a vascular loop for retraction (Fig. 15–16G).

After orbital surgery, hemostasis must be achieved before closure. Packing the orbit gently with gauze for 5 minutes usually provides adequate hemostasis. Hypotensive anesthesia should be reversed before closure to ensure that bleeding does not start when systemic blood pressure is elevated.

Periorbita is closed at the junction of the T with interrupted 5-0 chromic catgut sutures (Fig. 15–16H). The T is not closed water-tight so that any postoperative hemorrhage may escape through the incision. The bone fragment is cleaned and placed in position, after which it is sutured in place using a 2-0 Supramid suture. The ends are rotated into the holes. Stainless steel wire should be avoided so that MRI scanning can be performed in the

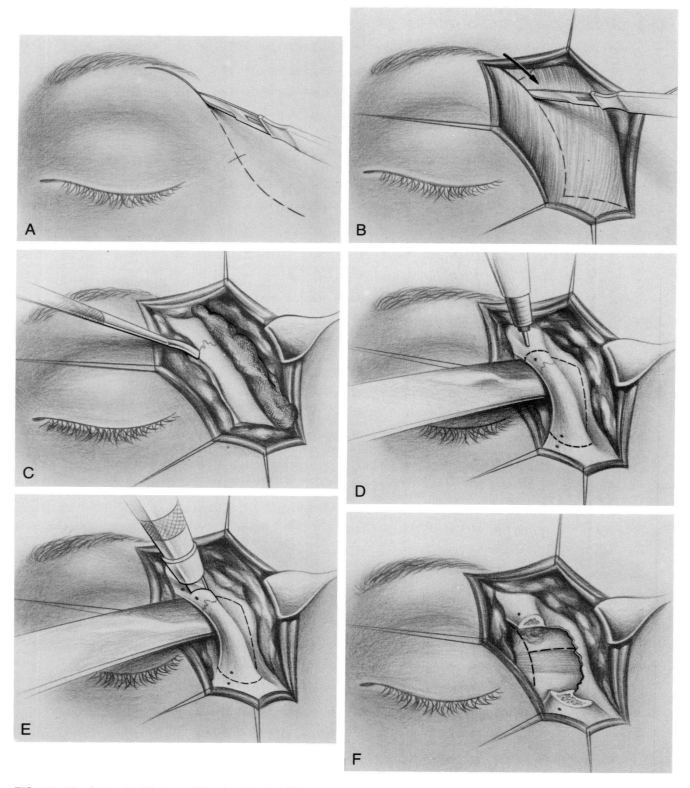

FIG. 15–16.   Lateral orbitotomy. (See text for details.)

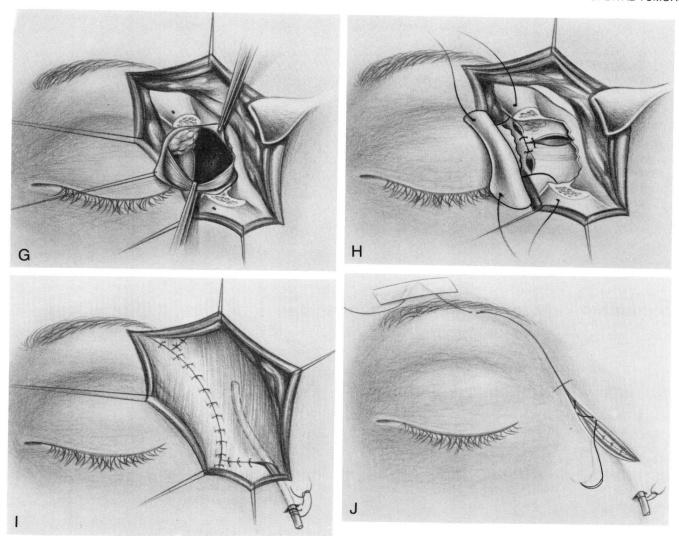

FIG. 15–16 *(Continued)*.

future. Periosteum is then closed over the lateral rim using interrupted 4-0 chromic sutures (Fig. 15–16I). A 3 mm round suction drain may be placed into the temporalis fossa at this time, if postoperative hemorrhage is likely, and brought through the cheek using a trochar supplied with the drain. The drain is sutured to the skin. The deep muscle layer is closed using interrupted 4-0 chromic sutures. The skin is then closed with a running 6-0 nylon subcuticular suture (Fig. 15–16J). The ends of the suture are secured with overlapping Steri-strips after application of tincture of benzoin. The drain is attached to suction.

Postoperatively, the patient is observed for visual function and evidence of hemorrhage. A pressure dressing is placed over the incision to reduce edema; however, the eye is not patched. The drain may be removed 24

to 48 hours later and the patient discharged from the hospital with instructions to call if pain becomes severe, hemorrhage occurs, or vision deteriorates significantly.

COMBINED LATERAL AND MEDIAL APPROACH

Masses lying posterior in the medial orbit may be reached from the medial aspect following displacement of the globe laterally into the bone defect produced by a lateral orbitotomy (Fig. 15–17). The combined medial and lateral orbitotomy is also helpful in exposing the optic nerve for decompression.

A lateral orbitotomy is first performed using either the S-shaped curvilinear incision previously described or the

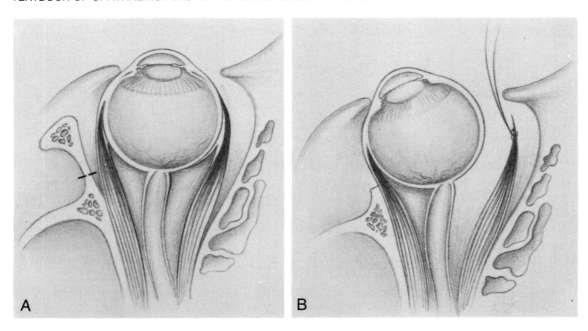

FIG. 15–17. Combined medial and lateral orbitotomy. (See text for details.)

Berke incision (Fig. 15–17A). The Berke incision is an extension of a lateral canthotomy approximately 2 to 3 cm beyond the lateral orbital wall. The incision is made through skin and muscle and opened, exposing the periosteum of the lateral orbital wall, which is incised along the lateral orbital rim. Periorbita is released from the orbital side of the lateral orbital wall, but not from the temporalis side. Vertical saw cuts are made, leaving the bone on a pedicle of temporalis muscle. The bone fragment is fractured into the temporalis fossa and covered with a wet gauze pack. The periorbita is incised, allowing displacement of the globe temporally.

A perilimbal transconjunctival incision is then made nasally. The medial rectus muscle is isolated, tagged with a 5-0 absorbable suture, and released from the globe. Pulling the muscle medially and retracting the globe temporally provides excellent visualization of the medial orbit (Fig. 15–17B).

Closure involves reattachment of the medial rectus muscle to its insertion using the 5-0 absorbable suture. The conjunctiva is closed with interrupted 6-0 plain chromic suture. The lateral periorbita is closed with 5-0 chromic catgut sutures and the bone fragment replaced. Periosteum is closed over the bone fragment, which rarely requires suturing in place because the bone remains attached to the temporalis periosteum. The lateral canthal tendon is reattached to the periorbita overlying the lateral orbital tubercle with 5-0 Mersilene or Polydek sutures. The muscle layer is closed using 4-0 interrupted

chromic sutures. The skin is closed with interrupted 6-0 silk or nylon sutures, reforming the lateral canthal angle.

Postoperative follow-up is as described for lateral orbitotomy. A drain is rarely needed because any postoperative hemorrhage drains from the conjunctival incision.

FINE NEEDLE ASPIRATION ORBITAL BIOPSY

Fine needle aspiration biopsy of orbital masses has been advocated for metastatic lesions, optic nerve lesions in blind or nearly blind eyes, inflammatory lesions, and lymphocytic lesions. Orbital apex lesions and fibrous masses are difficult to biopsy with this technique, which is performed in adults using a 22-gauge, 3.75 cm needle. The mass is localized by palpation if anterior and by CT scan or ultrasonography if posterior. The needle is placed into the mass and then attached to a 20 cc syringe in a pistol grip aspiration device (Fig. 15–18). Suction is generated by pulling on the pistol grip and the needle is gently moved back and forth to aspirate as much tissue as possible. Suction is released and the needle removed from the tissue. The needle is then removed from the syringe, and the syringe is filled with air and reattached to the needle. The biopsy is expressed from the needle, using the air in the syringe, onto a glass slide. The biopsy specimen is spread over the slide and fixed. The aid of the cytology technician is invaluable at this stage to en-

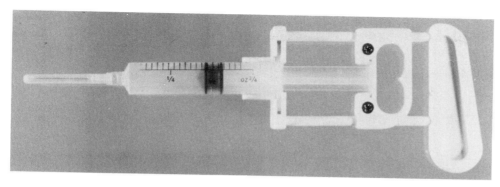

FIG. 15–18. Fine needle aspiration biopsy. A 20 cc syringe with a 22-gauge, 3.75 cm needle attached to a pistol grip aspiration device.

sure adequate fixation. The slide is then processed by the cytopathologist.

Positive identification of orbital tumors is reported as between 50% and 80%. The identification of metastatic or secondary tumors appears quite high, but may not be as successful for optic nerve tumors, inflammatory or lymphocytic lesions. The success rate may be lower due to sampling difficulties or inability to aspirate sufficient tissue.

Complications of fine needle aspiration biopsy are unusual in experienced hands. A review of complications experienced by oculoplastic or orbital surgeons discloses a 7% complication rate. The complications include orbital hemorrhage, motility disturbances, ptosis, and superficial scarring. All but the last resolved without treatment or sequelae.

A review of the literature discloses 156 reported cases of fine needle aspiration orbital biopsy. Two globe perforations occurred in an attempt to biopsy an apical mass through the superior orbit. Seven patients had permanent sequelae, four were blind, and three died. One death was caused by direct intracranial injury and two by either meningitis or brain abscess.

The length of the needle has been emphasized as an important parameter; in adults a 3.75 cm needle is used to avoid the risk of penetration of the superior orbital fissure. A shorter needle should be used in patients with shallow orbits or in infants. Apical masses should not be approached from the superior orbit, which appears to carry a greater risk of globe penetration. A potential complication of fine needle aspiration biopsy of malignant lesions is tumor seeding along the needle tract. While tumor cells can be found along the tract, a review of the literature apparently provides little proof of tumor spread. When lacrimal gland tumors are suspected of being pleomorphic adenomas, however, fine needle aspiration biopsy should not be undertaken because of the risk of tumor spread.

Endoscopic orbital biopsy can be a useful tool in orbital diagnosis. This technique requires experience, but avoids the disadvantage of insufficient tissue or sampling error. The orbital endoscope can also be useful in extracting intraorbital foreign bodies along the entry tract.

COMPLICATIONS OF ORBITAL SURGERY

Two major complications of orbital surgery, blindness and permanent diplopia, can be minimized by good surgical techniques. Meticulous hemostasis, knowledge of local anatomy, careful tissue manipulation, and adequate exposure are important.

Blindness can occur as an intraoperative or postoperative complication. Intraoperative vision loss may be due to disruption of optic nerve or ocular vasculature, excessive pressure on the globe, or direct trauma to the optic nerve or globe. The risk of disruption of the vasculature can be reduced by knowledge of orbital anatomy, gentle retraction of the globe and optic nerve, and use of the operating microscope. Excessive pressure on the globe can elevate the intraocular pressure, leading in some instances to a central retinal artery or vein occlusion. Marked elevation of intraocular pressure can lead to perilimbal globe rupture. Direct trauma to the globe or optic nerve can be avoided by using microscopic dissection near these structures and protecting the globe with a malleable retractor while drilling or sawing.

Postoperative vision loss is usually attributed to an intraorbital hemorrhage. Meticulous hemostasis during surgery and delayed wound closure until a dry field is obtained help to prevent postoperative hemorrhage. A drain placed into the surgical area helps to decompress a postoperative hemorrhage. Postoperative orders should instruct the nursing staff to check for hemorrhage by noting vision, proptosis, relative afferent pupil defect, and severe pain. These findings should be reported to the surgeon immediately. If a hemorrhage is present, it should be decompressed, usually through the original incision. The patient should be informed of these danger signs and told to call immediately should they occur. Obviously, patching the eye after surgery is undesirable because it prevents evaluation of the visual status and may increase orbital pressure.

Permanent diplopia is usually caused by direct damage to the extraocular muscles or their nerves. Transient diplopia is common and is usually ascribed to edema or muscle hemorrhage. Transient diplopia usually resolves over the first 3 to 4 weeks. Permanent diplopia can be avoided by gently retracting muscles from the operative field and using the dissecting microscope to stay clear of the nerves if possible.

Cerebrospinal fluid leakage is another potentially serious complication. Dural tears can occur on opening the lateral orbital wall above the frontozygomatic suture or operating in the supramedial orbit near the cribriform plate. Should leakage occur, the leak can be closed with sutures or a dermis or muscle patch. Up to 25% of patients with CSF leaks may develop meningitis or brain abcess; therefore parenteral antibiotics should be administered. The patient should be followed closely for symptoms of meningitis.

Additional complications of orbital surgery include blepharoptosis, scarring, dry eye, periocular anesthesia, corneal anesthesia, and pupil abnormalities. Such complications are minimized by attention to meticulous surgical principles.

The risks discussed above should be thoroughly discussed with the patient before surgery. In addition, the patient should be aware that not every surgical procedure results in a definitive diagnosis. The problems of sampling error and inadequate sample size are not absolutely avoided by direct biopsy. Monoclonal antibody techniques may improve the accuracy of diagnosis in such instances.

COMMON ORBITAL DISORDERS

The incidence of orbital disease varies among institutions, depending upon the referral population. Common orbital diseases are discussed in the following paragraphs. Graves' ophthalmopathy is discussed in Chapter 6 and orbital fractures in Chapter 16. Orbital disorders included in this section are:

A. Cellulitis
B. Idiopathic inflammatory orbital pseudotumor
C. Cavernous hemangioma
D. Lacrimal gland tumors
E. Optic nerve tumors (meningioma and glioma)
F. Metastatic tumors
G. Capillary hemangioma

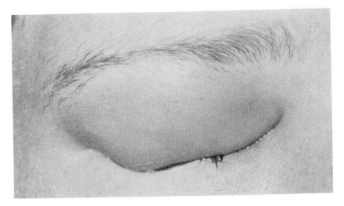

FIG. 15–19.   Preseptal cellulitis. A 17-year-old man reported a 3-day history of a purulent nasal discharge from ethmoid sinusitis before development of an edematous, erythematous, and mildly painful right upper eyelid preseptal cellulitis.

CELLULITIS

Infections can occur within the tissues of the eyelids (preseptal cellulitis) or within the orbit (orbital cellulitis). Preseptal and orbital cellulitis will be discussed separately. In many cases, however, it is difficult to determine whether the infection is only preseptal or orbital because the orbital septum does not provide an absolute barrier to the spread of infection.

Preseptal cellulitis presents with eyelid edema, erythema, and warmth of overlying skin (Fig. 15–19). Areas of skin breakage may release a purulent discharge. This condition may be secondary to trauma, a retained foreign body, external ocular infections, or upper respiratory tract infections. Rarely is it secondary to hematogenous spread. Dacryocystitis or dacryoadenitis may present as a preseptal cellulitis localized to the general vicinity of the lacrimal sac or lacrimal gland, respectively. The patient is usually febrile, with an elevated white blood cell count. Orbital findings are not present.

Common organisms responsible for preseptal cellulitis differ from children to adults. Childhood preseptal cellulitis is commonly due to Hemophilus influenzae, Staphylococcus, or Streptococcus. Mild childhood preseptal cellulitis can be treated with oral antibiotics with a spectrum covering H. influenzae, such as cefaclor 40 mg/kg/day. Children over age 4 with severe preseptal cellulitis or mild cellulitis that is not improving or worsening should be treated with intravenous antibiotics. Chloramphenicol, 100 mg/kg/day, and ampicillin, 200 mg/kg/day, are administered while awaiting culture results. Oxacillin, 100 mg/kg/day, can be used if a penicillinase-resistant Staphylococcus infection is suspected. Intravenous antibiotics should be continued for 1 week, followed by an additional week of oral treatment with an antibiotic to which the organism is sensitive.

Positive cultures in adults with preseptal cellulitis usually demonstrate Staphylococcus, Streptococcus, or anaerobes. Cultures can be obtained by draining lesions or subcutaneous aspirates. Any abscess must be drained for the cellulitis to resolve. Preseptal cellulitis in adults can be treated with oral antibiotics. Usually a penicillinase-resistant antibiotic is chosen, such as dicloxacillin, 250 mg qid, while awaiting culture results. Parenteral antibiotics may be required if the infection does not respond or becomes worse. Nafcillin, 1.5 g q4h and penicillin G, 2 to 3 million units q4h, provide coverage for most adult infections. Intravenous antibiotics should be continued for 1 week, followed by an additional week of oral treatment with an antibiotic to which the organism is sensitive.

Orbital cellulitis presents with pain, proptosis, external ophthalmoplegia, chemosis, eyelid edema, erythema, and limited acuity in severe cases (Fig. 15–20A). Etiologies include trauma, retained intraorbital foreign bodies, or contiguous sinusitis. Rarely is the infection derived from hematogenous spread. Patients are usually febrile and have an elevated white blood cell count. The organisms responsible for orbital cellulitis are similar to those in preseptal cellulitis. The workup for patients with suspected orbital cellulitis should include a CT scan (Fig. 15–20B), complete blood count, cultures of any drainage, blood cultures, and an otolaryngologic consultation with appropriate cultures of the nasopharynx. The possibility of an intraorbital foreign body must be considered.

Treatment of orbital cellulitis involves rapid institution of intravenous antibiotics after culture. Children over 4 years should be started on choramphenicol, 100 mg/kg/day, and ampicillin, 200 mg/kg/day. Chloramphenicol can be dropped from the regimen if cultures show that the organism is sensitive to ampicillin. Treatment is continued for 7 days and followed by oral ampicillin or cefaclor 40 mg/kg/day for one week. Adults should be started on nafcillin, 1.5 gm q4h, and penicillin G, 2 to 3 million units q4h. Treatment is continued for one week, followed by another week of oral treatment. Patients allergic to penicillin may be treated with cephalosporin, clindamycin, chloramphenicol, or vancomycin.

Surgical drainage of an associated sinusitis may be required before the infection responds to antibiotic therapy. Foreign bodies require removal through the entry path if possible, or through an appropriate approach to adequately expose the foreign body. Patients who develop an afferent visual defect indicated by decreased visual acuity, visual field loss, or development of a relative afferent pupillary defect may need rapid decompression of the orbit to restore visual function.

Complications of orbital cellulitis include orbital abscess formation, cavernous sinus thrombosis, meningitis,

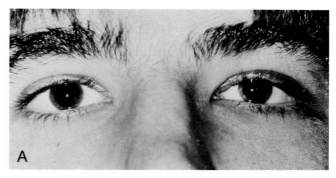

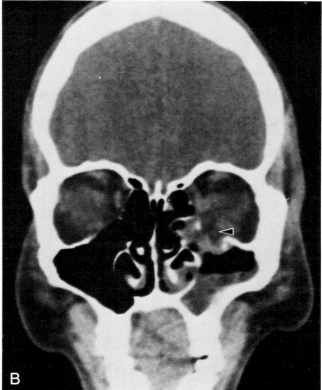

FIG. 15–20. Orbital cellulitis. A, A 19-year-old man suffered a blowout fracture of the left orbit without diplopia 2 weeks previously. Three days before admission the patient developed pain, eyelid erythema, fever, and diplopia. B, The CT scan discloses soft tissue swelling within the inferior orbit (arrow) and an air fluid level in the maxillary sinus.

extradural abscess, brain abscess, or osteomyelitis of the skull. An orbital abscess may develop, either acutely in patients who demonstrate signs of infection or insidiously in patients who are afebrile, have normal white blood cell counts, and may not have pain. Patients usually present with proptosis, chemosis, external ophthalmoplegia, and reduced visual acuity. An abscess may develop in patients who are inadequately treated with oral antibiotics. A CT scan is necessary to diagnose and localize

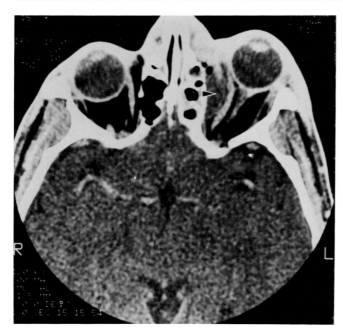

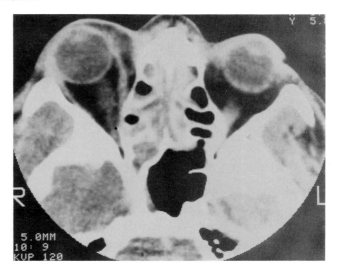

FIG. 15–22.   A patient with rhino-orbital mucormycosis demonstrating on CT scan a right ethmoidal sinusitis and subperiosteal abscess extending into the right medial orbit.

FIG. 15–21.   Orbital abscess. A 35-year-old man with symptoms of sinusitis for 2 weeks developed proptosis, diplopia, chemosis, and pain lasting more than 3 days. The CT scan discloses a left-sided subperiosteal abscess (arrow), which was drained through a medial ethmoidectomy.

the abscess within the orbit (Fig. 15–21). Treatment involves prompt surgical drainage of the abscess, cultures, systemic antibiotics, and placement of a drain for 4 to 7 days after surgery.

Diabetic or immunosuppressed patients with the symptoms described must be suspected of harboring fungal cellulitis. The severe morbidity and mortality associated with mucormycosis warrants a separate discussion of this subject.

RHINO-ORBITAL MUCORMYCOSIS
ROGER KOHN, M.D.

Rhino-orbital mucormycosis is a fungal infection of class phycomycetes and order mucorales that is notable for its high morbidity and mortality. Phycomycetes are ubiquitous fungi occurring in soil, air, skin, and food. Inoculation is by inhalation reaching the nasopharynx and oropharynx. At this early stage, most patients can generate phagocytic containment of the organisms. Individuals whose cellular and/or humoral defense mechanisms have been compromised by disease or immunosuppressive treatment may not generate adequate response. The fungus may then spread to the paranasal sinuses and subsequently to the orbit, meninges, and brain by direct extension.

Mucormycosis preferentially invades the walls of blood vessels, causing vascular occlusion, thrombosis, and infarction. This frequently affects the ophthalmic artery and, in more serious cases, may involve the internal carotid artery and cavernous sinus.

Mucormycosis infections are opportunistic, rarely occurring in healthy individuals. They are most commonly seen in diabetics, particularly those in ketoacidosis. Other predisposing conditions include various carcinomas (leukemia, lymphoma, multiple myeloma), anemia, generalized infections (septicemia, tuberculosis), fluid-electrolyte imbalance (thermal burns, extensive wounds, malnutrition, dehydration, severe diarrhea), and disorders of the following systems: gastrointestinal (gastroenteritis, hepatitis, and cirrhosis); renal (glomerulonephritis, acute tubular necrosis, uremia); pulmonary (alveolar proteinosis); and cardiovascular (congenital heart disease). Patients treated with antibiotics, folic acid antagonists, chemotherapeutic agents, corticosteroids, or ionizing radiation may also be predisposed to these infections.

Symptoms that may suggest mucormycosis in susceptible individuals include multiple cranial nerve palsies, unilateral periorbital or facial pain, orbital inflammation, eyelid edema, acquired blepharoptosis, proptosis, acute motility changes, internal or external ophthalmoplegia, headache, and acute loss of vision.

Evaluation should include radiologic studies of the paranasal sinuses and either a CT scan or MRI study of the orbit, sinuses, and anterior cranial areas (Fig. 15–22). Tissue should be obtained for fungal culture, microscopic examination, and for histopathologic examination. The

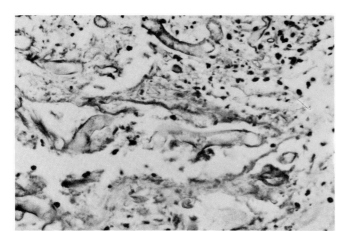

FIG. 15–23. Large, branching, nonseptate hyphae characteristic of mucormycosis (hematoxylin and eosin ×40).

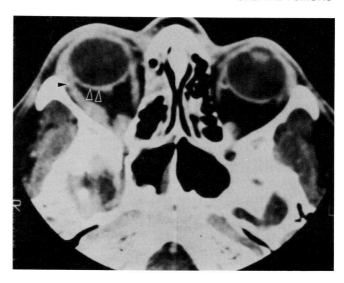

FIG. 15–24. Orbital pseudotumor: myositis. A 37-year-old woman presented with a 1-week history of pain with right eye movement and diplopia in right gaze. A contrast-enhanced CT scan reveals enlarged lateral, superior, and inferior rectus muscles. The enlargement of the lateral rectus muscle extends into the muscle tendon (arrow). Contiguous posterior scleritis is noted with contrast enhancement (double arrows).

fungus may be seen with routine hematoxylin and eosin stains, while special fungal stains (KOH, methenamine silver) may also prove helpful. Although the characteristic large, branching, nonseptate hyphae of mucormycosis (Fig. 15–23) are often recovered on paraffin section studies, absolute reliance on this modality may result in diagnostic delay. Therefore, frozen sections at the time of original biopsy are also recommended to afford earlier diagnosis and institution of appropriate management.

Optimal treatment includes: (1) early recognition of this disorder, particularly in medically compromised patients, (2) correction of any underlying metabolic derangement, (3) wide local excision and debridement of all involved and devitalized oral, nasal, sinus, and orbital tissue, (4) establishment of adequate sinus and orbital drainage, (5) daily irrigation and packing of the involved orbital and paranasal areas with amphotericin B, (6) intravenous amphotericin B.

The adjunctive use of daily irrigation and packing of the involved orbital and sinus areas with amphotericin B (1 mg/ml) should not be overlooked. Mucormycosis has a vaso-occlusive characteristic which diminishes the effective delivery of intravenous amphotericin B. Irrigation and packing may augment local delivery of this fungistatic agent.

The extent of surgical excision should balance the degree of morbidity and mutilation against the life-threatening risk this organism may represent. In limited cases, surgical excision may be confined to the tissues that are clearly infarcted. Should infection be extensive, as demonstrated by widespread necrosis, aggressive surgery, including exenteration of the orbit and any involved paranasal sinuses, may prove necessary and life-saving.

IDIOPATHIC INFLAMMATORY ORBITAL PSEUDOTUMOR

Inflammatory orbital pseudotumor is a definite clinical entity of unknown etiology with variable clinical expression. Sarcoidosis, foreign bodies, amyloidosis, and other etiologies have been related in rare cases.

Numerous classification schemes have been developed for orbital pseudotumors: etiologic, anatomic, histologic, radiologic, and by clinical course. Each classification is useful, but none provides a complete description of all clinical and pathologic aspects of orbital pseudotumors. Orbital pseudotumors may best be described in terms of a disease spectrum.

Orbital pseudotumor may be classified in an anatomic spectrum including muscle involvement (myositis) (Fig. 15–24), globe involvement (posterior scleritis), fat involvement (lipogranuloma), optic nerve involvement (optic neuritis or perineuritis), lacrimal gland involvement (dacryoadenitis), or orbital apex involvement (orbital apex syndrome). Histologically, the spectrum extends from lesions which are lymphocytic disorders of indeterminate etiology to a polymorphous infiltrate composed of plasma cells, histiocytes, monocytes, polymorphonuclear leukocytes, lymphocytes, and eosinophils with or without a fibrous component. Lymphocytic lesions of the orbit may be either inflammatory or lymphomatous. Inflammatory lesions usually contain germinal follicles, vascular channels, and a polymorphous infiltrate, while lymphomas may contain sheets of lymphocytes with atypical features, mitoses, and immature lymphocytes. Some lymphocytic lesions, however, remain indeterminate in their histologic appearance, demonstrating sheets of monomorphous lymphocytes. Indeterminate lesions may be divided into two groups using monoclonal antibodies to T and B cells and to the light chain portion of the immunoglobulins. Monoclonal lesions are probably lymphomas and the polyclonal lesions are probably reactive. Lymphomas, however, may occasionally demonstrate polyclonal reactions.

Radiologically, orbital pseudotumors may be defined as diffuse or localized and anterior or posterior (Fig. 15–25). Finally, orbital pseudotumor may be classified clinically as either acute or chronic. Acute inflammatory pseudotumor may present with pain, proptosis, chemosis, and erythema. The clinical course may be so short as to mimic orbital cellulitis. The clinical course of chronic orbital pseudotumor may be prolonged to mimic a slowly expanding orbital mass without pain or chemosis.

CT scanning with contrast enhancement is the most useful radiologic examination in evaluating patients with

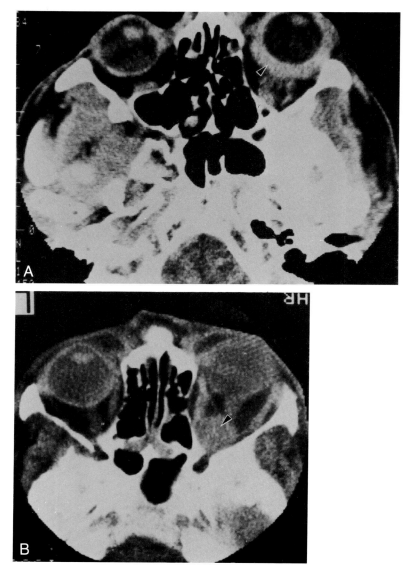

FIG. 15–25. Orbital pseudotumor: location. A, Biopsy-proven orbital pseudotumor, localized in the anterior orbit (arrow), encircling the globe. B, Biopsy-proven orbital pseudotumor, in the posterior orbit (arrow), presenting as an intraconal mass.

suspected orbital pseudotumor. Characteristics that strongly suggest orbital pseudotumor include a ragged border to the inflamed tissue (sclera, muscle, or optic nerve), extension of the inflammation along tissue planes such as muscle tendon to the contiguous sclera (Fig. 15–24), and contrast enhancement. Multiple tissue involvement is also highly suggestive of pseudotumor. Thyroid eye disease, by comparison, does not show contiguous tissue involvement associated with enlargement of the extraocular muscles.

Idiopathic orbital pseudotumor is initially managed with close follow-up, or systemic corticosteroids. Oral prednisone, 60 to 100 mg daily, is usually required as an initial dose. Tapering at a rate of 5 mg per week results in resolution in 50 to 80% of patients. The remaining patients may have a recurrence while the corticosteroids are being tapered or become intolerant of corticosteroids. Some of the patients with recurrent symptoms may again respond to corticosteroids and can be tapered more slowly (2.5 mg per week) over several months without disease recurrence.

Recurrent pseudotumors, corticosteroid-unresponsive pseudotumors, or lesions suspected of being lymphomas should be biopsied. Biopsy not only provides a histologic diagnosis, but also aids in predicting steroid response, radiotherapy response, and malignancy risk. Patients with lymphocytic lesions of indeterminate cause should be examined for systemic lymphoma and the younger population treated with radiotherapy. Corticosteroid-unresponsive orbital pseudotumor can often be controlled with 1000 to 2500 rads of radiotherapy. Patients who are unable to take corticosteroids, or who are controlled on oral corticosteroids but have recurrences when these are tapered off, can be treated with radiotherapy if the effects of steroids outweigh the risks of radiotherapy. Chemotherapy has been proposed as either an adjunct to corticosteroids or radiotherapy or an alternative to other forms of therapy.

CAVERNOUS HEMANGIOMA

Cavernous hemangiomas are venous hamartomas presenting between the ages of 35 and 70. Patients commonly complain of increasing proptosis, visual distortion, or, less commonly, diplopia. Rarely, the patient may present with sudden gaze-evoked vision loss which resolves within seconds of resuming primary gaze. The clinical course is protracted, slowly progressing over months to years. The orbital contents accommodate slow expansion of the orbital mass so that the volume of the hemangioma may be greater than the volume of the globe, yet the eye retains normal vision (Fig. 15–26).

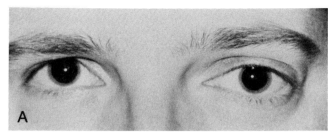
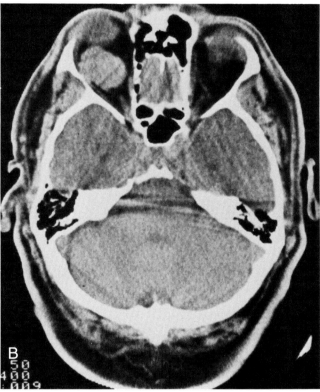

FIG. 15–26. Cavernous hemangioma. A, A 47-year-old woman has been followed for 7 years with slowly progressive axial proptosis of the right eye with retention of normal vision. B, The CT scan shows a large homogeneous intraconal mass consistent with cavernous hemangioma.

On the other hand, small cavernous hemangiomas located immediately behind the globe may present with retinal striae, optic disc edema, or gaze-evoked vision loss. The natural history of cavernous hemangiomas is inexorable slow growth over years, eventually leading to visual difficulties.

CT scanning discloses an encapsulated, well demarcated mass, usually within the muscle cone (Fig. 15–26B). Cavernous hemangiomas can, however, occur anywhere within the orbit or eyelids. Cavernous hemangiomas have very little arterial blood flow. Contrast enhancement is variable, and an arteriogram may show vessel displacement, but usually no detectable flow into the mass. B-scan ultrasound discloses a sharp capsule border with multiple internal reflections.

Treatment of orbital cavernous hemangiomas can be either conservative or by surgical removal. Surgery usually requires a lateral orbitotomy. The tumors are well encapsulated and can usually be removed without damage to adjacent orbital structures. Asymptomatic patients with cavernous hemangiomas may be treated nonsurgically; however, the hemangioma may eventually require excision as vision fails. Early surgery may be contemplated before vision loss because small tumors may be more easily and safely removed. Gaze-evoked vision loss does not in itself appear to be an indication for surgical removal. A case described by Unsold and Hoyt has been observed for 8 years without visual deterioration.

LACRIMAL FOSSA MASSES

Differential diagnosis of a mass arising within the lacrimal fossa includes dermoid cysts, inflammatory lesions of the lacrimal gland (dacryoadenitis), lymphomas, and primary lacrimal gland tumors.

DERMOID CYST

The majority of patients with dermoid cysts present before age 20. A dermoid cyst is usually palpable at the orbital rim and commonly causes a smooth indentation of the lacrimal fossa or orbital rim, often with a sclerotic margin. CT scanning may disclose a well encapsulated mass, often with a centrally shifting fat density (Fig. 15–27). The cyst may penetrate bone in the region of a suture. Occasionally, the cyst may leak its contents resulting in an acute inflammatory episode. Treatment involves complete surgical removal including the cyst wall. Either anterior or lateral orbitotomy is usually required.

DACRYOADENITIS

Inflammatory lesions of the lacrimal gland may be idiopathic, granulomatous, or infectious. The clinical course is usually short (days to weeks). The patient commonly presents with pain, tenderness, erythema, edema, and chemosis. The CT scan shows a diffuse enlargement of the lacrimal gland, which is often molded around tissue planes without overlying bone changes. Idiopathic lacrimal gland inflammation is a pseudotumor localized to the lacrimal gland. The most common granulomatous etiology is sarcoidosis. Infectious dacryoadenitis may follow a flu-like syndrome, or is occasionally bacterial in origin. The majority of these cases will respond either spontaneously or following a course of antibiotics or corticosteroids.

LYMPHOMA

Lymphomas of the lacrimal gland present in the fifth decade or later as a painless mass that has been present

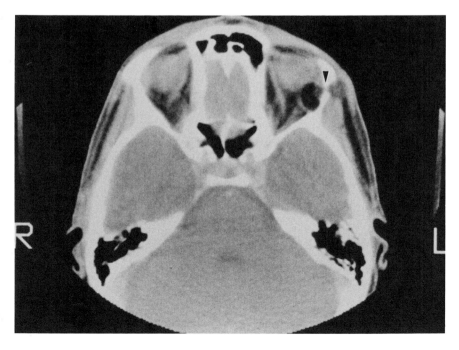

FIG. 15–27. Dermoid cyst. A 28-year-old woman presented with a palpable mass in the left temporal fossa, which periodically became inflamed over 6 years. The CT scan shows a dumbbell-shaped dermoid cyst extending from the temporal fossa into the intraorbital space through a hole in the lateral orbital wall (arrow). The intraorbital portion of the mass demonstrates a shifting fat density.

for less than a year. A diffuse oblong enlargement of the lacrimal gland, which molds to the orbital bone and globe, is seen on the CT scan. Overlying bone changes are rarely present. Of patients with lacrimal lymphomas, 15 to 20% have, or will develop, a systemic lymphoma. Patients with either a definite or possible lacrimal lymphoma should be evaluated for the presence of systemic disease. Radiotherapy is usually recommended in younger patients with localized lacrimal lymphomas, especially those with more aggressive histologic findings. There is, however, no evidence that radiotherapy prevents later systemic lymphoma. Older patients with lymphoma localized to the lacrimal gland may be followed without treatment, especially if the histologic type is favorable.

PRIMARY LACRIMAL GLAND TUMORS

The forms of primary epithelial lacrimal gland tumors are divided equally between benign and malignant. Distinguishing between benign and malignant lacrimal gland tumors is important to avoid incisional biopsy of a pleomorphic adenoma (benign mixed tumor), with its predilection for recurrence. Pleomorphic adenomas usually present as a painless mass in the lacrimal fossa. Symptoms have usually been present for a year or more and almost always for more than 6 months. Radiologically, pleomorphic adenomas usually show an enlargement of the lacrimal fossa, without destructive changes in the bone. CT scanning shows a well-demarcated mass lying in the lacrimal fossa (Fig. 15–28). Surgical management is appropriate if its intent is excisional biopsy of the mass by lateral orbitotomy. The mass should be excised completely, and an attempt should be made not to open the pseudocapsule surrounding the mass. Piecemeal removal of pleomorphic adenoma is associated with a high recurrence risk of 30% or more. Pleomorphic adenomas may undergo malignant transformation over a period of years, in either the primary tumor or in an area of recurrence.

Malignant epithelial lacrimal gland tumors are composed of adenoid cystic carcinoma, adenocarcinoma, pleomorphic adenocarcinoma (malignant mixed tumor), and other rare malignancies. Malignant lacrimal gland tumors usually present with pain and a mass in the lacrimal fossa. Symptoms have usually been present for less than 12 months. CT scanning commonly discloses enlargement of the lacrimal fossa associated with destructive changes in the bone. The margins of the mass are not as well defined as in pleomorphic adenomas. Malignant lacrimal gland tumors are aggressive and commonly have extended beyond resectable margins by the time of presentation. Early incisional biopsy and radical local resection may provide cure in some cases. Radiation and chemotherapy are of little value.

Management of lacrimal fossa masses depends upon what class the mass can be placed into: dermoid cysts, dacryoadenitis, lymphoma, benign tumors, or malignant tumors. The differential diagnosis depends on the duration of symptoms, presence or absence of pain, radiologic changes, and biopsy. Table 15–6 lists each of the various diagnoses and relates them to their common findings and appropriate treatment.

PRIMARY OPTIC NERVE TUMORS (MENINGIOMA AND GLIOMA)

Two primary optic nerve tumors are optic nerve glioma and optic nerve sheath meningioma. Optic nerve gliomas are derived from glial cells within the optic nerve, while meningiomas are derived from the arachnoid cap cells surrounding the optic nerve. Gliomas and meningiomas can usually be differentiated on historical, clinical, and radiologic grounds.

Optic Nerve Glioma. Optic nerve gliomas most commonly present in the first or second decade, although they may present up to middle age. The most common presenting findings include proptosis, vision loss, relative afferent pupillary defect, and an atrophic or edematous optic disc. Visual acuity is generally restricted to counting fingers or worse; however, an occasional patient may have visual acuity of 20/80 or better. CT evaluation usually shows a diffusely enlarged optic nerve with well-defined margins. The nerve can show kinks and demonstrate lucent central areas (Fig. 15–29A). The optic canal is commonly enlarged (Fig. 15–29B), although an enlarged canal is not helpful in delineating the posterior extent of the tumor. Patients with optic nerve gliomas may demonstrate stigmata of neurofibromatosis. Gliomas in patients with neurofibromatosis may not be as aggressive as gliomas in patients without it.

Management of optic nerve gliomas remains controversial. Several authors feel that removal of a glioma does not influence the clinical course, and therefore the glioma should not be excised. Optic nerve gliomas may be followed without treatment if significant vision remains and the clinical course remains static. Rapidly growing gliomas with significant visual loss should be excised from the globe to the chiasm through an orbital roof approach.

Optic Nerve Sheath Meningiomas. Optic nerve sheath meningiomas present most commonly in middle age, and

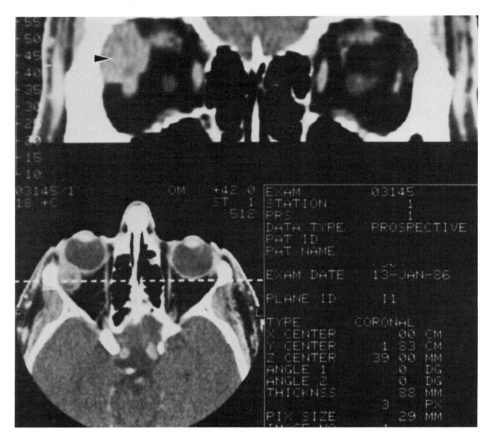

FIG. 15–28. Pleomorphic adenoma of the lacrimal gland (benign mixed tumor). A 36-year-old man presented with a 12-month history of fullness in the right supratemporal eyelid and a 3-month history of metamorphopsia. The CT scan shows a well-demarcated mass in the lacrimal fossa (arrow) with minimal bone reformation in the lacrimal fossa.

only rarely in children. The usual clinical picture is a female patient presenting with visual loss and minimal proptosis. The vision may vary with gaze position and the optic discs are usually pale or edematous and commonly demonstrate opticociliary shunt vessels (Fig. 15–30A). Visual acuity is poor, usually less than 20/50, but generally better than in patients with optic nerve gliomas. CT scanning shows narrowly or diffusely enlarged optic nerves with polar extensions, calcification, negative optic nerve shadows (railroad tracks), and irregular outlines (Fig. 15–30B). Rarely is the optic canal enlarged; more commonly it is normal or small, with bony erosion at the orbital apex.

Optic nerve sheath meningiomas can be followed with-

out treatment if vision remains and the clinical course is not rapidly progressive. The primary risk is that the tumor may seed into the cranial cavity if left untreated. Radiotherapy has been recommended in some progressive cases to retard the tendency to extend intracranially. This application of radiotherapy, however, is not universally accepted. Enlarging meningiomas with significant vision loss should be excised through a craniotomy following removal of the orbital roof. Optic nerve sheath meningiomas in children are probably more aggressive than in adults. Total excision through a craniotomy is necessary in children to remove the meningioma completely if it has significantly decreased vision and is enlarging.

TABLE 15–6. Diagnosis and Management of Lacrimal Fossa Masses

Type of Mass	Duration	Pain	Radiology (Bone)	Treatment
Dermoid	>12 months	No	Sclerotic enlargement	Excision
Dacryoadenitis	1–3 weeks	Yes	Normal	Antibiotic Steroid
Lymphoma	1–12 months	No	Normal	Biopsy Radiotherapy
Benign	>12 months	No	Fossa enlargement	Excision
Malignant	<12 months	Yes	Bone destruction	Incisional biopsy

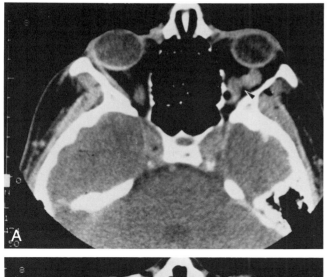

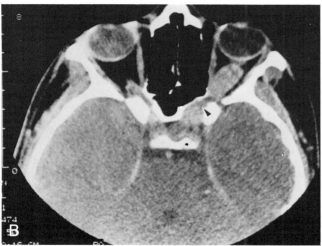

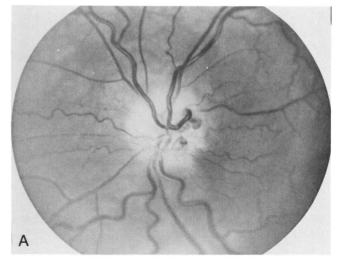

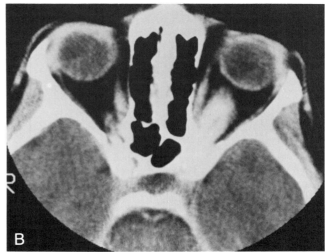

FIG. 15–29. Optic nerve glioma. A 26-year-old woman complained of decreasing visual acuity in the left eye for the past 3 years. 3 mm of axial proptosis, optic nerve pallor, and a central scotoma were noted on the left. The CT scan reveals an enlarged optic nerve with well-demarcated borders. A, Kinking can be observed in the optic nerve (arrow). B, The nerve extends intracranially through an enlarged optic canal (arrow).

FIG. 15–30. Optic nerve sheath meningioma. A, An 11-year-old boy was referred with a 3-month history of decreased vision in the left eye, now reduced to finger counting. Funduscopic examination disclosed an atrophic optic disc with opticociliary shunt vessels. B, The CT scan shows an enlarged optic nerve with indistinct margins, a central lucent optic nerve shadow, and calcification.

METASTATIC TUMORS

Carcinomas can metastasize to the orbit. The most common metastatic tumors in women are from the breast and lung, and in men from the lung, kidney, and prostate. Presenting findings include proptosis, diplopia, periorbital swelling, a palpable mass, or vision loss. Pain is usually not present. CT scan findings are varied, depending on the metastatic site. Metastases next to bone may show overlying bone erosion, while soft tissue metastases disclose an irregular margin, indicating infiltration which does not obey tissue planes.

An orbital metastasis may be the initial presentation of a carcinoma (Fig. 15–31A). Patients who harbor orbital tumors suspected of being metastatic should undergo a general work-up to rule out a primary carcinoma or other metastases (Fig. 15–31B). Women should specifically have a breast examination, mammography, and chest x-rays. Males should undergo a chest x-ray, rectal examination, and urinalysis. These studies are best coordinated with an oncologist. The orbit should be biopsied to determine the nature of the mass if no primary or other metastases are found. Rarely is the orbit the only metastatic site, even if the systemic work-up is normal,

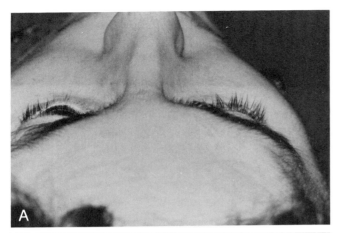

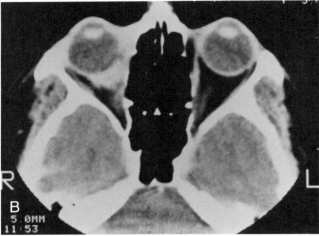

FIG. 15–31. Orbital metastatic scirrhous breast carcinoma. A, A 51-year-old woman had a palpable mass in the right orbit for 6 months. The right eye was 2 mm enophthalmic. B, The CT scan shows a mass completely surrounding the globe in the anterior orbit. Biopsy disclosed a scirrhous breast carcinoma.

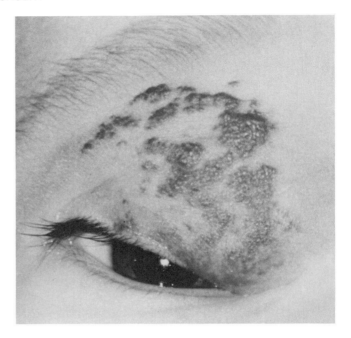

FIG. 15–32. Capillary hemangioma. A 9-month-old boy developed a large strawberry hemangioma of the right supranasal eyelid at age 3 months.

implying that the patient will need systemic therapy for control. Orbital metastases are treated with local radiotherapy, while the primary neoplasm is treated according to the recommendations of the oncologist. Orbital radiotherapy is palliative and the mean life expectancy is 1 year. Radical excision by exenteration or other mutilating surgery is not indicated.

CAPILLARY HEMANGIOMA

Capillary hemangiomas are vascular lesions that may be present at birth or appear within the first six months of life. They have a predilection for the supranasal orbit, but may occur in other cutaneous or orbital distributions. The lesions generally present as a bright red elevated cutaneous lesion (strawberry hemangioma) (Fig. 15–32). Additional lesions, commonly present around the neck or lower back, aid in diagnosis. Occasionally, the vascular mass may occur deep within the eyelids, producing a violaceous hue to the overlying skin, or more rarely, within the orbit, presenting with progressive proptosis. The vascular mass characteristically increases in size when the child cries.

The mass enlarges over the first 6 months, followed by a stationary period of several months. The mass then undergoes spontaneous reduction in size after a year of age, with maximal reduction at age 4 to 7. Complications that may ensue over the time required for the mass to involute spontaneously include: amblyopia, strabismus, ulceration, and spontaneous hemorrhage. Amblyopia may be the result of visual occlusion by the mass (deprivation amblyopia) or astigmatism induced by the hemangioma (anisometropic amblyopia). Treatment of the mass is indicated if amblyopia occurs before spontaneous resolution.

Because of their tendency toward involution, most capillary hemangiomas require no treatment. Of those that do require treatment, radiotherapy, surgical debulking, and systemic steroids are rarely indicated because they afford high risk with limited benefit. Instead, intralesional steroid injection has proven to be the safest and most effective therapeutic modality in persistent cases.

Low-dose radiotherapy reduces the mass; however, radiation in childhood may have deleterious side effects. The mass may be surgically debulked, but this should not be attempted by every surgeon because the lesions are vascular and a large percentage of the patient's blood volume may be lost before bleeding is controlled. Scarring is commonly caused by surgical debulking. Systemic steroids reduce the mass volume if given in sufficient doses (2 to 3 mg/kg/day). Steroid side effects may limit the usefulness of this form of therapy.

Intralesional steroid injection reduces tumor size in over 80% of cases. A mixture of triamcinolone and betamethazone sodium phosphate, 2 to 5 cc, is injected into numerous sites within the mass using a 27 gauge needle. The mass generally shows a reduction in size within 1 week. Repeat injections may be required for sufficient effect. Occasional complications of intralesional steroid injection include hemorrhage and cutaneous atrophy.

BIBLIOGRAPHY

Char, D., Sobel, D., Kelly, W., Kjos, B., and Norman, D.: Magnetic resonance scanning in orbital tumor diagnosis. Ophthalmology 92:1305–1310, 1985.

Chavis, R., Garner, A., and Wright, J.: Inflammatory orbital pseudotumor. Arch. Ophthalmol. 96:1817–1822, 1978.

Collins, W.: Dural Fistulae and Their Repair. In Neurological Surgery, Vol. 2 (Houmans, J., ed.), Philadelphia, W.B. Saunders, 1973, 981–992.

Dresner, S., Kennerdell, J., and Dekker, A.: Fine needle aspiration biopsy of metastatic orbital tumors. Surv. Ophthalmol. 27:397–398, 1983.

Dutton, J.: Radiographic Evaluation of the Orbit. In: Clinical Orbital Anatomy (Doxanas, M. and Anderson R., eds.). Baltimore, Williams & Wilkins, 1984, Chapter 3, 35–56.

Ellis, J., Banks, P., Campell, R., and Liesegang, T.: Lymphoid tumors of the ocular adnexa: clinical correlation with the working formulation classification and immunoperoxidase staining of paraffin sections. Ophthalmology 92:1311–1324, 1985.

Flanagan, J.: Vascular problems of the orbit. Ophthalmology 86:896–913, 1979.

Font, R. and Ferry, A.: Carcinoma metastatic to the eye and orbit. Cancer 38:1326–1335, 1976.

Font, R. and Gammel, J.: Epithelial Tumors of the Lacrimal Gland: An Analysis of 265 Cases. In Ocular and Adnexal Tumors (Jakobiec, F., ed.). Birmingham, Aesculapius, 1978, 787–805.

Gamblin, G., Harper, D., Galentine, P., Buck, D., Chernow, B., and Eil, C.: Prevalence of increased intraocular pressure in Graves' disease—evidence of frequent subclinical ophthalmopathy. N. England. J. Med. 308:420–424, 1983.

Garner, A., Rahi, A., and Wright, J.: Lymphoproliferative disorders of the orbit: an immunological approach to diagnosis and pathogenesis. Br. J. Ophthalmol. 67:561–569, 1983.

Glassburn, J., Klionsky, M., and Brady, L.: Radiation therapy for metastatic disease involving the orbit. Am. J. Clin. Oncol. 7:145–148, 1984.

Goldhammer, T. and Smith, J.: Optic nerve anomalies in basal encephalocele. Arch. Ophthalmol. 93:115–118, 1975.

Haik, G., Jakobiec, F., Wallsworth, R., and Jones, I.: Capillary hemangioma of the lids and orbit: an analysis of clinical features and therapeutic results in 101 cases. Ophthalmology 86:760–789, 1979.

Henderson, J.: Diagnosis of Orbital Tumors. In Orbital Tumors. Philadelphia, W.B. Saunders, 1973, 25–74.

Hitchings, R.: The symptom of ocular pain. Trans. Ophthalmol. Soc. U.K. 100:257–259, 1980.

Howard, G.: Cystic Tumors. In Clinical Ophthalmology, Vol. 2. Philadelphia, Harper and Row, Chapter 31, 1985.

Hoyt, W. and Baghdassarian, S.: Optic glioma of childhood: natural history and rationale for conservative management. Brit. J. Ophthalmol. 53:793–798, 1969.

Jakobiec, F., Yeo, J., Trokel, S., and Abbott, G.: Combined clinical and computed tomographic diagnosis of primary lacrimal fossa lesions. Am. J. Ophthalmol. 94:785–807, 1982.

Jakobiec, F., Depot, M., Kennerdell, J., Shults, W., Anderson, R., Alper, M., Citrin, C., Housepian, E., and Trokel, S.: Combined clinical and computed tomographic diagnosis of orbital glioma and meningioma. Ophthalmology 91:137–155, 1984.

Johnson, L., Krohel, G., Yeon, E., and Parnes, S.: Sinus tumors invading the orbit. Ophthalmology 91:209–217, 1984.

Kennerdell, J. and Dresner, S.: The nonspecific orbital inflammatory syndromes. Surv. Ophthalmol. 29:93–103, 1984.

Kennerdell, J., Slamovits, T., Dekker, A., and Johnson, B.L.: Orbital fine-needle aspiration biopsy. Am. J. Ophthalmol. 99:547–551, 1985.

Knowles, D. and Jakobiec, F.: Orbital lymphoid neoplasms: a clinicopathologic study of 60 patients. Cancer 46:576–589, 1980.

Knowles, D. and Jakobiec, F.: Ocular adnexal lymphoid neoplasms: clinical, histopathologic, electron microscopic, and immunology characteristics. Hum. Pathol. 13:148–162, 1982.

Kohn, R. and Hepler, R.: Management of limited rhino-orbital mucormycosis without exenteration. Ophthalmology 92:1440–1444, 1985.

Krohel, G. and Wright, J.: Orbital hemorrhage. Am. J. Ophthalmol. 88:254–258, 1979.

Krohel, G., Stewart, W., and Chavis, R.: Orbital Diagnosis. A Practical Approach. New York, Grune & Stratton, 1981.

Krohel, G., Krauss, H., and Winnick, J.: Orbital abscess: presentation, diagnosis, therapy and sequelae. Ophthalmology 89:492–498, 1982.

Krohel, G., Tobin, D., and Chavis, R.: Inaccuracy of fine needle aspiration biopsy. Ophthalmology 92:666–670, 1985.

Krohel, G.: Orbital Cellulitis and Abscess. In Current Ocular Therapy 2 (Fraunfelder, F. and Roy, H., ed.). Philadelphia, W.B. Saunders Co. 1985, 451–452.

Kushner, B.: Intralesional corticosteroid injection for infantile adnexal hemangioma. Am. J. Ophthalmol. 93:496–506, 1982.

Leone, C. and Lloyd, W.: Treatment protocol for orbital inflammatory disease. Ophthalmology 92:1325–1331, 1985.

Linberg, J., Orcutt, J., and Van Dyk, H.: Orbital surgery in clinical ophthalmology, Vol. 5 (Duane, T., ed.). Philadelphia, Harper & Row, 1985, Chapter 14.

Liu, D.: Complications of fine needle aspiration biopsy of the orbit. Ophthalmology 92:1768–1771, 1985.

Lloyd, G.: Primary orbital meningioma: A review of 41 patients investigated radiologically. Clin. Radiol. 33:181–187, 1982.

McCord, L. and Moses, J.: Orbital Fractures and Late Reconstruction. In Oculoplastic Surgery. New York, Raven Press, 1981, 244–248.

McDonald, W.: Pain around the eye, inflammatory and neoplastic causes. Trans. Ophthalmol. Soc. U.K. 100:260–262, 1980.

Norris, J. and Stewart, W.: Bimanual endoscopic orbital biopsy: an emerging technique. Ophthalmology 92:34–38, 1985.

Nowinski, T. and Anderson, R.: Advances in orbital surgery. Ophthalmic Plast. Reconstr. Surg. 1:211–217, 1985.

Orcutt, J., Garner, A., Henk, J., and Wright, J.: Treatment of idiopathic inflammatory orbital pseudotumors by radiotherapy. Brit. J. Ophthalmol. 67:570–574, 1983.

Reeh, M., Beyer, C., and Shannon, G.: Practical Ophthalmic Plastic and Reconstructive Surgery. Philadelphia, Lea and Febiger, 1976.

Rodrigues, M.: Monoclonal antibodies in ophthalmology. Am. J. Ophthalmol. 99:720–722, 1985.

Rootman, J. and Nugent, R.: The classification and management of acute orbital pseudotumors. Ophthalmology 89:1040–1048, 1982.

Rootman, J. and Nugent, R.: The classification and management of acute orbital pseudotumors. Ophthalmology 89:1040–1048, 1982.

Ross Russell, R.: Vascular causes of ocular pain. Trans. Ophthalmol. Soc. U.K., 100:251–252, 1980.

Sergott, R., Glaser, J., and Charyulu, K.: Radiotherapy for idiopathic inflammatory orbital pseudotumor: indications and results. Arch. Ophthalmol. 99:853–856, 1981.

Sherman, R., Rootman, J., and La Pointe, J.: Orbital dermoids: clinical presentation and management. Brit. J. Ophthalmol. 68:642–652, 1984.

Stewart, W., Krohel, G., and Wright, J.: Lacrimal gland and fossa lesions: an approach to diagnosis and management. Ophthalmology 86:886–895, 1979.

Stigmar, G., Crawford, J., Ward, C., and Thomson, H.: Ophthalmic sequelae of infantile hemangiomas of the eyelids and orbit. Am. J. Ophthalmol. 85:806–813, 1978.

Trobe, J., Glaser, J., and Post, J.: Meningiomas and aneurysms of the cavernous sinus. Arch. Ophthalmol. 96:457–467, 1978.

Unsold, R. and Hoyt, W.: Blickinduzierte Monokulare Obskurationen bei Orbitalem Hamangiom. Klin. Monatsbl. Augenheilkd. 174:715–721, 1979.

Weiss, A., Friendly, D., Eglin, K., Chang, M., and Gold, B.: Bacterial periorbital and orbital cellulitis in childhood. Ophthalmology 90:195–203, 1983.

Wright, J.: Orbital vascular anomalies. Trans. Am. Acad. Ophthalmol. Otolaryngol. 78:606–616, 1974.

Wright, J., Stewart, W., and Krohel, G.: Clinical presentation and management of lacrimal gland tumors. Brit. J. Ophthalmol. 63:600–606, 1979.

Wright, J., Call, N., and Liaricos, S.: Primary optic nerve meningioma. Brit. J. Ophthalmol. 64:553–558, 1980.

Wright, J., McDonald, W., and Call, N.: Management of optic nerve gliomas. Brit. J. Ophthalmol. 64:545–552, 1980.

Wright, J.: Factors affecting the survival of patients with lacrimal gland tumors. Can. J. Ophthalmol. 17:3–9, 1982.

Wright, J.: Surgical Exploration of the Orbit in Ophthalmic Plastic and Reconstructive Surgery. (Stewart, W., ed.). San Francisco, Am. Acad. Ophthalmol. Manuals Program, 1984, 310–311.

16

ORBITAL AND PERIORBITAL FRACTURES

Fractures are frequent components of orbital trauma and are related to the intensity, direction, and duration of mechanical force applied against the orbit and/or surrounding structures. The trauma may have caused extensive damage to the globe. Evaluation, recognition, and treatment of such ocular injury should always be the highest priority.

The clinical examination should be done as soon as possible, however, because soft tissue swelling and hemorrhage may rapidly mask such important features as visual acuity, pupillary changes, corneal and scleral laceration, intraocular hemorrhage (hyphema or vitreous hemorrhage), foreign bodies, traumatic glaucoma, recession of the anterior chamber angle, iridodialysis, lens subluxation, choroidal or scleral rupture, vitreous detachment, or retinal pathology (hemorrhage, edema, tears, or detachment), or optic nerve avulsion. Treatment of an ocular laceration should always be the highest surgical priority.

Bleeding is frequently associated with periorbital fracture. Blood may be found in the eyelid anterior to the orbital septum due to direct soft tissue injury. These tissues are not confining, affording extensive hemorrhage anterior to tarsus which may extend down to the eyelid margin and across the nasal bridge to uninvolved eyelids. Blood may also accumulate posterior to the orbital septum.

Bleeding after severe orbital trauma associated with an intact globe must be promptly assessed (Fig. 16–1). Injury to branches of the ophthalmic artery or vein may result in hemorrhage within the muscle cone. This may cause significant proptosis and/or temporary motility dysfunction. Such retrobulbar hemorrhage may spread through the connective tissue septae between the extraocular muscles into the peripheral orbital space.

In subperiosteal hemorrhages, the extent of blood accumulation is limited by bony suture lines, where periorbita becomes firmly adherent. If the subperiosteal space is intact, only mild proptosis will ensue. Disruption of periorbita allows the hemorrhage to become more extensive and move forward toward the orbital septum and bulbar conjunctiva. At the orbital margins, subperiosteal hematomas may assume a crescentic configuration.

Bleeding within the intracranial compartment may spread to the orbit by way of the supraorbital fissure or along the optic nerve sheath.

Vision loss after orbital trauma may result from orbital hemorrhage compromising the central retinal artery or apical fracture compromising the optic nerve at the optic canal. If complete loss of vision was concurrent with trauma, little will be gained from optic nerve or orbital decompression. If vision loss gradually worsened after trauma, evaluation should be directed at the optic canal and orbit. In fracture, surgical unroofing of the canal (transethmoidal or transfrontal) may restore some visual function. In hemorrhage, surgical orbital decompression may likewise restore some visual function.

The fracture itself mandates assessment of motility, levator action, enophthalmos or exophthalmos, intercanthal distance, nerve hypesthesia, and orbital emphysema (crepitus).

Infraorbital nerve hypesthesia suggests fracture of the infraorbital rim and/or floor. Supraorbital nerve hypesthesia suggests fracture of the orbital roof. Dysfunction of the zygomaticotemporal and zygomaticofacial nerve in zygoma fracture is a more subtle finding because of variable and overlapping nerve distribution.

Enophthalmos from displacement of orbital contents may initially present as exophthalmos because of orbital edema and ecchymosis. The orbital rims should be palpated. A fracture may be tender and demonstrate discontinuity or displacemnt of the orbital margin. Orbital emphysema is seen particularly in orbital floor and medial wall fracture due to fracture-induced communication with the paranasal sinuses. Air is forced through the fracture site and periosteal defect, accumulating in the peripheral orbital space, posterior to the orbital septum. Subcutaneous emphysema may also occur.

Supraorbital, glabellar, and naso-orbital fracture should prompt careful neurologic evaluation. This should include assessment of anosmia, suggestive of cribriform plate or olfactory nerve involvement. Inspection for a cerebrospinal fluid leak may be performed in the emergency room when the fracture is associated with a laceration, or in the operating room when it is associated with intact skin. Cerebrospinal fluid rhinorrhea indicates

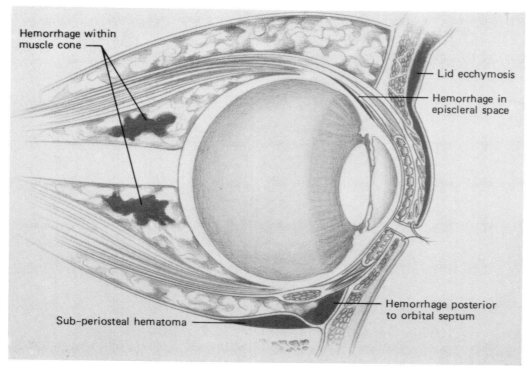

Hemorrhage within muscle cone

Lid ecchymosis

Hemorrhage in episcleral space

Sub-periosteal hematoma

Hemorrhage posterior to orbital septum

FIG. 16–1. Five common hemorrhage sites after severe orbital trauma.

a communication between the nasal cavity and the intracranial space from disruption of the cribriform plate or frontal sinus.

The orbital rims are relatively sturdy, providing a protective ring around the globe. Particularly weak areas in the rim include the frontozygomatic suture at the lateral orbital rim, the infraorbital fissure and foramen at the infraorbital rim, and the various suture lines in the region of the frontomaxillary and nasal bones. Flattening of the nasal bridge is best appreciated from a lateral viewpoint.

The orbital walls are somewhat less sturdy, particularly the inferior (orbital floor) and medial walls. Fractures of several walls may sometimes coexist.

RADIOLOGIC EVALUATION

Clinical examination must be aided by roentgenographic studies (Fig. 16–2). Retained opaque foreign bodies should also be visible on plain films. The Caldwell frontal view, taken in the nose-forehead position, superimposes the petrous portions of the temporal bones upon the superior maxillae. It provides an excellent view of the superior orbital fissures, sphenoid ridges, and lines of the temporal fossae while providing clear definitions of the frontal and ethmoid sinuses and nasal fossae.

The Waters view is set in the nose-chin position to view the maxilla without superimposition of the petrous bones. This study is particularly useful in stereoscopic form. In a Waters view, the maxillary sinuses appear distorted because of the inclined position. The orbital roofs and floors (Fig. 16–3), zygomatic bones, sphenoid ridges, and temporal arches are well visualized. A fracture along the orbital roof or medial orbital wall should be followed by skull roentgenograms to rule out an associated fracture over the anterior cranial fossa.

The lateral orbital view is useful in defining anterior-posterior displacement as in naso-orbital fracture and fracture of the anterior wall of the maxillary sinus.

Zygomatic arch views delineate the extent of arch displacement from fracture.

Optic foramina views are set in the nose-chin position with 38 degrees of rotation. This is an excellent way to ascertain potential traumatic compromise of this canal. It also provides information on the orbital apex, medial orbital wall and ethmoid air cells, and zygomatic bone and arch. Further definition may require tomography.

Polytomography is useful in ascertaining the presence and extent of an orbital floor fracture. It should be used if routing radiographs are confusing or if additional detail is desired for surgery.

Coronal CT scans accurately represent the relationship between orbital bone and soft tissue. Their expense, however, often precludes their use, and the information

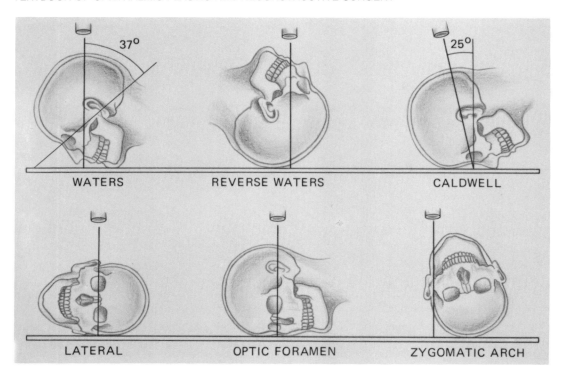

WATERS   REVERSE WATERS   CALDWELL

LATERAL   OPTIC FORAMEN   ZYGOMATIC ARCH

FIG. 16–2.   Positioning of head and x-ray beam for six common orbital projections.

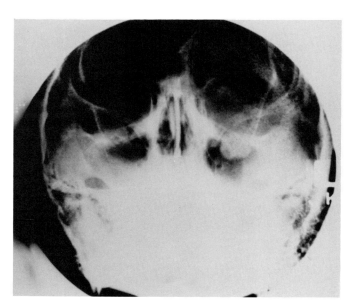

FIG. 16–3.   Waters view of orbit demonstrating left orbital floor blowout fracture with hanging-drop defect into the maxillary antrum.

derived from the preceding studies often makes them unnecessary.

General indications for surgical correction of orbital fracture include bony displacement, disfigurement, functional impairment, enophthalmos, and maintained and clinically significant diplopia. Many of these fractures, particularly blowout fracture, can be repaired 10 to 14 days after trauma to allow for complete assessment and diminution of tissue swelling. Further delay may make surgery more difficult as bony union becomes established. Zygomatic bone fractures are an exception to this. The mass of this bone necessitates earlier repair, within 7 days following trauma. Further delay may make surgical reduction much more difficult.

TRIMALAR (TRIPOD OR TRIPARTITE) FRACTURES

The trimalar (tripod or tripartite) fracture may result from a lateral blow to the cheek resulting in a fracture of the zygomatic bone (Fig. 16–4). Most commonly, the zygoma is fractured at its sutural junction with the frontal bone superiorly, the zygomatic arch laterally, and maxilla medially. This combination may be incomplete, with perhaps one or two of these junctions fractured. Trimalar fractures may present with the bone fragments either

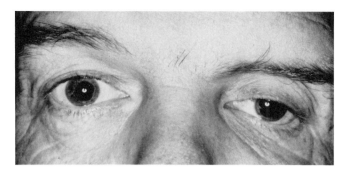

FIG. 16–4. Left trimalar fracture with zygoma hinged at the maxilla. The outer canthus and globe are inferiorly displaced.

displaced or properly positioned. Non-displaced zygoma fractures do not require surgery.

In complete fracture (Fig. 16–5), the bone fragment is usually displaced posteriorly. This causes a steplike deformity of the infraorbital rim at the zygomaticomaxillary suture, a flattened malar eminence, an elevated zygomatic arch laterally, and a depression at the zygomaticofrontal suture superior to the lateral canthus. Hypesthesia over the distribution of the infraorbital nerve is commonly present in trimalar fractures. Local ecchymosis and edema often occur. Difficulty in opening the mouth may be a manifestation of a displaced zygomatic arch impinging on the coronoid process of the temporalis muscle. Extraocular muscle imbalance is typically absent or transient.

The inferiorly displaced zygoma is usually incompletely detached and is hinged at either its frontal or

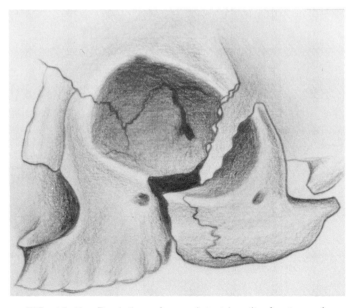

FIG. 16–5. Depiction of complete tripartite fracture of zygoma.

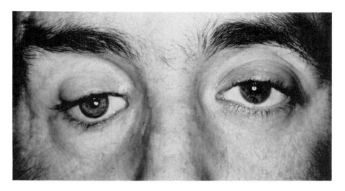

FIG. 16–6. Right trimalar fracture with zygoma hinged at the maxilla. The outer canthus and globe are inferiorly displaced.

maxillary attachment. If it is hinged to the frontal bone, there is usually no canthal displacement because the lateral canthal tendon and Lockwood's ligament remain attached to the lateral orbital retinaculum and lateral orbital tubercle. The principal displacement is in the region of the zygomaticomaxillary suture. This causes the lower eyelid to retract inferolaterally due to the downward pull on the orbital septum. In this situation, the globe remains in relatively normal position.

When the zygoma is hinged at the maxilla, the principal displacement is in the region of the zygomaticofrontal suture. The lateral orbital tubercle is inferiorly displaced, commensurately displacing the outer canthus and globe (Fig. 16–6). This situation is not usually associated with diplopia because the extraocular muscles are not entrapped. The lower eyelid is not displaced (except adjacent to the outer canthus) and there is no step-off deformity at the infraorbital margin.

If the zygoma is not hinged at either location, the globe drops and the eyelid follows. A pronounced step-off deformity is evident at the infraorbital rim.

Surgical Correction of Trimalar (Tripod) Fractures. Surgical repair of trimalar fractures requires general anesthesia. The fracture can sometimes be reduced by using a towel clip by means of closed reduction technique. This grasps the central portion of the fractured bone, elevating it into position. The fragment may be felt to "pop" into place.

An intraoral buccal sulcus incision may also be used. A blunt instrument is positioned beneath the zygoma, restoring the bone to proper position by applying upward and outward pressure (Fig. 16–7).

The most commonly used closed method is the Gillies approach (Fig. 16–8), which entails a 4 cm incision placed at the temporal fossa hairline. This incision is carried down through the temporalis fascia and muscle to the

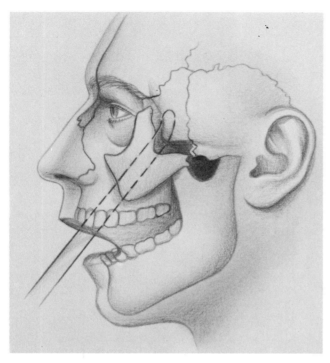

FIG. 16–7.   Lateral view of intraoral buccal sulcus approach in tripod fracture repair.

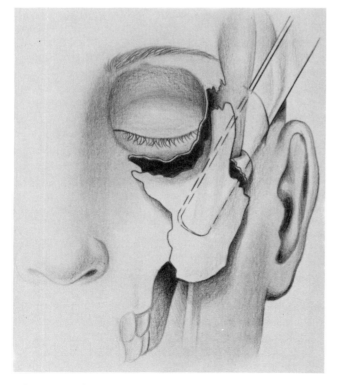

FIG. 16–8.   Gillies approach in tripod fracture repair.

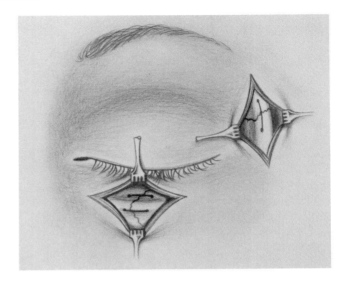

FIG. 16–9.   Sites of incision and wiring in open reduction of tripod fracture.

periosteal level with blunt and sharp dissection with curved Metzenbaum scissors. A Gillies elevator bar or periosteal elevator is inserted beneath the temporalis fascia and passed gently downward to a position below the zygoma. Leverage is then applied to the instrument in an upward and outward direction, reducing the fracture. The fragment may be guided into place by the surgeon's other hand. Excessive pressure on the temporal bone and overlying tissue should be avoided in this maneuver. In a fresh fracture, the zygomatic bone, once repositioned, usually maintains its position. The temporalis fascia is closed with interrupted 4-0 Vicryl sutures, while the subcutaneous layer is approximated with 5-0 Vicryl sutures in a vertical mattress fashion. Skin is closed with a running 6-0 silk suture. If instability persists, open and direct interosseous wiring may be added.

Open reduction methods involve a superolateral eyebrow incision and a horizontal incision directly over the infraorbital rim fracture site (Fig. 16–9). The dissection is carried to the respective fracture sites. A periosteal elevator is inserted through the inferior incision, rotating the zygoma up into its normal position. In more tenacious fractures, it may be necessary to pull the fragment carefully, using a towel clip through the temporal incision while the periosteal elevator upwardly rotates the fragment from below. All entrapped soft tissue should be removed from the fracture sites before wiring.

Small drill holes are placed on each side of the fractured zygomaticomaxillary and zygomaticofrontal sutures. Orbital structures must be protected in this process. The bone fragments are united with 27-gauge wire. The wire should be positioned and tightened with a wire twister, avoiding excessive tightening. The wire ends are cut and left approximately 5 mm long, reposited in a drill hole or pressed flat upon bone to avoid trauma to overlying soft tissue. Supramid sutures may not be strong enough to support relatively unstable trimalar fractures. The zygomatic arch rarely requires wiring.

If sufficient periosteum remains, it should be closed with interrupted 5-0 Vicryl sutures. The muscle and subcutaneous layers are closed with interrupted 5-0 Vicryl mattress sutures, and the skin is closed with running 6-0 or 7-0 silk.

NASO-ORBITAL AND MEDIAL ORBITAL WALL FRACTURES

Naso-orbital fractures result from force delivered to the nasal bridge or medial orbital rim. These are the weakest of the midface bones. This often results from sudden impact and deceleration such as a dashboard injury in an automobile accident. In mild cases, the fracture may be limited to the nasal bones and the frontal process of the maxillae. In more severe cases, the lacrimal and ethmoid bones may crack and splay laterally, causing traumatic telecanthus (increased distance between the medial canthi). This often severs the intraosseous nasolacrimal duct, causing lacrimal obstruction.

Characteristic findings in patients with acute naso-orbital fracture include traumatic telecanthus, rounding of the medial canthus, epistaxis, intraorbital and periorbital ecchymosis, subcutaneous emphysema (from fracture-induced communication with the ethmoid air cells), flattening and widening of the midface, epiphora, and possible cerebrospinal fluid rhinorrhea. The medial rectus muscle is rarely entrapped within a medial orbital wall fracture.

CSF rhinorrhea suggests a cribriform plate fracture. Most of these are managed conservatively with bed rest, head elevation to 60 degrees, and intravenous antibiotics. The patient should be cautioned not to blow his nose or smoke. If the cerebrospinal fluid leak does not readily abate, neurosurgical consultation is mandatory. Hemorrhage may be severe if the anterior and/or posterior ethmoidal arteries are disrupted. This bleeding must be stopped promptly. Direct ligation may occasionally be required if nasal packing and cautery prove insufficient. Coexistent airway obstruction should be rectified, and broken teeth and blood removed.

These fractures may result in lateral splaying of the medial orbital walls, along with their attached medial canthal tendons. The fracture often extends posteriorly into the lacrimal and ethmoid bones. Such cases may require repositioning the bony fragments, along with

transnasal wiring combined with inner canthal Y- to V- or C- to U-plasty. If dacryostenosis is present, this procedure may be further combined with dacryocystorhinostomy. Fracture of the nasal bones should be repaired with the assistance of an otolaryngologist or plastic surgeon.

In some cases, the available bone is insufficient to support a medial canthal reconstruction. This problem may be managed by one of several methods of transnasal wiring. Surgical reconstruction of naso-orbital fractures should proceed as soon as clinical stability permits.

Transnasal Wiring. If the contralateral nasal bone is intact, it may be used as the point of fixation. Under general endotracheal anesthesia, a vertical incision is made through the involved inner canthal skin. This may take on a Y-to-V or C-to-U configuration if skin muscle advancement is also required in the reconstruction (see Chapter 3).

With blunt and sharp dissection, the incision is carried to the fracture site, contiguous with the medial canthal tendon. Either a 2-0 Supramid suture or 27-gauge wire is used to engage the superficial head of the tendon. If insufficient tendon remains, the Supramid or wire may be positioned in the medial portion of tarsus of both the upper and lower eyelids.

On the intact contralateral side, a 15 mm vertical incision is made through the skin and subcutaneous tissues, just anterior to the insertion of the superficial head of the medial canthal tendon. The periosteum is opened vertically at the anterior lacrimal crest and reflected anteriorly. With a Hall drill, a 5 mm opening is made through the bone and nasal mucosa anterior to the attachment. With a Burr tip, a small groove is carved directly above and below this opening to accommodate placement of a supportive piton (Fig. 16–10).

A Wright needle is passed from the surgically drilled opening through the nasal septum, emerging at the fracture site. Some pressure is required to penetrate the septum. Careful attention must be paid to prevent momentum from carrying the needle immediately through the fracture site; the medial globe is in close approximation. The Supramid suture or wire should be placed through the eyelet opening of the Wright needle, and this material becomes properly positioned as the Wright needle is withdrawn. The two ends of Supramid or wire are passed through the two openings in the piton. As the piton is positioned over the hole and within the carved grooves, the traumatized canthus is quantitatively drawn medially as the Supramid or wire is secured. The Wilkins bar is an equivalent alternative to the piton for this purpose. The deeper layers are closed with 5-0 Vicryl

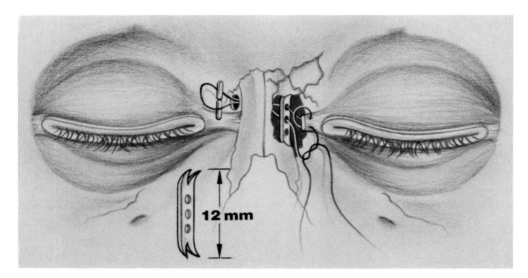

FIG. 16–10.   Depiction of left inner canthal reconstruction with the use of various supportive pitons. This device may be placed on the ipsilateral side if sufficient bone remains on the left, or on the contralateral side if insufficient bone remains on the left.

mattress sutures, followed by skin closure with running 7-0 silk sutures.

In bilateral naso-orbital fractures, the bone may be insufficient on either side to support the reconstruction. Such circumstances require standard transnasal wiring techniques (see Chapter 3).

BLOWOUT FRACTURE

A traumatic disruption of the orbital floor, not necessarily involving the infraorbital rim, denotes a blowout fracture. This is the most common periorbital fracture seen in ophthalmic plastic surgical practice. It is caused by impact of an object (usually spherical) larger than the orbit, striking the globe or anterior orbital contents (Fig. 16–11). The force generates increased hydraulic pressure within the orbit. This causes the orbital floor to blow out at its weakest point, usually posteromedially at a thin portion of the maxillary bone near the infraorbital groove. Under these traumatic circumstances, the medial orbital wall may also fracture because of its relative fragility. Rarely will the orbital roof and lateral wall "blow out" in this process.

A recent alternative theory suggests that the orbital floor is directly fractured at impact. The degree of increased intraorbital pressure determines the extent to which orbital contents are pushed through this fracture.

Clinical findings that support the diagnosis of orbital blowout fracture include a suggestible history, infraorbital nerve hypesthesia (from the lower eyelid to the cheek and canine teeth), periorbital ecchymosis, orbital emphysema (crepitus on palpation as the fracture may allow air from the maxillary antrum to enter soft tissue), enophthalmos, blepharoptosis, and characteristic motility disturbances. Ptosis of the globe is occasionally encountered.

Patients with blowout fracture should be instructed to refrain from blowing the nose or sneezing, to avoid exacerbating orbital emphysema.

In a blowout fracture, the bony disruption may allow inferior orbital contents to herniate through the fracture site into the maxillary antrum (Fig. 16–12). These contents are principally periorbita, orbital fat, and/or various connective tissue septae. The inferior oblique and inferior rectus muscles rarely extend through the fracture. Instead, the entrapment of orbital fat and connective tissue partially immobilizes one or both of these muscles due to their various interconnections. A vertical tropia results, and may cause limitation of supraduction, infraduction, or both. If inferior rectus restriction is anterior to the equator, hypotropia results. If inferior rectus restriction is posterior to the equator, hypertropia results. Characteristically, this immobility causes hypotropia on upgaze and hypertropia on downgaze (Fig. 16–13). Forced duction testing usually corroborates restricted vertical gaze.

Radiologic studies are helpful in establishing the diagnosis of orbital blowout fracture. Waters views provide an excellent view of the orbital floor, demonstrating bony disruption and/or orbital contents herniated into the maxillary antrum (Fig. 16–3). Tomography and CT scan techniques (coronal and/or sagittal views) may add further definition and clarity to the relationship between

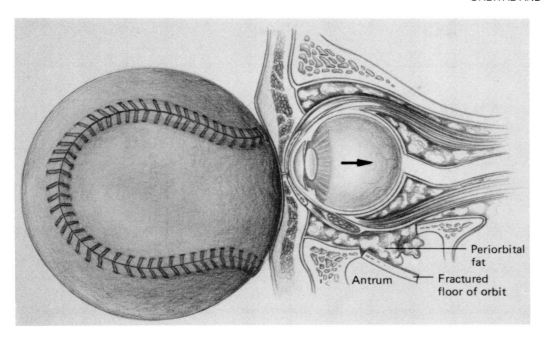

FIG. 16–11. Traumatic blowout fracture often results from the impact of a spherical object against the globe or anterior orbit. This transiently increases intraorbital pressure and may fracture the orbital floor at its weakest point.

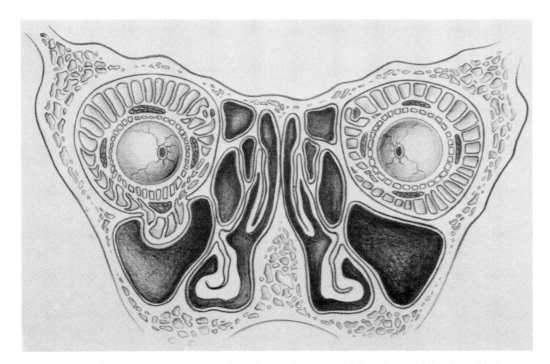

FIG. 16–12. Coronal view demonstrating blowout fracture with herniation of inferior orbital contents into the maxillary antrum.

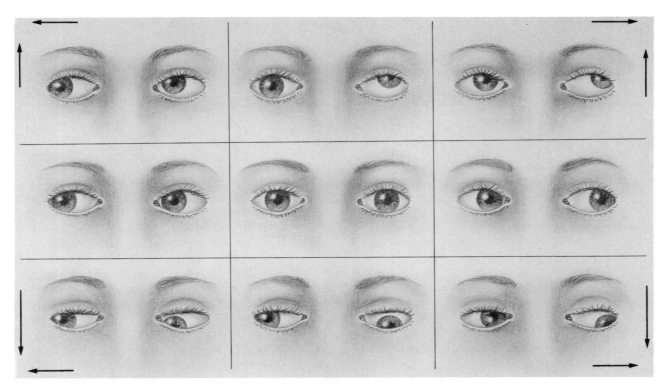

FIG. 16–13. Characteristic motility dysfunction in blowout fracture: hypotropia (diminished supraduction) on upgaze and hypertropia (diminished infraduction) on downgaze.

the orbital floor fracture and contiguous orbital soft tissues.

The mere radiologic presence of a blowout fracture is not an indication for surgical repair. Instead, treatment should be based on clinically significant and maintained diplopia and/or enophthalmos. The former is followed serially by diplopia field recordings and forced ductions. Diplopia from a blowout fracture is most clinically significant in the primary position and downgaze (reading position). Enophthalmos is followed serially by exophthalmometry. A Hertel recording demonstrating 1.5 mm or more of enophthalmos is considered abnormal. In most cases, enophthalmos is a delayed and progressive finding.

Forced duction testing is carried out under topical anesthesia. If several drops of proparacaine HCl (Ophthetic) are insufficient, placing a cotton pledget soaked in a 4% cocaine solution in the lower fornix will produce adequate analgesia. The conjunctiva at the lower limbus is grasped with toothed forceps and the globe is gently rotated vertically to evaluate its upward and downward excursion (Fig. 16–14). Both the ease of movement and the extent of excursion should be noted. Limitations suggest entrapment, although in the first few days after

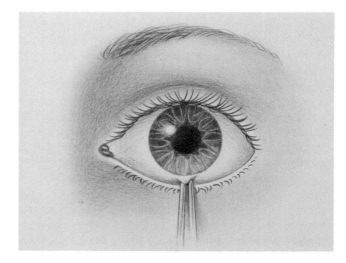

FIG. 16–14. Proper position of forceps in forced duction testing.

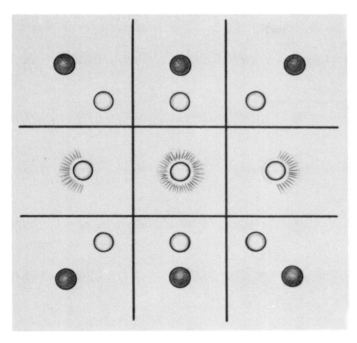

FIG. 16–15. Diplopia fields (as seen from examiner's perspective with red glass over patient's right eye) corresponding to motility dysfunction of Fig. 16–13.

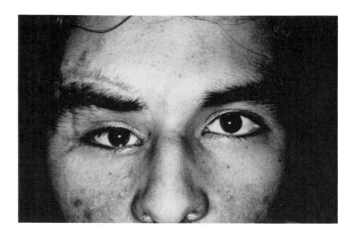

FIG. 16–16. Severe ptosis of globe resulting from a large orbital floor fracture. Right brow laceration was previously repaired.

trauma, orbital hemorrhage and swelling may produce similar restrictions.

During forced duction testing, the functional capacity of the inferior rectus muscle may be evaluated by the active generation force (AGF) test. With the inferior limbus held by toothed forceps and the globe raised to a position of supraduction, the patient is asked to look down. The force generated in this infraduction maneuver is a barometer of inferior rectus function. The more limited the AGF test results, the more likely will vertical motility surgery be required to restore single vision.

Diplopia fields are charted in the nine cardinal positions of gaze (Fig. 16–15). A red glass is placed before one eye and the patient is asked to look directly at a penlight. He is to respond, indicating whether he sees one or two lights, and if two are seen to indicate their spatial positions. The chart should be recorded from the examiner's perspective, and notation should be made as to which eye is covered by the red glass. Single vision should be recorded as a solitary circle. Double vision should be recorded as one red and one white circle, positioned corresponding to the patient's spatial designation. Diplopia testing may be further quantified by using horizontal and vertical free prisms to ascertain specific diopteric separation. Each endpoint is the position where prisms produce a solitary light.

After motility and enophthalmos parameters are followed for 10 days to 2 weeks, if either the enophthalmos

or diplopia is clinically significant and not improving, surgery should be considered. A decision before this time may be based on erroneous information caused by soft tissue and muscle cone hemorrhage and swelling, or neuromuscular injury. A decision after this time may make surgery more difficult because the tissues may become more tenaciously entrapped.

Ptosis of the globe is an uncommon sequela of large orbital floor fractures (Fig. 16–16). It results from significant diminution of support by Lockwood's ligament and other supportive structures. Its presence is a third indication for orbital floor repair.

Generally, larger blowout fractures cause greater tissue displacement into the antrum. Yet, the smaller fractures are the ones that are most impacted because they become entrapped within a much more confined space.

Surgical repair of blowout fractures can proceed from either an orbital (subciliary or fornix) approach (Fig. 16–17) or an antral (Caldwell-Luc) approach. The orbital approach is recommended because it is more effective and safer. In selected cases with large orbital floor defects, or those with tenaciously herniated orbital contents, a combined orbital and antral approach may be advisable.

Subciliary Approach to Blowout Fracture Repair. Under general anesthesia, forced ductions are performed initially to confirm the degree of preoperative tissue entrapment. It may be useful to dilate the pupil and intermittently check optic nerve perfusion. A horizontal incision is made in the lower eyelid just below the tarsal border, approximately 3 to 4 mm below the eyelid margin. To avoid lymphatic compromise, the incision should not extend too far laterally. The dissection is carried to the infraorbital rim by blunt and sharp dissection with

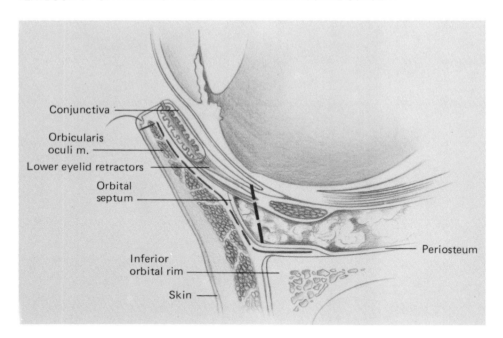

FIG. 16–17. Surgical approaches to orbital floor (solid line) repair: subciliary approach (lighter dashed line), inferior fornix approach (darker dashed line).

Stevens scissors. Care is taken not to enter the orbital septum, thus keeping fat out of the dissection. The periosteum is opened 1.5 mm below the orbital rim and elevated from the orbital floor. Periosteal edges may be tagged with 5-0 Vicryl sutures to facilitate later identification.

A fiberoptic headlight aids visualization of the orbital floor. With a periosteal elevator separating the periosteum from the orbital floor posteriorly, the fracture site is located (usually positioned nasally) and completely exposed (Fig. 16–18A). The infraorbital neurovascular bundle should be carefully preserved in this process. It should not be confused with herniated orbital contents. Likewise, the infraorbital groove must not be confused with the fracture. Unattached bony fragments should be removed.

Incarcerated tissues are gently freed from the fracture by a hand-over-hand maneuver with Addson forceps, malleable retractors, or a periosteal elevator. Occasional upward traction on a bridle suture placed in the inferior rectus muscle belly may facilitate identification of the fracture and disimpacting entrapped tissues (Fig. 16–18B). Care must be taken in freeing incarcerated tissues to avoid undue bleeding and trauma to the nearby optic nerve. Forced ductions should be repeated to ensure no residual entrapment. Before the defect is covered, bone fragments and blood should be aspirated from the maxillary antrum.

A sterile alloplastic sheet is fashioned to cover the defect completely, overlapping the surrounding intact bone by 3 to 4 mm circumferentially (Fig. 16–18C). This sheet should not be too large. The edges of the plate are smoothed to minimize trauma to adjacent structures. It should be notched posteriorly to accommodate the optic nerve. Before placement, the alloplastic material is soaked in an antibiotic solution.

Choices of material include Supramid, silicone, cranioplast (methyl methacrylate), proplast, Teflon, and Silastic. Iliac crest cancellous bone and rib cartilage grafts are not recommended because they unnecessarily involve a second surgical site and may partially or completely resorb.

Supramid is an excellent choice because it is biologically inert, sterilizes easily, has adequate tensile strength, and can be readily trimmed to the desired configuration. Supramid sheeting ranges in thickness from 0.05 to 2.0 mm. Generally, thicknesses ranging from 0.4 to 0.6 mm are suitable in most cases. The thicker implants are indicated to improve cases with significant enophthalmos. Yet, thicker implants run the risk of inducing or exacerbating vertical extraocular muscle imbalance. The more posterior the implant material is placed, the more it reduces enophthalmos. The more anterior the material is placed, the more it reduces hypoophthalmos.

Two small fixation holes are drilled in the infraorbital rim just anterior to the defect. Comparable holes are placed in the anterior edge of the implant. Using these

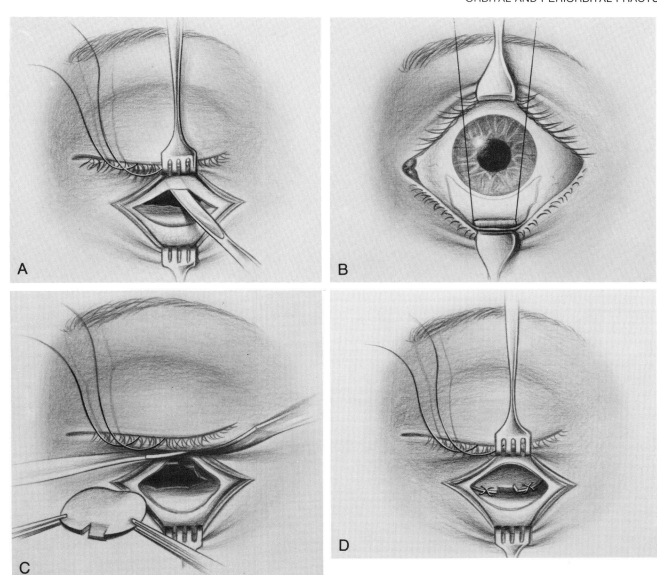

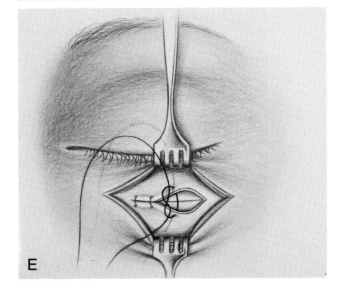

FIG. 16–18. Blowout fracture repair. Subciliary approach. A, A horizontal incision is made in the lower eyelid below the tarsal border. The dissection is carried to the infraorbital rim. Periosteum is opened and elevated posteriorly, exposing the fracture site. B, Inferior rectus bridle suture may facilitate identification of the fracture. C, Incarcerated tissues are freed from the fracture. A sterile alloplastic plate is fashioned to cover the defect completely in the orbital floor. The plate should have its edges smoothed and its posterior surface notched to avoid trauma to orbital tissues. A tongue of this plate may be fashioned anteriorly to fit into the fracture to discourage forward migration. D, The implant is fixated to the orbital rim with two 2-0 Supramid sutures. E, Periosteum is sutured, followed by a two-layer eyelid closure.

holes, the implant is secured to the orbital floor anteriorly with two 2-0 Supramid sutures (Fig. 16–18D). To further reduce implant migration at times, a small "tongue" of the implant can be fashioned and positioned in the fracture (Fig. 16–18C). It is imperative that no orbital contents become incarcerated between the implant and the orbital floor or fall back into the antrum. Forced ductions should be repeated to ensure restoration of full excursion. Coexistent fractures of the medial orbital wall or infraorbital rim may be repaired at the same time.

Once adequate hemostasis is established, periosteum is closed over the implant (Fig. 16–18E). This is accomplished using the previously placed 5-0 Vicryl sutures in an interrupted fashion. The orbicularis oculi muscle and subcutaneous layers are then closed with 6-0 Vicryl sutures using vertical and horizontal mattress techniques. Skin is closed with a running 7-0 silk suture. No dressing is applied to the wound so that it can be observed for postoperative bleeding and visual acuity assessed when the patient awakens from anesthesia. Postoperative systemic antibiotics may prove useful.

Inferior Fornix Approach to Blowout Fracture Repair. A variant of this technique uses an inferior fornix approach. Under general anesthesia, a lateral canthotomy is carried through the skin and lateral canthal tendon to periosteum at the lateral orbital rim. The inferior crus of the tendon is disinserted from the rim. Placing a 4-0 silk modified Frost suture at the central margin of the lower eyelid allows downward traction to expose the inferior fornix. The fornix is incised with Stevens scissors (Fig. 16–19A). The incision is carried to the infraorbital rim with blunt and sharp dissection.

The fornix technique then proceeds in a manner similar to the subciliary approach. Once periosteum is closed over the implant, the fornix is closed with running 6-0 chromic catgut sutures (Fig. 16–19B). This reapproximates inferior eyelid retractors. The inferior crus of the lateral canthal tendon is reattached to periosteum at the lateral orbital tubercle with a 2-0 Supramid suture. Running 7-0 silk is then used to complete the outer canthal closure.

If the implant is too thin, diplopia, enophthalmos, or hypo-ophthalmos may persist. If it is too thick, diplopia, exophthalmos, or hyperophthalmos may occur. Implant extrusion may induce infection, and vice versa. Extensive hemorrhage may increase intraorbital pressure and compromise vision. The implant should be carefully fixated to avoid impingement on adjacent structures.

Antral (Caldwell-Luc) Approach to Blowout Fracture Repair. Under general anesthesia, an incision is made in the gingival margin of the canine fossa. Periosteum is then separated from the anterior surface of the exposed maxilla. A periosteal elevator is used to create an osteotomy opening into the maxillary sinus. Blood and free-floating bone fragments are evacuated from the maxillary sinus and antrum. In conjunction with an orbital approach, herniated orbital contents are gently reposited superior to the plane of the orbital floor. The maxillary antrum may then be packed either with petroleum gauze imbricated with antibiotic ointment or a catheter balloon. The other end of the pack or catheter is brought out through an antrostomy opening into the nose to afford its postoperative removal.

Disadvantages of the antral approach include limited visualization, poor access for placement and securing of an orbital floor implant, increased infection rate, increased intraorbital pressure from the antral pack, and the hazard of forcing bony spicules toward the globe and optic nerve.

Complications After Blowout Fracture Repair. Vision loss after blowout fracture surgery is fortunately rare. Gradual loss of vision may result from extensive intraorbital hemorrhage causing central retinal artery or optic nerve ischemia. Immediate loss of vision may be caused by direct trauma to the optic nerve. Such trauma may result from an orbital floor implant impinging upon the optic nerve or upward extension of a bony spicule from an antral approach.

Extraocular muscle imbalance and diplopia may persist, though improved, after orbital fracture repair. Motility surgery should be delayed 6 to 12 months, if possible, to allow for postoperative improvement. This delay may obviate the need for surgery, or at least diminish the amount of such correction. During this waiting period, the impact of diplopia may be lessened by the use of prism glasses (Fresnel or fixed prism) or a frosted glass. When motility surgery is performed, it can be best quantified using adjustable suture techniques.

Residual enophthalmos may be mild and require no treatment. Minimal elevation of the upper eyelid with a Fasanella-Servat procedure can sometimes effectively camouflage the defect and normalize the patient's appearance. More extensive enophthalmos requires exchanging the original floor implant for a thicker one, possibly inducing hypertropia and further compromising motility. The patient and physician should clearly discuss this issue thoroughly. If the patient desires such a revision, orienting the thickest portion of a wedge-shaped implant posteriorly helps to improve enophthalmos with less effect upon motility.

Lower eyelid retraction may result from adhesions between the orbital septum and the infraorbital rim. This retraction may be corrected by recessing the inferior

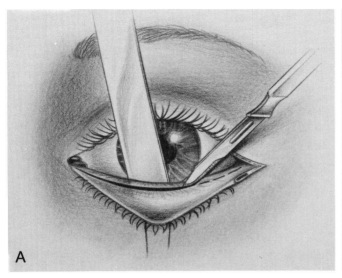 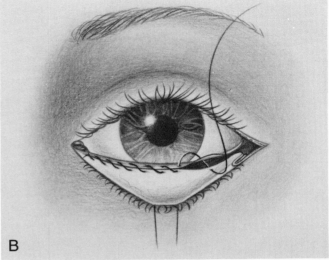

FIG. 16–19. Blowout fracture repair. Inferior fornix approach. A, Inferior fornix is incised with either Stevens scissors or #64 Beaver blade. The incision is carried to the infraorbital rim and proceeds in a manner similar to the subciliary approach. B, Once periosteum is closed over the implant, the fornix is closed with chromic catgut sutures.

eyelid retractors. Techniques for this surgery are presented in Chapter 6.

Migration of an orbital floor implant may damage contiguous structures. This migration may result from poor reapproximation of the periosteum or failure to anchor the plate to underlying bone. Anterior migration may cause partial or complete extrusion through the skin, or infraorbital neuralgia (pain and paresthesia). Extension of an implant through the skin is likely to cause infection. Posterior migration may cause loss of vision from impingement upon the optic nerve. Medial migration may cause dacryostenosis from impingement of the implant upon the lacrimal sac at its junction with the nasolacrimal duct.

Implant infection and extrusion often occur together. An infection in the presence of an alloplastic material usually defies antibiotic treatment. It usually requires removal of the implant, after which the infection often readily abates. If cicatricial tissue sufficient to cover the defect has formed since the original surgery, the implant may not require later replacement.

Lymphedema is principally seen with a skin incision curved upward laterally toward the outer canthus. Most cases gradually resolve over several months.

Infraorbital nerve dysfunction may result from the original fracture, surgical manipulation of the infraorbital neurovascular bundle, or postoperative encroachment by a migrating orbital floor implant. Sensory function of the infraorbital nerve gradually returns over the first year after surgery.

LE FORT FRACTURES

Le Fort fractures involve the maxilla and are usually complex, asymmetric, and incomplete (Fig. 16–20). Pure Le Fort fractures are uncommon. Le Fort I is a low transverse maxillary fracture that does not extend to the orbit. The fragment of maxilla containing the teeth is separated from the remainder of the facial bones. In severe cases, this fragment may be free-floating.

Le Fort II fractures are pyramidal, involving the maxilla, nasal bones, and medial orbital floor. This fracture begins at the lower portion of the nasal bones, across the naso-orbital margin above the nasolacrimal canal, through the medial portion of the orbital floor (at times associated with a blowout fracture), over the infraorbital rim, through the inferior orbital canal, involving the anterior and posterior walls of the maxillary sinus. The fracture crosses the posterior pillar of the upper jaw, the pyramidal and pterygoid processes, and pterygomandibular fissure, ending at the medial orbital margin and lateral wall of the nose. This extensive fracture of the upper jaw, medial orbit, and lower segment of the nose may be partially displaced or free-floating.

Le Fort III fractures create a craniofacial dysjunction involving both orbits, separating the maxilla from the skull. The facial skeleton is free-floating, attached to the cranium by soft tissue alone. This fracture extends from the upper portion of the nasal bones, across the orbital margin near the frontomaxillary suture, through the ethmoid bone and lamina papyracea, passing posteriorly and

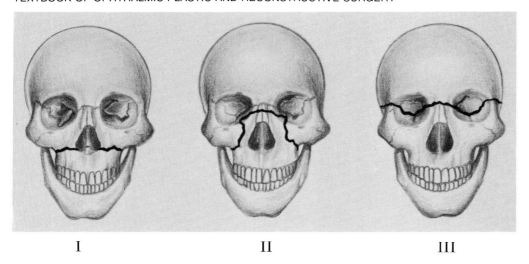

I   II   III

FIG. 16–20.   Depiction of fracture sites in Le Fort I, II, and III fractures, respectively.

inferiorly below the optic foramina to the infraorbital fissure. It then separates into two segments. One portion extends upward along the zygomaticosphenoid suture between the orbital roof and the lateral orbital wall, crossing the lateral orbital rim at the zygomaticofrontal suture. The second portion extends inferiorly and posteriorly crossing the pterygoid process. The zygomatic arch is also fractured.

Le Fort II and III fractures may occasionally extend to the orbital apex, compromising vision from optic canal involvement. Surgical management of these fractures requires open reduction, often with the use of arch bars. They may present with concomitant skull fracture, necessitating neurosurgical care.

ORBITAL ROOF FRACTURES

The strength of the supraorbital rim makes isolated orbital roof fractures uncommon. They are seen principally in conjunction with wounds inflicted by sharp instruments (Fig. 16–21) or gunshots and may also occur in conjunction with LeForte III fractures (craniofacial disjunction).

Coexistent findings may include brow and eyelid ecchymosis, forehead hypesthesia, and diminution of superior rectus, superior oblique, or levator muscle function. Diplopia may result from extraocular muscle injury and injury to the trochlea. The levator muscle may be compromised from third cranial nerve injury, mechanical entrapment, or direct injury. Sensory loss from supraorbital nerve damage may also occur. These fractures may extend into the superior orbital fissure and optic canal with resultant damage to the optic, oculomotor, trochlear, and/or abducens nerve.

Superior orbital rim, frontal sinus, and glabellar fractures may remain extracranial, or may communicate with the intracranial compartment. Air detected within the anterior cranial fossa in an orbital roof fracture suggests a dural tear. Cerebrospinal fluid rhinorrhea further suggests involvement of the posterior wall of the frontal sinus or the cribriform plate.

Unless significant displacement is present, superior orbital rim fractures do not require surgical reduction. Displaced fractures that are limited in size, do not involve the orbital roof, and have not violated the intra-

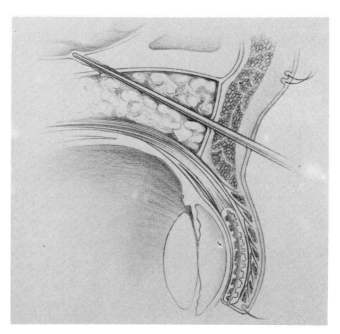

FIG. 16–21.   Orbital roof fracture from a penetrating sharp instrument.

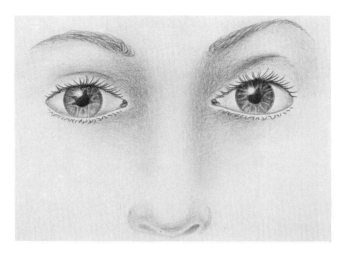

FIG. 16–22. Large contour deformity of superolateral orbital rim from previous fracture.

cranial space may be carefully repositioned and wired under microscopic control. At times, periosteal closure alone provides adequate support. All other superior orbital rim or roof fractures and those associated with CSF leakage should be evaluated and managed in conjunction with a neurosurgeon.

DELAYED ORBITAL CONTOUR DEFORMITY

Patients may present with orbital rim contour deformities that arose from previous trauma that was either inadequately repaired or untreated. If these defects are mild, no further surgery is required. Larger defects may require subperiosteal placement of custom implants (Fig. 16–22). Methyl methacrylate and proplast are efficacious implant materials (Fig. 16–23). Bone grafts undergo variable absorption and are not recommended.

Skull and orbital radiographs define the extent of bony deformity. Radiography must be correlated with the clinical findings. With the help of an experienced ocularist, a mold of this region is made, incorporating the defect. From this mold, a positive impression is fashioned, using the desired alloplastic material.

The implant is sterilized and surgically placed under general anesthesia. One or two small incisions should be placed adjacent to, but not overlying, the contour deformity in an adjacent hairline or in conformity with Langer's lines. This diminishes the likelihood of postoperative extrusion. The incision is carried down to the defect with blunt and sharp dissection with either Stevens or small Metzenbaum scissors. If intact periosteum remains, a periosteal pocket should be fashioned and elevated to receive the implant.

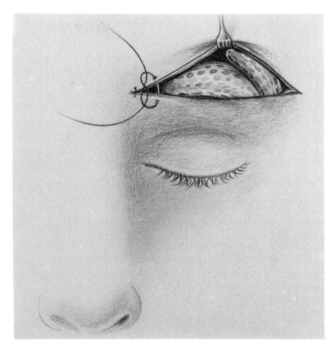

FIG. 16–23. Proplast implants may be placed in subperiosteal space to correct contour deformity of the orbital rim.

Alloplastic materials must be soaked in an antibiotic solution before placement. Minor modifications in the implant may be performed with scissors. Minor modifications in the surrounding bone may be achieved using a Hall drill with fine burr tip. Once the configuration and fit are optimal, small corresponding drill holes are made in the recipient bone and implant. The alloplastic material is placed within the periosteal pocket and secured with 2-0 Supramid sutures. The wound is closed in two or three layers with interrupted sutures.

BIBLIOGRAPHY

Allen, L.: Modified impression fitting. Int. Ophthalmol. Clin. 10:747, 1979.

Berkowitz, R., Putterman, A., and Patel, D.: Prolapse of the globe into the maxillary sinus after orbital floor fracture. Am. J. Ophthalmol. 91:253, 1981.

Beyer, C. and Smith, B.: Naso-orbital fractures: complications and treatment. Ophthalmologica, 163:418–427, 1971.

Browning, C. and Waller, R.: The use of alloplastics in 45 cases of orbital floor reconstruction. Am. J. Ophthalmol. 60:684, 1965.

Callahan, M., Cox, C., and Callahan, A.: Correction of facial contour deformities resulting from loss of soft tissue or bone. Trans. Am. Acad. Ophthalmol. Otolaryngol. 83:641, 1977.

Callahan, M. and Callahan, A.: Ophthalmic Plastic and Orbital Surgery. Birmingham, Aesculapius, 1979, 156–182.

Converse, J., Smith, B., Obear, M., and Wood-Smith, D.: Orbital blowout fractures: a ten year survey. Plast. Reconstr. Surg., 39:20–36, 1967.

Converse, J. and Smith, B.: On the treatment of blowout fractures of the orbit. Plast. Reconstr. Surg. 62:100–104, 1978.

Crikelair, G., Rein, J., and Potter, G.: A critical look at the blowout fracture. Plast. Reconstr. Surg. 49:374, 1972.

Cullen, G., Luce, C., and Shannon, G.: Blindness following blowout orbital fractures. Ophthalmic Surg. 8:60, 1977.

Dodick, J., Galin, M., and Littleton, J.L.: Concomitant medial wall fracture and blowout fracture of the orbit. Arch. Ophthalmol. 85:273, 1971.

Dortzbach, R. and Segrest, D.: Blow-out Fractures of the Orbital Floor. In Stewart, W.: Ophthalmic Plastic and Reconstructive Surgery. San Francisco, American Academy of Ophthalmology, 1984, 387–389.

Edwards, W. and Ridley, R.: Blowout fracture of medial orbital wall. Am. J. Ophthalmol. 65:248, 1968.

Emery, J., vonNoorden, G., and Schlernitzauer, D.: Management of orbital floor fractures. Am. J. Ophthalmol. 74:299–306, 1972.

Epstein, L.: Clinical experiences with proplast as an implant. Plast. Reconstr. Surg. 63:219–233, 1979.

Fischbein, F. and Lesko, W.: Blowout fracture of the medial orbital wall. Arch. Ophthalmol. 81:162, 1969.

Greenwald, H., Keeney, A., and Shannon, G.: A review of 128 patients with orbital fractures. Am. J. Ophthalmol. 78:655–664, 1974.

Grove, A.: Orbital trauma and computed tomography. Ophthalmology 87:403–411, 1980.

Kohn, R., Romano, P., and Puklin, J.: Lacrimal obstruction after migration of orbital floor implant. Am. J. Ophthalmol. 82:934–936, 1976.

McCord, C. and Moses, J.: Exposure of the inferior orbit with fornix incision and lateral canthotomy. Ophthalmic Surg., 10:53–63, 1979.

McCord, C.: Oculoplastic Surgery. New York, Raven Press, 1981.

Morgan, D., Madan, D., and Bergerot, J.: Fractures of the middle third of the face: a review of 300 cases. Br. J. Plast. Surg. 25:147, 1972.

Nicholson, D. and Guzak, S.: Visual loss complicating repairs of orbital floor fractures. Arch. Ophthalmol. 86:369–375, 1971.

Putterman, A., Stevens, T., and Urist, M.: Nonsurgical management of blow-out fractures of the orbital floor. Am. J. Ophthalmol. 77:232, 1974.

Putterman, A.: Late management of blow-out fractures of the orbital floor. Trans. Am. Acad. Ophthalmol. Otolaryngol. 83:650, 1977.

Rumelt, M. and Ernest, J.: Isolated blowout fracture of the medial orbital wall with medial rectus muscle entrapment. Am. J. Ophthalmol. 43:451, 1972.

Reeh, M., Beyer, C., and Shannon, G.: Practical Ophthalmic Plastic and Reconstructive Surgery. Philadelphia, Lea and Febiger, 1976, 182–189.

Smith, B. and Regan, W.: Blow-out fracture of the orbit: mechanism and correction of internal orbital fracture. Am. J. Ophthalmol. 44:733, 1957.

Soll, D.: Orbital Trauma. In Stewart, W.: Ophthalmic Plastic and Reconstructive Surgery. San Francisco, American Academy of Ophthalmology, 1984, 360–386.

Stasior, O. and Apt, R.: Orbital Fractures. In Soll, D.: Management of Complications in Ophthalmic Plastic Surgery. Birmingham, Aesculapius, 1976.

Tenzel, R. and Miller, G.: Orbital blowout fracture repair, conjunctival approach. Am. J. Ophthalmol. 71:1141, 1971.

Trokel, S.: The orbit: annual review. Arch. Ophthalmol. 91:233–234, 1974.

INDEX